A Jerry Baker Good Health Book

Grandma Putt's
Home Health
REMEDIES

www.jerrybaker.com

A Jerry Baker Good Health Book

Grandma Putt's
Home Health
REMEDIES

972 Teas, Tonics, and Treatments for Arthritis, Back Pain, Headaches, Nausea, Sore Throats, and more!

Executive Editor: Kim Adam Gasior   **Interior Design and Layout:** Trish Field
Managing Editor: Cheryl Winters-Tetreau   **Cover Design:** Kitty Pierce Mace
Production Editor: Stacy Mulka   **Indexer:** Nan Badgett

Publisher's Cataloging-in-Publication
(Provided by Quality Books, Inc.)

Baker, Jerry.
    Grandma Putt's home health remedies : 972 teas, tonics, and treatments for arthritis, back pain, headaches, nausea, sore throats, and more! / by Jerry Baker.
    p. cm. – (Jerry Baker's good health series)
    Includes index.
    ISBN-13: 978-0-922433-89-6
    ISBN-10: 0-922433-89-5

    1. Self-care, Health. 2. Traditional medicine. I. Title. II. Title: Home health remedies.
III. Series: Jerry Baker good health series.

    RA776.95.B35 2008   615.8'8

         QBI08-600115

Published by American Master Products, Inc. / Jerry Baker
Printed in the United States of America
2 4 6 8 10 9 7 5 3 1 hardcover

Contents

Introduction

Back before stores were stocked with aisles of cough syrups, pain relievers, and supplements, folks relied on home remedies to get well. They didn't rush off to clinics or doctor's offices, but consulted wise women like my Grandma Putt, who used time-tested remedies, no-nonsense treatments, and do-it-yourself cures to set things right.

For instance, I'll never forget the day Grandma and I stopped by Mr. Schuster's roadside stand for some fresh honey. Unfortunately, Mr. Schuster had hurt his back and couldn't even get out of bed, much less tend to his hives. Grandma hated to see him suffer, so she gathered up some thyme, arnica, and willow bark from her garden, and showed Mrs. Schuster how to use 'em to soothe her husband's sore back.

Well, a week later, there was a knock at our door. Mr. Schuster stood there, grinnin' like a kid in a candy store—with a jar of fresh honey in one hand and one of Mrs. Schuster's blackberry pies in the other. He was pain-free and up-and-at-'em again, thanks to Grandma Putt.

After that, we had visitors stopping in with one ailment after another, desperate for relief. There were Mrs. McKinney's migraines, old farmer Benson's arthritis, my classmate Betty Sue's acne, and an assortment of bumps, bruises, rashes, and stings. And you know what? Grandma Putt had a good old-fashioned home remedy to take care of 'em all!

So last year, as I stood in line at my local pharmacy, about to plunk down big bucks for a bottle of pain relievers, I got to thinking about Grandma Putt and her terrific treatments. As I recall, we didn't have much money back then, but our health sure didn't suffer. Yet here we are today, spending a small fortune on pricey prescriptions and medical treatments—only to get temporary relief at best. So, I decided it was time to dig up those old-time remedies and put them to use again.

Our team gathered up all of Grandma Putt's great tips, tonics, and teas, as well as all of the other amazing old-time healers we could find. Not only did we discover a ton of remarkable home treatments, but also the scientific reasons why those remedies worked. That's right—our grandmas really *did* know what they were doing. So we packed all this homespun health wisdom into the treasure trove of remarkable remedies you're holding in your hands.

In *Grandma Putt's Home Health Remedies,* you'll discover hundreds of tried-and-true treatments for arthritis, headaches, sore throats, rashes, high blood pressure, bites and stings, indigestion, and much, much more using the very same back-to-basics, commonsense know-how that kept our grandparents…*and their grandparents*…in the pink of health. Even better—I've made it super easy for you to find relief by listing each ailment alphabetically, along with the best ways to treat it.

But sometimes, there's just no substitute for modern medicine. So to make sure that you've got the very best information at your fingertips, I've included many *Modern Marvels* sidebars throughout the book that highlight the latest medical breakthroughs.

And of course, some health problems are too serious to treat at home. If that's the case, then it's time to *Dial the Doctor.* In these boxes, you'll learn what to look for so you can get the professional help you need.

I also want you to always remember that this book can never (and should never) replace your doctor's advice. But it can help you stay out of the local clinic and neighborhood pharmacy if you've got minor problems. So with that in mind, dig into all the wonderful health hints, tips, and D.I.Y. recipes that Grandma Putt and other wise old women used way back when to keep their loved ones in good health.

Acne

No matter how much you hate pimples, you have to give them credit for timing. You could go months or years without an outbreak, but as soon as you want to look your best—for your 15-year high school reunion or a meeting with the company hotshots, for example—they make a sudden appearance.

Here's where the problem begins. Every now and then, the sebaceous glands under your skin work overtime and produce more oil than your skin needs or your oil ducts can handle. The excess collects under the skin's surface. Add some dead skin cells to the mix, and a hard plug forms. If it stays under the skin, it's a whitehead. If it enlarges and pushes out to the surface, it's a blackhead. If it ruptures the wall of a pore, invading bacteria jump in, and there's your zit. If more than one zit erupts— and let's face it, zits travel in groups—you've got yourself an acne breakout.

Tea Time

An effective remedy for a painful pimple is to cover it with a tea bag. Black tea contains tannins, compounds that help pimples drain, and have antibacterial properties. Soak a tea bag in hot water just to soften it. Let it cool slightly, then hold it on the pimple for 10 minutes or so.

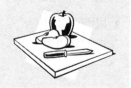
Blame Internal Chemistry

Acne usually comes about as a result of the increased hormonal activity that occurs during adolescence. Unfortunately, this process sometimes ends up clogging pores and blocking the flow of sebum. In grownups, the sudden appearance of acne is often either a sign of a hormone imbalance or a side effect of certain drugs, such as steroids, lithium, anticonvulsants, and medications containing iodine. If you take any of these medicines, ask your doctor if you can change prescriptions.

Thankfully, most acne is more of an embarrassment than a serious medical problem. But if it persists into adulthood or is particularly severe, you may need medical treatment to prevent scarring. The most effective medications—for both topical and oral use—are derivatives of vitamin A. These drugs are safe when used under the supervision of a dermatologist, but they shouldn't be taken casually, because they can be irritating and toxic. And, since infection isn't the primary cause of acne, long-term treatment with antibiotics should be avoided.

Keep Your Skin Crystal Clear

While you can't prevent acne entirely, there are a number of simple strategies for keeping outbreaks under control, and preventing them from coming back. So before you hand over your

Modern Marvel

OTC Acne Aids

Over-the-counter acne creams contain ingredients, such as benzoyl peroxide and salicylic acid, that can be helpful in reducing acne flare-ups in some people. Use a cream at night and, after a week or so, add a morning application. You should notice an improvement in about three weeks.

hard-earned dough to a dermatologist, here are a few things to try:

- **Baby your skin.** All the scrubbing in the world won't make those zits disappear—in fact, it may just cause them to spread. So when you wash your skin, do it gently.

- **Be a clean machine.** Pimples can be literally overflowing with bacteria, and the last thing you need is for stray germs to cause an infection elsewhere. The most important home treatment is to keep pimples, and the surrounding skin, clean and dry. Wash the area with soap and water a few times a day. If you touch one of the foul bumps, wash your hands immediately afterward.

- **Lavender is lovely.** Steam your pores open and prevent acne with an herbal antiseptic. Just place 1 tablespoon of lavender flowers in a pot of hot, steaming water. Place a towel over your head to trap the steam, then bend over the pot (but not so close that you burn your face). Let the lavender vapors steam your face for 15 minutes, then rinse with cool water and pat dry.

- **Stay cool and calm.** Try to arrange your life so you're under as little stress as possible (easier said than done, we know!). Stress alters hormone levels, which can trigger zit outbreaks.

- **Erase 'em with eggs.** Egg white draws the oils away from your skin. It's also a mild astringent and may contain some anti–inflammatory proteins as well. So when a nasty pimple appears, use a cotton swab to apply a little to the area.

- **Refresh with an herbal rinse.** Calendula's bright orange flowers can be made into a refreshing facial wash. Just steep 1 teaspoon of flowers in 1 cup of hot water for 10 minutes, strain, and let cool. After cleansing your face as usual, rinse with the calendula solution.

- **Wash with the witch.** Witch hazel, an excellent oil remover, has long been a popular item in medicine cabinets. Use a clean cotton ball to dab some on your skin to help keep it oil-free.

- **Apply a sweet soother.** Mix 1 teaspoon of onion juice with 2 tablespoons of honey. Apply it to your face, and leave it on for 10 to 15 minutes. Rinse with warm water followed by cool water. This combination has a soothing effect on irritated skin.

- **Drain away infection.** Buy some dried yarrow, an astringent herb, from a local herbalist or

> ## Nature's Bacteria Killer
>
> Tea tree oil, available at health food stores, is one of the most powerful herbal oils for killing the bacteria that make pimples painful. Add a few drops of oil to a cup of warm water. Moisten a washcloth with the water, and hold it on the pimple for about 10 minutes several times a day.

health food store. Crumble the leaves, add a little water to make a paste, and apply it to the pimple. Leave it on for about 20 minutes, then wash the area well.

Say Goodbye to Iodine

Most dermatologists insist that chocolate and pizza don't cause zits. However, doctors do warn that the *iodine* in a hot fudge sundae or a slice of anchovy and extra-cheese pizza just might. Known to trigger angry red pimples, iodine is abundant in dairy products because iodine cleansers are used on milking machines. Fast food, salty foods, and shellfish can aggravate acne for the same reason.

Beware of Boils

Boils are similar to pimples in some ways. They appear as red or pinkish, pus-filled bumps on the skin, sometimes with a white or yellow spot in the center. They're unsightly, but that's not why they're worrisome. When bacteria colonize a hair follicle, they can multiply to harmful levels. Your immune system tries to keep them in check, but if it fails, the organisms can trigger a potentially serious infection. At the very least, they can cause boils, along with a lot of inflammation and pain.

If you're generally healthy, a boil is unlikely to be serious. The pus will usually drain on its own, and the boil should disappear within one to two weeks. Keep the area clean and help the boil drain in the same way you take care of bad pimples. Large or painful boils, on the other hand, should always be treated by a doctor, especially if you have other signs of infection, such as a fever, chills, or fatigue.

Age Spots

You already know that unrestrained sunbathing can trigger the development of premature wrinkles. What you may not know is that the sun's strong rays can also produce a bunch of flat, freckle-like age spots that make you look like a speckled frog. Technically, they're called lentigines, although folks sometimes call them (wrongly) liver spots.

While lentigines usually debut—often on the hands, face, or shoulders—around age 40, they're a long time in the making. If you spend years enjoying the sun's golden rays, your body tries to protect your skin from solar damage by producing an excess of protective melanin. Over time, however, the melanin turns to cellular debris that bunches up in irregular patches, and voilà—age spots! While they're completely harmless, much like freckles, they're almost never as cute. In fact, they practically scream "I'm old!"

dial the DOCTOR

Spots to Watch

While age spots are harmless, precancerous lesions may not be. Consult a dermatologist immediately if one of your age spots suddenly darkens to a deep brown or black, changes shape, becomes raised, or bleeds.

Tea Time

Traditional herbal blood purifiers are said to clear the skin of blemishes and spots. To try one, mix equal parts of the dried roots of burdock, yellow dock, and dandelion. Steep 1 tablespoon of the mixture in 1 cup of boiling water for 20 minutes, then strain and drink. You can add honey and lemon to taste. *Caution:* Dandelion greens should not be used if you're taking diuretics or potassium supplements. Consult your doctor if you have any concerns.

No More Spots

If you want to fade your spots, your doctor is likely to suggest that you try one of the many vitamin A skin creams, called retinoids, on the market. They peel off the top layer of skin—and possibly those vexing spots with it. But if the over-the-counter retinol products don't do the job, you may need to up the ante and use a prescription-strength retinoid such as tretinoin (Retin-A). These drugs slough off old age spots and stop new ones from forming. Their only drawback is that they can be quite harsh, especially if you have very fair skin. In fact, if you use a prescription-strength retinoid, you may trade your age spots for a nasty sunburn with only the slightest exposure to the sun. And wasn't it too much sun that sent you scurrying for the stuff in the first place?

Out, Out, Darned Spots!

In truth, you probably don't have to spend a lot of money to get rid of age spots. Sometimes the very best remedies are the most basic. Here are some low-tech but highly effective ways to coax those pesky spots into the background:

- **Do the fade.** Acid-based exfoliants will slough off the top layer of your skin, along with the lentigines. The spots will seem lighter on the underneath layers, and eventually, as skin layers are replaced, the lentigines will no longer be there. Most dermatologists recommend alpha hydroxy acids, commonly known as AHAs, for this job. These natural acids come from milk (lactic acid), sugarcane (glycolic acid), and fruit (citric acid). The glycolic acid in sugarcane is the most common AHA. It loosens those dead cells and motivates new cells from lower layers of the epidermis to get busy growing some new skin.

■ **Cream 'em with kinerase.** This plant growth hormone stops leaves from turning brown—and it may help diminish brown spots on your skin with little or no irritation. Look for it in over-the-counter lotions, then use it twice a day.

■ **Wash your face with flowers.** Elderflowers have long been known to keep the complexion clear and free of blemishes. In fact, they are used today in many commercial skin creams. Make your own elderflower water by steeping 1 ounce of fresh flowers in 1 pint of distilled water overnight. Strain, then use as a rinse after your daily cleansing regimen.

■ **Erase them with aloe.** Best known for its ability to heal burns, aloe gel may help fade skin spots by boosting cell turnover so the pigmented cells eventually slough off. Apply the gel directly to the spots twice a day for a month or two. The smell's a bit pungent, but the results are worth it.

■ **Make room for mushrooms.** Their juice contains kojic acid, a lightening agent that has been found to block the overproduction of melanin.

Grandma Says:

Cover your head. Folks in Grandma Putt's day would not dream of going outdoors without a hat—and neither should you. A wide-brimmed hat or visor can actually block half the sunlight that would otherwise reach parts of your face. So slap on a chapeau—you'll be stylish and skin savvy, too!

Bet on Buttermilk

The next time you grocery shop, grab a quart of buttermilk. For ages, women have enjoyed lolling in milk baths and, more specifically, in buttermilk baths because of buttermilk's high lactic acid content. Unfortunately, to buy enough for a tubful would probably equal the price of a cow, so do what my Grandma Putt always did—simply bathe your face and/or hands in buttermilk once or twice a day.

It's just as effective as those over-the-counter treatments for fading age spots without over-lightening or irritating skin. Mind you, juice from your portobello burger probably won't do the trick, but any over-the-counter skin lotion that contains kojic acid will. Simply apply it twice daily, and your age spots may fade significantly in less than two months.

■ **Mix up some 'radish.** The enzyme activity of horseradish and yogurt may help decrease age spots. Mix 1 tablespoon of grated horseradish in ¼ cup of plain yogurt, then refrigerate. Dab the mixture on daily until you see your spots fade. Follow each application with a smear of vitamin E oil or wheat germ oil.

■ **Get some lemon aid.** Lemon is a mild bleaching aid that works as well on age spots as it does on stains in fabrics. Mix equal parts lemon juice and water and apply to each spot. Leave it on for 5 minutes before rinsing. Repeat three times a week, and the brown spots may fade to taupe. Add more lemon juice and less water as your skin gets used to the preparation. Your goal is to be able to apply the juice "straight up."

Save Your Skin with Sunscreen

By far, the best way to prevent age spots is to apply sunscreen every time you go outside. Be sure to slather it on all exposed skin—not only your face but also your legs, arms, and hands. If you have a fetching short haircut, don't forget

MODERN MARVEL

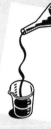

Skin A-Peel

If, despite your best efforts, you find yourself applying your foundation with a putty knife, you may want to consider pulling out all the stops with one or more skin-stripping medical procedures. Your doctor may suggest removing your spots with a chemical peel, which uses strong acids to dissolve the skin surface; a liquid nitrogen peel, which "freezes" spots for easier removal; or a laser peel, in which your doctor actually lifts off age spots using a high-intensity light. All of these methods can erase age spots as completely as paint stripper peels off unwanted varnish—but they're expensive, and the recovery can be painful.

your ears! And reapplying sunscreen every time you wash your hands really makes a difference, so always carry a small bottle with you.

Avoid the Danger Times

The sun is most damaging at its highest peak. The force of ultraviolet (UV) rays is 10 times stronger at noon than it is 3 hours earlier or later. Even if you spend all day out in the sun, you'll get the biggest dose of UV radiation from 11 a.m. to 1 p.m.—when the sun is directly overhead.

Anal Pain

dial the DOCTOR

The Bottom Line Is...

Call your doctor if you have anal pain accompanied by fever, chills, sweating, or other signs of infection, or if it hurts so much that you can't have a bowel movement.

The anus is the last link in the digestive chain, and for the most part, it's pretty tough. But it's not invulnerable to problems, and most of them seem to cause either pain or itching. Pain in your nether regions can be caused by several things. Anal fissures, which are small tears in the tissue, are rarely serious, but they can hurt like the dickens for the couple of weeks it takes them to heal. An anal abscess, an infection of a gland inside the anus, can make the area sore and tender. And then there are hemorrhoids, those pesky protuberances that can make even sitting an agonizing experience.

It's not a pleasant prospect, but anal pain generally requires a trip to the doctor. Otherwise, there's really no way to tell what's causing the problem. Anal abscesses, for example, will sometimes go away on their own. Other times, however, the infection gets worse, and the doctor needs to step in. An untreated abscess can also progress to a dangerous, tunnel-like growth called a fistula that requires surgery. Even anal fissures, which almost always heal on their own, can cause so much pain that they require a doctor's care.

Soothing Solutions

While you're waiting to get in to see your doctor about anal pain, here are some easy remedies that will make your life a lot more comfortable—and you don't have to bust the bank to try 'em:

- **Soak that bottom.** No matter what's making your bottom hurt, soaking in a warm bath for 10 to 20 minutes will almost certainly make you feel better. It helps soothe the area and relaxes tight muscles.

- **Get over-the-counter help.** Don't ignore the benefits of common pain relievers, such as aspirin and ibuprofen. They block chemicals in the body that cause pain, and they help control inflammation.

- **Drink and keep drinking.** No kidding: By the time you're feeling thirsty, your body is already running low on water, which means that you're more likely to have hard stools or other causes of anal pain. Most people need about 6 glasses of water daily. If you're active or live in a warm climate, drink 8 to 10 glasses, and don't wait until you're parched. Keep water nearby and sip it throughout the day.

Tea Time

A daily cup of slippery elm tea will help keep your digestive tract, including the back end, running smoothly. It also soothes aggravated tissues throughout the intestine. Mix a teaspoon of slippery elm powder, available at health food stores, in a glass of warm water or juice and drink one to three times a day.

Helpful Supplements

If you can't seem to get adequate fiber from foods, take advantage of the fiber supplements that are available at drugstores and health food stores. Just follow the directions on the label. Products that contain psyllium, for example, are loaded with fiber. They make stools soft and slippery, and therefore, less likely to cause anal pain.

Just don't confuse fiber supplements with stimulant laxatives, which can irritate tissues and worsen the pain. Laxatives should be used only under a doctor's supervision.

■ **Some like it hot.** A little gentle heat makes everything feel better, and your rear end is no exception. Cover a heating pad with a towel, set the heat on low, and sit and relax for as long as it feels comfortable.

Inspect the Medicine Chest

Some prescription drugs increase the risk of constipation, which can cause or aggravate anal pain. Among the likely suspects are prescription analgesics, antidepressants, tranquilizers, blood pressure drugs, iron and calcium supplements, and antacids. If you've noticed any change in your usual bowel habits, or you're constipated more than occasionally, ask your doctor or pharmacist if any of your medications could be to blame. But don't, under any circumstances, stop taking any medicines without your doctor's permission.

Arthritis

Are your hinges so creaky in the morning that you feel like the Tin Woodman without his trusty oilcan? Do your fingers, knees, and hips get so stiff that even simple activities, such as working in the garden, make you feel like you're doing hard time in the mines?

Mother Nature doesn't mess up very often, but she sure could have done a better job of joint design. By age 40 or 50, many of us begin to notice some joint tightness. It's usually caused by osteoarthritis, the "wear and tear" arthritis that occurs when the spongy cartilage that covers and protects the bones of our joints becomes thinner due to age and daily friction.

When Your Joints Are Out of Joint

Without their protective cushioning, bones may start to grind against each other, which can damage the tissue surrounding the joint. The

Tea Time

My Grandma Putt knew that ginger is a powerful anti-inflammatory herb that can take the edge off arthritis pain. So she often made this healing tea: grate about an inch of fresh ginger and steep it in hot water for 10 minutes, then strain. Drink it once or twice a day, hot or cold.

immune system attempts to come to the rescue, but instead, the white blood cells overreact and release inflammatory proteins. These in turn cause swelling, pain, and further damage to the tissue. Joints become stiff and sore, although not all at once and maybe never more than a few.

Osteoarthritis usually announces itself with pain and stiffness, especially in weight-bearing joints such as your hips and knees. Repetitive motion is often the culprit. If you spent your youth hurling a ball, you may be at risk for arthritis in your shoulders. Even relatively young skiers and runners can develop severe knee problems.

MODERN MARVEL

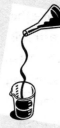

Poked and Prodded

Research directed by the National Institutes of Health indicates that people with osteoarthritis of the knee who receive acupuncture have less pain and better function than those who don't—even weeks after the treatment. Ask your doctor to recommend a reputable acupuncturist near you. And if getting the needle makes you nervous, transcutaneous electrical nerve stimulation (TENS) is an attractive alternative. A TENS unit is a battery-powered device, smaller than a deck of cards, that you attach to your belt or waistband. It delivers electrical impulses through the skin. Although TENS doesn't offer a cure, it may relieve chronic pain. It increases endorphins—naturally occurring narcotics in the body—that inhibit pain impulses arising from the spinal cord. Ask your doctor about TENS.

Move with Ease

You should call your doctor at the first sign of joint pain. It's always possible that you have rheumatoid arthritis or another kind of joint disease. In most cases, though, your joints are simply wearing out a bit. But don't panic and throw a lot of money at the problem right away. In many cases, you can use home remedies such as these to eliminate most—if not all—of your pain:

- **Watch the clock.** If you take an occasional pain reliever, it's best to take it before noon. Since the pain and inflammation tend to be worst in the late afternoon and evening, you can get a jump on them by starting your treatment in the morning or at midday.

- **Hide the high heels.** Skinny stilettos are murder on your knees—but they're not the only culprits. In fact, high, wide-heeled pumps may predispose you to osteoarthritis of the knee, too. The problem, it seems, isn't the stability of the platform but the height of the heel. Women who regularly wear heels higher than 2 inches are twice as likely to develop arthritis as women who don't. Heels shift your body weight away from your ankles and onto your hips and the inner part of your knee joints, and arthritis is often the result.

- **Exercise as much as you can.** Exercise is a tricky issue if you have arthritis. You obviously don't want to push yourself too hard when you're hurting. On the other hand, regular exercise lubricates your joints and helps with weight loss. Walking is almost always a good choice. If you have too much knee or ankle pain to walk, ride a stationary bike. Set the seat high so you don't have to bend your knees as much.

- **Cut those calories.** The next time your bathroom scale sneaks up a hair, don't fret about your fanny—it's your knees that deserve your pity! Each time you gain a single pound of body fat, experts say it feels like four times that much on your knees. The strain is especially hard on your muscles and tendons—your built-in shock absorbers. The good news is, studies show that if you lose as few as 11 pounds, you can reduce the stiffness and pain in your knees by half.

- **Get action with attraction.** Although scientists aren't sure why, studies show that wearing knee wraps embedded with magnets may help you get out of a chair more easily, walk faster and less stiffly, and even sleep better. Attracted to the possibilities? Look for wraps with "unipolar" magnets, then place the positive end of the magnet directly over your sore knee. You should feel relief within 30 minutes.

- **Oil your joints.** Trout, salmon, and other cold-water fish contain an abundance of omega-3 essential fatty acids, which ease swollen, stiff joints by reducing both inflammation and cartilage destruction. So serve 'em up often.

- **Pepper the pain.** A quick way to ease arthritis pain is to apply a topical cream that contains capsaicin, the hot chemical compound that's found in red pepper. Most drugstores carry the cream, which comes in concentrations from 0.025 to 0.075%; if you have sensitive skin, try a lower strength first. Follow the label directions and be careful not to get it near your eyes or on any areas of broken skin. Wash your hands after using it.

- **Add some arnica.** To soothe aching joints, add a few drops of arnica oil to your favorite healing salve. Try using a warming wintergreen, lavender, or rosemary salve as a base. All three can help increase circulation to the painful area. For every ½ teaspoon of salve, add 3 or 4 drops of arnica oil. Apply to sore joints three or four times per day. Arnica is for external use only, though, and don't use it on broken skin.

- **Put cold on heat.** When an arthritic joint is inflamed, it may be painful, swollen, or even feel hot. Put some ice on that fire. Put an ice pack on the sore joint for about 20 minutes at a time. Repeat the treatment once an hour, continuing for as long as it seems to help.

- **Warm the stiffness.** When your joints are achy, but there's no swelling, heat works better than cold. It feels good, for one thing, and it promotes the flow of healing nutrients into the joint. Moist heat seems to work best, so you may want to use a warm compress instead of

From Grandma's Kitchen

Whenever my Grandma Putt's arthritic knee started acting up, she went to the garden and cut a head of cabbage. Cabbage leaves have been used for centuries to soothe inflammation, and a sturdy outer leaf is just the right shape to place over a bent knee or an elbow. Blanch a leaf or two, then apply it, either warm or cool, to inflamed joints. Wrap it with gauze or an elastic bandage to hold it in place.

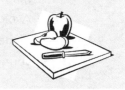

a heating pad. Soak a small towel in hot water, wring it out, and drape it over your painful joint. When the towel cools, soak it again and reapply it.

- **Stop pain with licorice.** Licorice root is a friend indeed when your arthritis flares up, because it can counteract the inflammation. Licorice root is available in capsules and tablets at health food stores (don't bother with licorice candy; unfortunately it contains little or no real licorice). Since a substance in licorice called glycyrrhizic acid can cause high blood pressure in some people, look for deglycyrrhizinated licorice (DGL) products, then follow the label directions.

- **Spice up your menu.** The herb turmeric is aromatic and spicy, and research suggests that it's

MODERN MARVEL

Rebuild with Glucosamine

One of the most effective treatments for osteoarthritis is glucosamine sulfate, a supplement produced from shellfish. It combats cartilage-destroying enzymes and halts cartilage loss in the knee and hip. Start with 500 to 1,000 milligrams three times a day. It takes two to four weeks to get relief from pain—and twice that long to ease functioning in your joint. Avoid it if you have a seafood allergy. *Caution:* If you have diabetes or are on blood-sugar-lowering medication, consult your doctor before taking.

a great inflammation fighter. You can add it to rice, stews, and meat dishes.

- **Lay off the lattes.** If you drink more than four cups of coffee a day, you're doubling your risk of developing arthritis. Caffeine not only alters the mineral balance that's needed to make cartilage, it's dehydrating and may prevent joints from being adequately lubricated.

- **Drink up.** Like most people, you probably don't drink enough water, and that could be making your arthritis symptoms worse. Drink at least eight full glasses every day—and don't wait until you're thirsty. The fact is, by the time you feel thirsty, your body's water levels have already dropped too low.

Get Prescription Relief

If your joints are so swollen and painfully stiff that you can barely climb out of your car, and you're popping aspirin or ibuprofen tablets as if they were breath mints, it's time to visit your doctor. He or she can prescribe a medication for you that will ease your pain, perhaps with fewer side effects than aspirin or ibuprofen.

Asthma

It's no accident that asthma flare-ups are called attacks. When asthma sufferers' airways narrow or shut down, they literally feel as if they're fighting for their lives—and in many cases, they are. Even very mild asthma can flare up as instantly and seriously as severe asthma—and prove to be just as fatal.

Even though many people still think of asthma as a childhood disease, increasing numbers of adults—more women than men—are developing it. Researchers aren't sure of the exact reason. They suspect that several factors come into play. The usual triggers (such as pollen, dust, and frigid air) can inflame airways and cause them to fill with mucus. But both increased body weight (which can literally weigh on the chest wall, making it more difficult to breathe), and the surges and drops in hormones associated with menstruation and menopause, may also play a role.

Fighting for Breath

Our airways naturally narrow a bit when we're exposed to smoke, pollutants, very cold air, or substances that can harm us if we breathe them in. But in people with asthma, perhaps due to a glitch in their genes, this response is exaggerated. Luckily most people can quickly reverse an asthma attack using prescription medication—usually an inhaled bronchodilator—to open the constricted airways. When an attack is more prolonged, however, the inhaler doesn't do much. As airways become more inflamed and often clogged with mucus, it gets harder and harder to breathe. This type of episode is a medical emergency, and you need to get to the nearest hospital emergency room—fast.

Breathe Easy

The bottom line? Never fool around with asthma. People can and do die from this disease. While nearly everyone with asthma uses inhalers and other medications, there are drug-free ways to tackle it as well. Here are the best ones to discuss with your doctor:

■ **Put your trust in fish.** Tuna, salmon, trout, and other cold-water fish contain loads of omega-3 essential fatty acids (EFAs), which not only inhibit inflammation but may also promote healing. Eat fish regularly or take 1 to 3 grams of fish oil daily to minimize asthma symptoms. If you don't eat fish often or are sensitive to it,

dial the
DOCTOR

Watch for Warning Signs

If you have wheezing, shortness of breath, or tightness in your chest that doesn't respond to inhaled or oral medications, head to the hospital immediately. Other serious signs include difficulty talking, rapid or shallow breathing, flared nostrils, tightly stretched skin on your neck and/or around your ribcage with each breath, and gray or bluish skin around your mouth or under your fingernails.

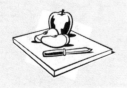
as many people with asthma are, down 1 to 3 tablespoons of flaxseed oil (another source of EFAs) a day. You can find both oils at health food stores and drugstores, but don't use them if you take aspirin, other nonsteroidal anti-inflammatory drugs, or prescription blood thinners.

Enjoy your daily brew. A few cups of strong coffee can sometimes reduce asthma symptoms. Nobody knows exactly why, but it may be because caffeine is a chemical that's similar to the theophylline in tea, which opens constricted bronchial tubes.

Watch for culinary culprits. Asthma is often caused by allergies, and in some cases, the problem is specific foods. Unfortunately, there is no handy list of food allergens—they vary with each individual. If you suspect that foods may be triggering your asthma, talk to your doctor immediately. Then keep a careful record of what you eat, when you eat it, and what kind of symptoms develop afterward. After a few weeks, a pattern may emerge. Take your record to your doctor and ask him or her to check your suspicions with skin or other allergy tests.

Get a cleaner vacuum. Vacuum cleaners can kick up 2 to 10 times the amount of allergens that normally float around your house. The extra onslaught can persist for up to an hour after you turn off the vac. If you have chronic asthma, look into special vacuums that eliminate this dusty "exhaust." (They're expensive but worth it to ease your symptoms.) You could also wear a dust mask when you vacuum or, better yet, swap housecleaning chores with someone else.

■ **Beat it with borage.** The star-shaped flowers of the borage plant are packed with gamma-lino-lenic acid (GLA), a fatty acid that fights asthma inflammation. Check your health food store for either borage or primrose oil (also packed with GLA) and take 3 grams (3,000 milligrams) daily. If you're pollen-sensitive, however, check with your doctor first.

■ **Sleep high.** Heading to a dude ranch or rustic retreat anytime soon? Be sure to get dibs on the upper bunk. It's well worth the climb. When you sleep in the bottom bunk, you're showered with dust bunnies and dust mites that fall from the bedding above when the sleeper tosses and turns—and asthma is more likely to flare.

■ **Exercise often.** It used to be that if exercise triggered your asthma, you could count on becoming a couch potato. Not anymore. For one thing, doctors now know the couch is home to billions of dust mites, so you can't hang out there. For another, proper exercise helps people with asthma. You need muscle tone, a stronger heart, and increased stamina to fight any disease, and asthma is no exception.

■ **Unload your stress.** Emotional stress doesn't cause asthma, but it can aggravate it. To reduce anxiety and perhaps improve your breathing, take 20 minutes a day to write nonstop about

Grandma Says:

Get steamed. To help me unclog my tight airways, Grandma would fill a pot with water, bring it to a boil, and remove it from the stove. Then I'd place a towel over my head to trap the steam, lean over the pot, and breathe deeply. These days, you can also turn on a hot shower and sit in the steamy bathroom for 10 to 15 minutes.

what's stressing you (don't edit yourself, just get it out). Studies show that after about four months, you may be breathing easier—which is less stressful by itself!

- **Breathe more slowly.** If you're a wheezer, experts say you're also an overbreather. That is, you breathe heavily or rapidly or inhale through your mouth—any one of which can promote irritation and inflammation of the airways. To slow your breathing, use your heart rate as a guide. For every seven heartbeats, breathe in once through your nose. For the next nine beats, breathe out through your mouth with your lips pursed until your air is gone.

- **Keep the air clean.** Because asthma is often triggered by airborne allergens, make your bedroom an allergy-free zone. It's easy: Simply keep the door and windows shut at all times.

MODERN MARVEL

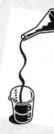

Maximize Magnesium

Studies show that if your diet is deficient in magnesium, your asthma may be more severe. The recommended supplement dose is 800 milligrams of magnesium gluconate (divided into two 400-milligram doses) along with 800 milligrams of calcium citrate a day, but check it with your doctor first. This much magnesium may cause diarrhea. If this occurs, reduce the dose, then increase it gradually.

Never allow your beloved terrier or tabby to enter. Remove all carpet and throw rugs. Get rid of dust-collecting knickknacks. And use an air cleaner with a HEPA filter (a high-efficiency particulate air filter, which can trap nearly 100 percent of all airborne particles).

- **Use a peak flow meter.** This little gadget costs only a few dollars at the drugstore, and it can save your life. The meter gauges how much air you're able to push out of your lungs, and it may help you predict when an asthma attack is sneaking up on you. Ask your doctor which readings may signal the need to take action, then blow into it twice a day and compare your readings against your "personal best" number.

An Apple a Day...

can keep asthma away. An apple's skin (as well as the skins of tomatoes and onions, and the Indian spice turmeric) contains quercetin, a potent bioflavonoid that may help keep your airways clear. If you aren't crazy about apples, you can take 500 to 1,000 milligrams of quercetin in capsule form three times a day, along with 100 to 200 milligrams of bromelain, a pineapple-derived enzyme that will boost its absorption. Avoid bromelain if you take blood thinners. And avoid quercetin if you are allergic to or sensitive to onions.

Athlete's Foot

dial the DOCTOR

Serious Stuff

While a normal case of Athlete's foot is nothing to fret about, it can become a serious infection. If the fungus has spread to your arches, or your feet are fiery red, swollen, and covered with blisters, contact your doctor—pronto.

The irony of athlete's foot is that while it's rarely serious, it sure feels (and looks) like it could be. The nasty fungus known as *Tinea pedis* that's behind athlete's foot thrives in the warmth and dampness created by the sauna inside your gym shoes or snug-fitting socks. It usually settles in the moist area between your fourth and fifth piggies, and feeds off dead skin cells. And, once the webs of your toes become cracked and red, they itch like the devil!

Tinea gains a foothold best in folks with weakened immune systems and those who have recently used antibiotics. (Those drugs kill off all bacteria, including the beneficial types that keep fungi in check.) People with diabetes are also at increased risk, because they tend to have more sugar in their systems. Fungal infections thrive in alkaline environments, so if your diet is high in sugar, yeast, and other alkaline foods, you can get the itch.

Treats for Your Feet

If you're on the ball, and you catch the infection in the early stages of itching, you can always fight back with an over-the-counter antifungal agent. But why spend the money if you don't have to? In most cases, you can tackle athlete's foot with simple, homemade cures—and your symptoms should clear up within a week. Here are some worth trying:

- **Soak those piggies.** To soothe the itch and start the healing process, place your feet in a basin of warm water spiked with 2 to 3 teaspoons of tea tree oil, and soak for about 15 minutes twice daily. This oil, from the Australian malaluca tree, is one of nature's best antifungals. Or, if you have sensitive skin, start with a gentler herb. Since tea tree oil may sting when applied topically, first try one of the gentler antifungal herbs, such as goldenseal, chamomile, or calendula. You can even look for over-the-counter antifungal creams that pack all three for more healing punch.

- **Zap it with zinc.** Not only will zinc increase immunity (and thereby quash fungi), but it will also help broken skin heal faster. Take 30 milligrams of supplemental zinc daily, with food, for as long as the fungus persists.

- **Be a clean machine.** Dodge this grungy fungus by meticulously cleaning under your toenails and between your toes during your daily bath or shower. Dry very well!

Tea Time

Tea made from fresh ginger provides more than 20 antifungal compounds that'll help soothe your itchy feet. To make the tea, add 1 teaspoon of grated ginger to a cup of boiling water, steep for 10 to 15 minutes, and strain. Sweeten with honey and drink a cup three times daily, then swab your hot, itchy feet with a cotton ball soaked in any leftover tea.

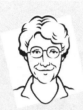

Grandma Says:

Gobble those berries! When we were hit with athlete's foot, Grandma Putt fed us loads of strawberries and blueberries. They're packed with vitamin C, which boosts your immune system to help fight infection. If the fruit's out of season, and if you don't have kidney or stomach problems, take 1,000 milligrams of vitamin C twice a day.

■ **Dry 'em well.** If you're prone to athlete's foot, dry each toe separately after you shower. Then use a paper towel between them to absorb every drop of moisture. Or use a blow dryer set on low. It may sound silly, but it'll feel good!

■ **Count on cotton.** While you're treating your athlete's foot, avoid wearing panty hose and stick to socks made of 100 percent cotton. Wash and dry your feet twice daily, then slip 'em into a fresh pair of all-cotton socks sprinkled with antifungal powder.

■ **Catch some air.** Let those tootsies hang out in the fresh air and sunshine if you're not going anywhere. Just don't walk barefoot around the house. Not only will you track foot powder all over your rugs, but you'll plant contagious little fungus seedlings wherever you go. And you don't want to be known as Johnny Fungusseed, do you?

Kitchen Cures

You can often find relief from athlete's foot right in your kitchen cabinets. So pull up a chair and try some of these:

■ **Go for garlic.** Garlic is a potent topical antifungal. Try placing a clove of raw, peeled garlic between all your toes every night for a week. (Apply a generous film of olive oil first.) Put on cotton socks before going to bed, then wash and dry your feet each morning. Although you may need to sleep in the guest room, this treatment should stop the itch in its tracks. *Caution:* Garlic can burn the skin, so if you feel any discomfort, remove the garlic and wash your feet immediately.

- **Take time for thyme.** A traditional remedy for athlete's foot is soaking your feet in hot water to which you've added a few drops of oil of thyme to relieve the itching and burning. Then dust your feet with a mixture of myrrh and goldenseal powder in any proportion and put on a pair of heavy cotton socks. Repeat daily for several days.

- **Soak in vinegar.** Fungi hate acids, and apple cider vinegar is one of the best acid soaks there is. Here's what to do: Simply fill a basin with equal parts vinegar and warm, soothing water, then soak your feet for 10 minutes daily. Dry each toe and the area between your toes thoroughly when you're done.

Lay on Some Licorice

Licorice contains a whopping total of 25 fungicidal substances. Too bad munching on licorice whips won't do the trick. What you need to do is add 6 teaspoons of powdered licorice to a cup of boiling water and simmer for 20 minutes. Strain out any residue and apply the clear tea to your inflamed toes three times a day.

Give Up on Cornstarch

This popular ingredient has replaced talc in many powdered anti-sweat products, but it can actually encourage fungus growth. You're better off using a medicated antifungal powder or a foot spray that combines calendula and witch hazel, an astringent herb that reduces moisture.

Back Pain

There aren't many good things to say about back pain, but here's a small bit of comfort: It usually doesn't last very long, and it's rarely serious. Most people recover in a few weeks without spending a dime at the doctor's office.

Okay, now for the lousy news: Sooner or later, just about everyone gets it. Sure, you can injure your back on the job or in a car crash, but by far the most frequent cause isn't anything catastrophic—it's everyday weakness and inflexibility in the muscles that support the back.

Weakness Equals Pain

The weaker your muscles (especially those in your upper back, hips, and hamstrings—the muscles at the backs of your thighs), the more apt you are to hurt your back. A sudden, uncharacteristic movement—something as simple as swinging a golf club—strains the stiff muscles, tendons, and ligaments, damaging tissue and causing swell-

Get in the Swim

Swimming is one of the fastest ways to take the kinks out of aching back muscles. For one thing, merely submerging yourself in warm water will help reduce muscle tension. More important, the water supports your weight, which allows you to exercise without putting additional strain on your back.

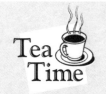

Tea Time

Willow bark is a natural source of aspirin-like salicylates, which ease pain. Unlike aspirin or ibuprofen, though, it won't irritate your stomach while it's easing your back pain. To make a tea, pick up some willow bark from a health food store, steep 2 teaspoons in a cup of boiling water, and strain. You can also take capsules or apply willow bark ointment directly to your back. Don't use it in any form, however, if you take aspirin; the double dose of salicylates may be too much.

ing and intense aching. Your muscles may even seize in spasms to protect your back from further movement and additional injury.

Ease the Ache

Don't twiddle your thumbs waiting for Father Time to cure your aching back—you can nudge him along. In fact, you should, because if you treat a back problem in the acute phase, you may reduce the likelihood of long-term pain and disability. Back pain that's severe or doesn't start getting better within a week or two should always be checked by a doctor. For garden-variety aches, though, here's what you need to do:

- **Move and keep moving.** The worst thing anyone with an achy back can do is to sit still. In fact, resting for more than a day or two reduces muscle flexibility and strength and can lead to further disability. On the other hand, movement keeps blood flowing into the site, waste products flowing out of it, and muscle spasms to a minimum. Let your pain be your guide and do everyday activities as you can tolerate them.

- **Do the ball stretch.** The more you work your back muscles, the faster you can return to normal activities. Grab an oversize exercise ball and give this mini-workout a try. First, lie face down across the ball with your hands and feet on the floor. Lift one arm and then the other as high as you can, raising your torso from the ball.

Pause for a count of 10, then return both hands to the floor. Next, place both hands behind your head and lift your torso as high as you can. Hold for 5 counts, then release. Repeat as many times as is comfortable.

- **Stretch and flex.** Even if your back pain has you lying on the floor, you can stretch your arms and legs, elongating the tissues in your back and drawing healing blood and oxygen to the area. Just remember to stay relaxed, cushion your back with a pad, and use slow, gentle movements as you extend your arms over your head and stretch your legs along the floor. Hold each stretch for about a minute, then relax.

- **Ease pain with Epsom.** A traditional Epsom salts bath can help ease spasms and relieve pain. Add 2 cups of the salts to a hot bath, sink down, and feel the relief. Afterward, place an ice pack on your back.

Lie Down and Say "Ahh..."

According to studies, weekly massages can cut the need for pain medication for back spasms and muscle tightness in half. As a general rule, a muscle spasm should relax when the therapist massages it. If it persists, you probably have some inflammation, too, and massage may not be the best therapy for you. You'll probably need at least four massage treatments to smooth out spasms, too, so be patient.

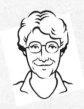

Grandma Says:

Roll over. When an aching back kept Grandpa Putt up at night, Grandma would have him lie on his side with a pillow between his knees. Try it yourself. Or, if you're a back-sleeper, put a pillow under your knees to reduce the arch in your back and relieve some of the strain.

Straighten Up that Spine

If your mother always nagged you to stand up straight, she had the right idea. Keep your shoulders back, chest out, stomach in, chin up! That's good posture, and correct posture means that your body is aligned so it puts less strain on your lower back. If you stand a lot, as a surgeon or supermarket clerk does, shift your weight from hip to hip to avoid back pain.

And while you're standing tall, take a load off your shoulders. When you carry a shoulder bag, you tend to tense your shoulder to keep the bag from slipping off. This scrunched-up posture causes all kinds of muscle strain and related pain. Pick up a short-handled purse or carryall. Since you can't sling the bag over your shoulder, you'll be more inclined to switch the weight from hand to hand.

Sit Smart

Don't focus on your posture only while you're standing. Sitting smart counts, too. If you sit at a desk all day, keep your feet flat on the floor. Your arms should be positioned so your elbows form right angles. Set your computer monitor at eye level. Your chair seat should be deep enough to support your hips, but the front edge should not touch the backs of your knees. The chair back should have an angle of about 10 degrees, and cradle the small of your back comfortably. If it doesn't, add a wedge-shaped cushion there.

Here's some back-happy news: An old-fashioned, straight-backed chair is better for your back than many of those high-tech, ergonomic extravaganzas that cost hundreds—or even thousands—of dollars. Or you can try a kneeler chair to see if it relieves your back pain.

Go Hot or Cold

It sounds contradictory, but some folks find that heat really eases their back pain, while others swear by cold. How to decide? Try both—heat one day and cold the next—and see what works best for you.

- **Apply instant heat.** Tiger Balm is a familiar remedy from ancient Chinese medicine. Rubbed into the skin, this potent salve creates heat to warm tight muscles and a tingling sensation to divert your attention from the pain.

MODERN MARVEL

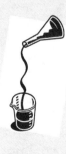

Knock Down Swelling

Studies have shown that aspirin, ibuprofen, and similar drugs often work as well for back pain as more powerful prescription drugs. They help in two ways: They're analgesics, which means they work directly on pain, and they have anti-inflammatory effects, which reduce swelling. Acetaminophen is fine for pain, but it has little or no effect on inflammation.

Consult a doctor if you have back pain that persists without abating for more than three days; if it's accompanied by fever, or bowel or bladder change; if you have pain at night or when resting; or if you are weak or can't stand on your tiptoes, which may indicate nerve damage. If you have a history of cancer or diabetes, you should see a doctor immediately to check for a tumor or nerve damage.

■ **Put cold to work.** Ice is a great analgesic and is preferable to aspirin or other nonsteroidal anti-inflammatory drugs like ibuprofen, which, in large doses, can upset your stomach. Simply fill a paper or Styrofoam cup with water and freeze it, then peel away the rim to expose the ice surface. Grasping the cup, lie on your side, then apply the ice directly to the painful area in a circular motion. Limit the massage to about 5 minutes, and don't place the ice directly on the bony portion of your spine.

Thyme for a Bath

Ease your aching back by tossing a handful of dried thyme into the tub as you run hot water for a bath. Soak for 10 to 15 minutes, letting the aromatic oils in this herb take your aches and pains down the drain.

Sore Back Soothers

Your local health food store has some excellent back-pain fighters on the shelf. Here's a quick rundown:

■ **Stop aches with arnica.** Arnica gel is a top-notch first-aid ointment for muscle or joint pain. For inflamed and irritated nerves, add several drops of St. John's wort oil and apply frequently. Note that arnica is for external use only. Do not use on broken skin.

- **Relax with an herbal mix.** Scour your health food store for herbal pain formulas that contain cramp bark, black cohosh, and oatstraw in capsule form. These herbs are all excellent antispasmodics and muscle relaxants. If valerian, which is a sedative, is also among the ingredients, the capsules will make a great nightcap for a bad back. Follow the dosage directions on the label. Skip the valerian if you're taking other medications, though.

- **Baby it with bromelain.** This anti-inflammatory enzyme, derived from the pineapple plant, may be especially helpful for relieving pain related to inflammation. As long as you're not taking blood thinners, check at a health food store for bromelain supplements, then follow the label directions.

Bad Breath

Do your friends lean wa-a-ay back the minute you start talking? Does your spouse burrow under the pillows when you lean in for a little smooch? If you answered "Yes!" to either of these questions, blame halitosis, the polite term for dragon breath. Bad breath is certainly better than no breath at all, and, truth be told, no one's breath is minty-fresh all the time. But if you have the impression that people are thinking "roadkill" every time you open your mouth, it's time to take a few steps to freshen things up a bit.

Start at the Sink

Bad breath is almost always the product of odor-causing bacteria in the mouth. But if your breath is *always* bad, you should talk to your doctor. All sorts of conditions, including digestive problems, can cause it. In most cases, though, you can fight the fumes with a few simple strategies:

- **Get those bristles moving.** Are you brushing twice a day with a soft brush? The bedtime brushing is important so plaque doesn't form during the night (when you have less saliva). Massage your gums with the brush, too, and floss before you brush. Flossing every day helps remove plaque—and bacteria—from between your teeth. The American Dental Association also recommends professional cleaning at least annually, and some dentists suggest twice a year.

- **Rake your tongue.** Most bad breath comes from the wet, boggy area in the back of your mouth, where bacteria breed a sulfurous-smelling plaque on your tongue. Before brushing, reach into your mouth as far as you can without gagging and scrape away the plaque. Most drugstores carry plastic tongue scrapers, or you can simply use your toothbrush.

- **Swish, swish, swish.** Some mouthwashes merely mask odor with a minty solution, so make sure you use an antiseptic mouthwash that kills bacteria. Or try making your own odor-fighting mouthwash with whole or powdered cloves steeped in hot water.

- **Try a myrrhvalous mouthwash.** Add 1 teaspoon of tincture of myrrh to ¼ cup of water, then swish and spit. It instantly freshens breath—and it tastes good, too. (Tinctures are potent liquid plant extracts; you can find them at many health food stores.)

From Grandma's Kitchen

Grandma Putt knew apples not only keep the doctor away, but they also keep bad breath at bay. In fact, an apple is a great remedy for garlic breath. In a healthy mouth, garlic odor usually goes away after a while, but you'll speed up the process if you dilute the pungent aroma by eating an apple, then brushing your teeth.

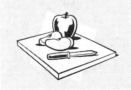

Bad breath is usually a result of poor dental hygiene, a poor diet, or a sinus or gum infection, but it can also signal something as serious as kidney failure, liver disease, or diabetes. Visit your doctor if you have persistent bad breath that you can't clear up with simple home care.

■ **Chug plenty of H2O.** Keeping yourself well hydrated is a good health practice in general, but it's especially important to help keep bad breath at bay. Drink those eight glasses a day to help keep saliva production going and reduce bacteria buildup.

Love those Leaves!

Some Native American traditions call for using spearmint or bergamot leaf as a quick and easy digestive aid and breath freshener. Chew a leaf or two slowly. Then make a cup of mild mint tea by steeping three leaves in a cup of boiling water for 10 minutes. Strain out the leaves, let the tea cool, and use it as a gargle, rinse, or spray. And to keep your breath smelling sweet, carry a sandwich bag or pouch of mint or parsley leaves so you can chew on them periodically throughout the day.

Bad Breath Rx

You can knock bad breath flat on its back with these kitchen counter cures:

■ **Refresh and brighten.** Here's a cleansing and refreshing mixture that clears up bad breath while brightening the teeth. You can use this tooth powder daily or alternate it with a commercial brand. In a small dish, mix 1 tablespoon baking soda, ½ teaspoon sea salt or kosher salt, ½ teaspoon powdered allspice, and ½ teaspoon ground sage. Sprinkle onto your toothbrush and brush, or stir 1 teaspoon into a cup of warm water and gargle.

- **Feel fresh with fennel.** Chewing fennel seeds after meals will help freshen breath and promote healthy digestion.

- **Pepper away mouth germs.** Red pepper (cayenne) not only kills germs, it leaves your breath spicy fresh as well. Just dilute 5 to 10 drops each of cayenne tincture and myrrh tincture (available at health food stores) in half a glass of warm water and use it to rinse your mouth.

Help from the Produce Aisle

Vegetables and fruits are not only valuable sources of vitamins and antioxidants, they also contain chlorophyll, a natural deodorant that sweetens your breath. Eat five to nine servings a day for a healthy body and healthy breath.

While you're at it, throw in some sour foods, such as pickles and lemons. They will jump-start the flow of saliva, helping to flush away those nasty halitosis bacteria.

Bites and Stings

Even if you live in a bustling city where the only lawns, meadows, or woods you're likely to see are on picture postcards, it's almost impossible to avoid the occasional close encounter of the insect kind. Biting and stinging bugs make themselves at home just about anywhere, and they all have one thing in common: They inject chemicals that often make your skin swell and hurt.

Bite Back

With a few dangerous exceptions (the black widow comes to mind), most bites and stings are only minor nuisances. See a doctor if you wind up with bad hives or other serious reactions. Otherwise, try these quick tips for relief:

■ **Freeze the bite.** As with other types of inflammation, some well-applied ice can freeze a painful insect sting in its tracks. Ice also soothes the itchiness of mosquito bites.

Wrap some ice cubes in a washcloth or small towel to make a cold pack, then hold it against the affected area for about 20 minutes. Remove it for at least 20 minutes, then continue applying it in this way until you're feeling better.

- **Cool it down.** Soak a washcloth in cool water, wring it out, and drape it over the bite. The cool compress will help reduce itching.

- **Take away the sting.** If the insect left a stinger embedded in your skin, remove it as quickly as possible. Otherwise, it will continue to irritate the skin; a bee's stinger will continue to release venom even after the insect is gone. Scrape the stinger out with your fingernail, or pull it out with your fingers or tweezers.

- **Soak in oats.** To instantly relieve itchy skin, place 1 cup of oats in a sock, and hang it from the faucet as you run your bathwater. (Very hot water can make the itch worse, so stick to warm water.) While you're soaking, squeeze the sock and let the milky water cascade over the bites.

- **Prepare to repair.** To help your skin repair itself, be sure to get plenty of vitamins C and E, two nutrients that are critical for skin health. You'll get both—along with other vitamins and minerals—by taking a multivitamin.

- **Think prevention.** Natural mosquito repellents are effective only if you use them frequently, and there aren't too many of the little blood-suckers around. Look for products that contain neem, lemongrass, or citronella oils. Test an

dial the DOCTOR

A Dangerous Reaction

If you have any sign of body swelling or difficulty breathing after a sting, call 911 or get to an emergency room immediately. Stings can cause a life-threatening reaction, called anaphylaxis, in some people. If you know you're allergic, your doctor will probably prescribe an epinephrine self-injector (epi-pen) so you can take fast action if you're bitten or stung.

area of your skin first to be sure the repellent doesn't irritate you, then spray or dab it directly on your skin, following the package directions. Studies show that neem oil provides significant protection against malaria-carrying mosquitoes for up to 12 hours; another study found that lemongrass and citronella oils are highly effective against most species of mosquitoes.

■ **Keep your shoes on.** Bees often hover just above the ground, gathering pollen from clover and ground flowers. So don't go barefoot across the lawn—you could step on a bee and get stung.

Soothing Sage Mash

Make a sting-soothing poultice of sage and vinegar. Run a rolling pin over a handful of freshly picked sage leaves to bruise them. Put the leaves in a pan, cover with apple cider vinegar, and simmer on low until they soften. Remove the leaves, carefully wrap them in a washcloth, and place it on stings and swellings.

Black Eyes

If you like old movies, you've probably seen some unfortunate character holding a steak to his injured eye after a run-in with a bully or a barn door. While no one really uses steaks to soothe black eyes (have you checked the price of beef lately?), the idea wasn't so far-fetched. Black eyes hurt, and putting something cool on it probably felt pretty good.

A hard knock can break blood vessels beneath the skin, causing swelling and a lot of tenderness. It takes a week or two for a black eye to heal completely, and in the meantime, chemical changes in the skin give it its astonishing range of hues.

Banish the Black-and-Blue

Since shiners always look terrible, you can't go by appearance alone in deciding whether you're seriously injured. If you have bleeding, pain in the eyeball (as opposed to the surrounding area),

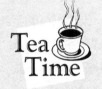

Tea Time

Soothe a black eye with a tea bag. Tea contains tannins, chemical compounds that help reduce swelling. After brewing, let the tea bag cool for a few minutes, then squeeze out the excess moisture. Lie back, close your eyes, and hold the tea bag against the injured area for 10 minutes.

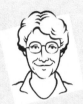

Grandma Says:

Repair with C.
Back in Grandma's day, folks would slap a raw steak on a black eye. Nowadays, we have better treatments. Vitamin C, for example, helps strengthen tiny blood vessels called capillaries. As long as you don't have stomach or kidney problems, take 2,000 to 3,000 milligrams daily in divided doses until the black eye is gone.

or vision changes (double vision, for example) after the injury, get to a doctor right away. Otherwise, you can speed healing without spending a bundle on fancy ointments. Here's how:

- **Start with cold.** Nothing is better for a black eye than applying ice right away. Cold causes blood vessels to constrict, or narrow, which reduces internal bleeding, swelling, and those unsightly color changes. Cold also numbs the area and helps ease the throbbing. Make yourself an ice pack by wrapping some ice cubes in a washcloth or small towel, then gently hold it against the area for 15 to 20 minutes every few hours during the 24 hours following the injury.

- **Then use heat.** You don't want to apply heat to a black eye right away because it may increase bleeding under the skin. From 24 to 48 hours after the injury, though, a warm compress is just the thing. The heat promotes circulation and helps flush pain-causing substances from the area. Soak a washcloth in warm water, wring it out, and apply it for a few minutes as often as necessary to reduce discomfort.

- **Run the hot-cold cycle.** You can also try a technique called contrast hydrotherapy, in which you alternate warm and cold compresses. The combination of heat and cold helps the body flush and clean the tissues and will help your eye heal more quickly. Start by applying a warm compress for about 3 minutes. Switch to cold for 30 seconds, then go back to heat. Repeat the process two or three times, always ending with the cold application. Use this technique three times a day until your black eye is completely healed.

Heal with Comfrey

The herb comfrey is among the best treatments for minor wounds and bruises, and it's perfect for a black eye. If you're using fresh leaves, mash them into a paste and apply it directly to the bruise. If you're using the dried form, crush the leaves between your fingers and add just enough water to moisten. Wrap the dampened powder in a piece of cheesecloth, then hold it on the area. Apply either form of the herb for about 20 minutes twice a day. Comfrey is available at health food stores.

Skip the Aspirin

Even though it's a great remedy for pain, aspirin reduces the ability of blood to clot normally, which could result in even more bruising in the days following the injury. A better choice is acetaminophen, which has the same painkilling properties as aspirin but is less likely to cause additional bleeding or bruising.

Blisters

Watch for Infection

The only time blisters are really dangerous is when they get infected. If the pain is getting worse, or if you notice the area is swelling or turning red, apply an over-the-counter triple antibiotic ointment a few times a day. If that doesn't help, see a doctor.

You have to give your skin credit: It's not only weather resistant, germ repellent, and self-healing, it also knows how to protect itself. When you exert too much pressure—by spending all day on your knees scrubbing floors, for example, or wearing tight shoes without socks—the skin responds to potentially damaging friction by forming a blister, a protective, fluid-filled pad that can be painful.

Most blisters go away on their own, usually within a few days to a week, but that doesn't mean you can ignore them. Blisters can easily become infected—and when that happens, they hurt like the dickens!

Hurry the Healing

Your doctor will charge a bundle to open and drain a blister. You might need the help—but probably not. Except when they get infected, there's no reason to pop blisters to drain out the fluid. Here are some easy, inexpensive steps to prevent infection and help blisters heal:

■ **Catch 'em quick.** Before a blister appears, you'll usually notice a hot spot—a red, tender area on your skin. Acting quickly at this stage may prevent a blister from forming. If you've had a burn, for example, quickly apply ice to the area and keep it there for about 20 minutes. If the hot spot is caused by friction, cushion the area with moleskin, gauze, or other padding.

■ **Wash away the germs.** The best way to keep infection-causing germs out of blisters is to clean them (and the surrounding skin) once or twice a day. Wash the area well with soap and water, then dry it thoroughly. Too much moisture will soften the blister and make it more likely to break open before it's ready.

■ **No worries with "wort."** The herb St. John's wort is great for killing germs and easing pain. Use an alcohol-based tincture, available at health food stores, to moisten a square of gauze, then apply it to the blister after you've washed it.

■ **Lay on some yarrow.** Big blisters sometimes take a long time to heal. You can speed things along by applying yarrow, an herb that naturally draws out the fluid. Chop or crumble fresh or dried yarrow (available at health food stores), as finely as you can, then add water to make a paste. Apply the paste to the blister, and cover it with an adhesive or gauze bandage. Replace once a day until the blister is gone.

Count on Clover

Red clover oil is a great choice for healing blisters. You can put the oil directly on the sore, then cover it with a bandage to promote healing. Repeat the treatment once a day until the blister's gone. The oil is available in most health food stores, but be sure the product you buy is made for topical use. What you don't want is an essential oil, which is too concentrated to apply directly to your skin.

Tone Up with Tannins

These compounds, which occur in many plants and trees, can strengthen the skin. To prevent blisters, soak your hands or feet in a strong, tannin-rich infusion of black tea, oak bark, or pine twigs. To make it, simply soak a handful of the tea, bark, or twigs in a basin of freshly boiled water. When the water cools, strain the solution,

Comfort from Calendula

To reduce blister tenderness and help speed healing, apply a salve that contains the herb calendula along with skin-protecting vitamins A and E. You can apply the salve, available at health food stores, once a day. Or buy dried calendula, crumble it between your fingers, and add enough water to make a paste. Cover the blister with the paste and leave it on for about 20 minutes, then rinse it off.

then soak your hands or feet for 10 to 15 minutes. One caveat: If you have diabetes, talk to your doctor before soaking your feet.

Blister Know-How

Even though blisters are a fairly common ailment, you'd be surprised at how many contradictory treatments there are for these irritations. Here's our best advice:

- **Let it breathe.** Even though it's good to protect a blister with a bandage, you want to expose it to the air for at least 20 minutes a day. A little air circulation will help protect the area from infection-causing bacteria, which thrive in dark, moist places.

- **Lace tight.** When putting on running or other sports shoes, be sure to lace them up properly, so your feet are held firmly in place. Otherwise, they'll rub around against the insides of the shoes and create blisters.

- **Take care of your hands.** Wear gloves when you work with household or construction tools. Likewise, wear gardening gloves when you're raking or pruning.

- **Lighten up.** A golf club, squash racket, or tennis racket is a blister machine, so loosen your fingers and change your grip as often as you can while playing.

- **Get tough.** If you are about to embark on a home improvement project or other activity that will be a shock to your soft hands, get them ready. Rub denatured alcohol on your hands three times a day for several weeks before doing the manual labor.

- **Fight the friction.** Blisters on the feet are most likely to develop if your feet are either too sweaty or too dry. If your socks are often soggy, the origin of your blister problem may be your sweaty skin. Try sprinkling a little cornstarch into your socks before you put them on, and dust some between your toes, too. If the skin on your feet is very dry, smooth a thin film of petroleum jelly over them before you pull on your socks and sneakers. Avoid this treatment if you are prone to or have athlete's foot.

Herbal Helpers

You probably have two of the strongest antiseptic herbs in your kitchen. Rosemary and thyme can help if you're worried about infection. Add a tablespoon of each herb to a cup of hot water and steep for about 10 minutes. Let the liquid cool to room temperature, pour some on a cloth, and hold it against your blister for about 20 minutes. Repeat once or twice a day until the blister is gone.

Bloating

The human body is naturally full of water, but that doesn't mean that more is necessarily better. At certain times of the month, or after pigging out on chips, pickles, or other salty foods, women can accumulate so much extra fluid that it makes their skin puffy. They may actually need to use soap to slip a ring off.

Bloating is mainly a problem for women because the increase in estrogen right before menstruation encourages water to accumulate in the spaces between the cells, making tissues swell and skin plump up. In fact, some women gain a whopping 10 pounds of water weight in the week prior to their periods, when higher estrogen levels spur the body to retain sodium, which in turn makes tissues hold onto more water.

Estrogen replacement drugs used to treat menopausal discomforts (such as hot flashes) can cause bloating. And bloating can be due

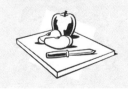

to steroid medications, blood pressure drugs, and inflammatory reactions to everything from insect bites to sunburn to bread. Belly bloating, in particular, can be an allergic reaction to foods (especially the gluten in wheat) or a result of lactose intolerance—a lack of the lactase enzyme that breaks down the milk sugar (lactose) in dairy foods. The lactose ferments and forms a gas, which puffs up your belly.

Beat the Bloat

The conventional treatment for bloating related to simple water retention is water pills, or diuretics. These drugs help the kidneys excrete excess sodium and water in the tissues, but they can also flush out important minerals, such as potassium, which actually battles fluid retention. If your problem is more occasional—such as when you've overdone it with the tortilla chips or you're about to menstruate—try these more natural ways to siphon off the fluid:

■**Prune water weight with herbs.** You can beat bloating (and retain ample potassium) by sipping potassium-rich teas. Parsley is a good choice. So is cleavers—an herb that, in the nineteenth-century, was known as bedstraw because it was used to stuff beds. Just be sure to have only one cup of either of these teas a day—too much can drain important minerals from your body.

- **Slim down with silk.** Next time you're shucking corn, don't chuck the silk—instead, dry it and save it to make cornsilk tea, an old-fashioned folk remedy that will help your kidneys flush out fluids. Because cornsilk is rich in potassium, it will also help balance the sodium in your system that may be making you hold water. To make the tea, steep 1 tablespoon of dried silk (also called stamens, which is available at health food stores) in 1 cup of boiling water for 5 minutes. You should see an effect within an hour or two, and you can continue to drink up to three cups a day for four days.

- **Add more water.** That's right: Believe it or not, drinking ample water—at least eight glasses daily—will combat fluid retention, especially the kind that pools in your belly after you eat. Drinking water helps the kidneys flush it all out.

- **Prowl the produce aisle.** That's where you'll find piles of potassium-rich foods that'll send puffiness packing. Among the best are sunflower seeds, dates, figs, oranges, peaches, bananas, tomatoes, and all the leafy greens—even the tops of celery stalks are rich in this precious mineral!

Win the Bloat Battle

Need more ammunition in your war against bloat? Here are five steps worth taking:

- **Read the label.** While you're shopping, check the labels on prepared and processed food with an eagle eye. Sodium, which promotes fluid

dial the DOCTOR

Trouble in the Water

Don't assume that bloating is normal. In some cases, it's a sign of underlying liver, heart, or kidney conditions, so you'll want to talk to your doctor. Likewise, talk to your physician if simply pressing on your skin leaves a dent. It's a sign of edema, which can be a sign of a serious condition.

retention, hides in everything from cereal to cheese to colas. Your goal is to keep sodium intake to 1,000 to 2,000 milligrams a day, but that can be tough. Just 2 ounces of American cheese packs 800 milligrams, and 3 cups of microwave popcorn contains 500 milligrams.

- **Try B$_6$.** Bloating can occur if you're deficient in vitamin B$_6$, which helps your body metabolize hormones—including the hormones that cause premenstrual bloat. Try taking a B-complex supplement regularly to balance out the B$_6$.

- **Do the dairy thing.** All dairy foods, especially milk, are loaded with calcium. A study of more than 400 women found that getting 1,200 milligrams of calcium daily cut bloating and other premenstrual symptoms by half.

- **Kick back.** If your ankles swell, it means that fluid is pooling in your legs. Sit with your legs raised to help your circulatory system move the fluid more easily. Of course, if ankle swelling is a chronic problem, you'll need to check with your doctor—and keep a footstool handy.

- **Wrap up with yarrow.** Make a strong infusion of yarrow and peppermint by steeping 2 tablespoons of each in 1 pint of water for 15 minutes, then strain, and chill. Meanwhile, prepare several lengths of gauze, muslin, or cheesecloth. When the infusion is thoroughly chilled, saturate the cloths, wrap them around your lower legs, and relax—with your legs

Drink It Black

Even if you're not a coffee drinker, have a cup now and then
when you have trouble with fluid retention. Why?
Because black coffee is a natural diuretic.

elevated—for 20 minutes or so. This will help discourage fluid retention while leaving your legs feeling refreshed.

Sip a Bloat-free Tea

To drop the excess water weight, combine equal parts of the following herbs: hawthorn, horse chestnut, ginkgo, cleavers, and dandelion leaf. Steep 2 tablespoons of the mixture in 1 quart of boiling water for 15 minutes, let cool, and drink throughout the day. Some caveats: Dandelion is rich in potassium, so don't ever take it with potassium tablets. And, if you take blood-thinning medications, consult your doctor before using ginkgo.

Feel Better with Melons

The Chinese use cucumbers and melons to reduce fluid retention. These foods contain a substance called cucurbocitrin, which is said to increase the natural leakiness of tiny blood vessels in the kidneys. This means that more water is processed and eliminated by the kidneys.

Eat "Lawn Salad"

Avid weed whackers may consider it a nuisance, but bloaters should think of it as a plus—the lowly dandelion, that is. The fresh, young leaves of the dandelion plant (which the French call pissenlit, or "urinate in bed") act as a natural diuretic. In fact, in head-to-head tests, dandelion leaf tea was shown to be just as effective as prescription diuretics.

If your fluid retention is due to heart problems, talk to your doctor about slowly adding dandelion to your diet and decreasing your dosage of diuretic drugs. *Do not* reduce your medications on your own.

Body Odor

We've all had occasions when no matter how frequently or ferociously we've scrubbed, it seems like we still smelled a little sour, and that odor has turned our favorite sweaters into instant rags. The culprits are bacteria that thrive on skin. When they devour the fatty sweat produced by the apocrine glands in your underarms, scalp, and genitals, the result is a very pungent smell.

Keep Odor at Bay

Strong body odor can sometimes be a sign of a serious medical condition or skin infection. That's why you should call your doctor if an unusual odor permeates your skin no matter what you do to get rid of it. In most cases, though, you can take care of body odor without chipping in for your doctor's new Lexus. Here are some tips:

- **Sweeten your diet.** Some body odor is caused by what you eat; the famous smells

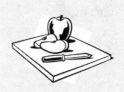

of garlic and onions can come right through your pores. But there's no need to boycott 'em. Just neutralize their potent scents by following them with parsley and other green leafy vegetables that contain chlorophyll, a natural deodorant. (That's the origin of the parsley-as-garnish tradition.) If you keep it up, you'll begin to notice the difference in just a few days.

■ **Change deodorants periodically.** After years of use, your usual deodorant may no longer work quite as well as it used to. It may have been altered by the manufacturer, your body chemistry may be changing, or you may have simply developed a tolerance for the brand. Try another—change is good! You'll be using a deodorant every day for years, so why have bored armpits? If you get a rash from one deodorant, try another designed for sensitive skin. You may also want to look for a plain deodorant rather than an antiperspirant, since antiperspirants contain aluminum chloride, which can be a skin irritant.

■ **Clean up your digestion.** Just as old garbage can stink up your whole house, the odor from decaying matter in your intestines can radiate throughout your body. For starters, cut back on red meat, which can sometimes create a stink. Beef protein is harder for your gut to break down, and the more food left hanging around, the more chance smelly bacterial by-products have to hang around, too.

- **Load up on yogurt.** The best way to control odor-causing "bad" bacteria in your gut is to fill it with "good" bacteria. You can get your supply of good guys by eating yogurt that contains live, active cultures of Lactobacillus acidophilus (check the label; frozen yogurt and yogurt-covered snacks don't have live cultures) or downing acidophilus capsules, which you can find at health food stores.

- **Munch your veggies.** Raw veggies and fruits provide roughage that helps escort smelly waste through—and out of—your intestinal tract. Cooked foods, on the other hand, are slower to move through your intestines. Plus, when you cook foods, you change the oxidation, which can prompt more odor during digestion.

- **Splash it on.** Splashing some rubbing alcohol under your arms may reduce the bacteria population. For a persistent odor problem, try using alcohol in place of deodorant—but whatever you do, don't apply it after shaving or if you have any nicks or cuts in your skin. That would sting like crazy!

Carve That Jack-o'-Lantern

A deficiency of zinc can prompt body odor. One way to get your zinc levels up is to munch on pumpkin seeds, which provide a good, concentrated source of the mineral. If you're not keen on the seeds, you can take 30 milligrams of supplemental zinc daily to help reduce body

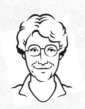

Freshen up with juice. Nobody in Grandma's house had a body odor problem, but maybe it's because we drank so much vegetable juice. Juices from chlorophyll-rich foods like kale, chard, and other dark green vegetables can restore the pH balance of blood that's too acidic—and therefore too friendly to bad bacteria—due to a diet heavy on proteins.

and foot odor—but not without your doctor's guidance. If taken continuously, zinc can deplete copper and other minerals, and it could be toxic. To be safe, don't exceed 15 milligrams of zinc a day without talking to your doctor first.

Sweet-Smelling Tactics

You can fight body odor by following some of these easy-to-digest maneuvers:

- **Try odor-killing herbs.** That tangy-smelling sage you use to season poultry stuffing contains compounds that can tame wetness, plus oils that fight bacteria. Pine-scented rosemary is another natural antibacterial herb. Mix 1 tablespoon of each with 1 cup of baking soda, and sprinkle the mix on any odor-causing body part.

- **Wear odor-fighting fibers.** Polyester and most synthetic fabrics keep odors close to your body. Cotton, silk, and some of the new wicking fabrics designed for athletes allow moisture to circulate, so it won't cling to your body or clothing. Look in sporting goods or camping stores for lightweight, wicking underwear.

- **Cut back on coffee.** You probably already know that the odorous oils in garlic, onions, fish, and exotic spices can linger in your body, but did you know that coffee and tea are also bad news? That's because they boost the activity of sweat glands. Try eliminating these offenders and see if that foul odor fades.

- **Feel fresh with fennel.** It makes a sweet post-meal drink, especially if you've had garlic, onions, or other smelly foods. In fact, fennel is such an excellent natural deodorizer that Indian restaurants often offer fennel seeds instead of after-dinner mints.

Rub on the "Magic Mineral"

If you're going through deodorants and antiperspirants like there's no tomorrow, consider trading your stick for a stone—a crystal deodorant stone, that is. Not only will one stone last much longer than a standard stick, it may be much kinder to your system. The aluminum chloride in antiperspirants completely plugs up the sweat glands, whereas crystal stones contain a natural astringent called alunogenite that may only partially block the glands.

Love That Lemon!

Giving your body a steady stream of water—no fewer than eight glasses a day—is one of the best ways to flush out toxins and eliminate the stink. Here's a twist on the standard advice: Each evening, add a squeeze of fresh lemon juice and 1 teaspoon of chlorophyll (available at health food stores) to your glass. Both will help eliminate odor-causing bacteria from your gut.

Breast Pain

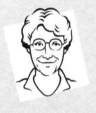
Women today are almost desperate for
more regularity in their lives. Soccer practice that ends when it's supposed to. Weekend
chores that get done on time. Friends who
show up for dinner at the appointed hour.
In today's high-octane world, a little predict-
ability just makes things easier. In many
women's lives, unfortunately, one of the
few things that happens like clockwork is
breast pain during their monthly
menstrual cycles.

Baby Your Breasts

Most women just live with breast pain
because they figure they can't do anything
about it. Nothing could be further from the
truth. You should certainly check with your
doctor just to be on the safe side, but there
are many simple strategies that are just as
effective as anything you'll find in a high-
priced specialist's office:

■ **Lighten up.** Some dark-colored foods may aggravate monthly breast pain. The worst offenders seem to be chocolate, black tea, cola, and coffee, so try avoiding these foods in the week or so prior to your period.

■ **Take a poke at pain.** The herb pokeroot is a favorite among herbalists for relieving breast pain. Health food stores carry pokeroot tincture and oil. Put either on a cotton ball and rub it all over your breasts for relief. The herb is for external use only.

■ **Toss a salad.** Dandelion greens have a pleasant, slightly bitter taste, and they contain compounds that reduce fluid retention. As long as you don't use pesticides on your lawn and you pick the leaves before the flowers bloom, you'll have the fixings for a fresh-tasting, wholesome salad that keeps breast pain at bay. Mix 'em up with spinach, which also helps reduce excess fluid. Go easy on the dandelion if you take diuretics or potassium supplements, though.

■ **Prime your body with primrose.** Evening primrose is a traditional remedy for breast pain, and there's some evidence that it works. It's rich in omega-6 fatty acids, which inhibit the body's production of inflammation-causing prostaglandins, natural chemicals that cause pain. Take 1,500 milligrams of evening primrose oil in capsule form twice a day to reduce the discomfort.

One problem with evening primrose oil supplements is that they're expensive. Some less costly supplements include borage oil, flaxseed oil, and black currant oil, all of which also contain beneficial omega-6 fatty acids.

- **Shop for color.** Fruits and vegetables with bright red, yellow, or orange hues are loaded with carotenoids, plant pigments that appear to prevent breast pain in some women. Add as many to your diet as you can.

Cut Back On Fat

You already know that dietary fat is loaded with calories, but there's another reason to cut back. There may be a connection between a diet rich in saturated fats (such as red meat and rich desserts) and high levels of estrogen, which can promote monthly breast pain.

Call For Cabbage And Clay

Long before there were doctors or corner drugstores, herbalists treated breast pain with a poultice made from green clay (available at health food stores) and cabbage. Cabbage and clay draw out the swelling, reducing monthly breast lumps and discomfort. Combine 4 parts shredded cabbage with 1 part clay, mix well, and apply it to your breasts at bedtime. Cover the poultice with a moist cloth, then wrap a layer of gauze bandage around your body or wear a loose-fitting, soft cotton bra to hold it in place. Your breasts will probably feel a whole lot better in the morning.

Painless Pain Fighters

When your breasts are sore and achy, the last thing you need is a complicated pain-relief formula that takes time and effort to make. Here are some simple recipes that will bring fast relief:

- **Sip away the pain.** Chasteberry, or vitex, can help to normalize hormone levels that, when unbalanced, can contribute to breast swelling and discomfort. To make chasteberry tea, add 1 teaspoon of dried berries to 1 cup of boiling water, steep for 15 minutes, and strain. Drink a cup twice a day.

- **Shake the salt habit.** When your breasts are sore and tender, any swelling can make them hurt even more. To reduce fluid retention, cut down on salt. Don't just set aside the saltshaker, though—read food labels, too. Many packaged foods contain high amounts of sodium.

- **Count on castor oil.** Castor oil packs are a soothing anti-inflammatory. To make one, saturate a clean cloth with castor oil, and cover your breasts with it. Top the cloth with plastic wrap (castor oil stains clothing), and then with a hot water bottle or a heating pad set on low. Leave everything in place for 1 hour. Repeat three or four times a week.

- **Ease it with E.** A number of scientific studies have shown that vitamin E supplements can help ease breast pain. The recommended dose is 400 to 800 IU daily. Be sure to get supplements

dial the DOCTOR

Monthly Trouble Signs

If you have regular breast pain, stay in touch with your doctor and report any changes in your monthly symptoms. You'll definitely want to make an appointment if the pain is severe or getting worse, affects only one breast, or is accompanied by signs of infection, such as redness, nipple discharge, a fever, or general aches.

that contain d–alpha tocopherols, which are thought to be more effective than other forms of vitamin E.

Get Support

Even if you're not an athlete, a sports bra is an important piece of equipment if your breasts are tender and sensitive. It will keep them in place so they don't rub against each other or your clothing. Also, avoid underwire bras, which can impede circulation.

Spoon Up Some Yogurt

The beneficial organisms in yogurt slightly decrease the time that stools—and the estrogen they contain—stay in your intestine, and eliminating excess estrogen from the body can help reduce monthly breast pain. Check the label to be sure that the yogurt contains live cultures of Lactobacillus acidophilus, which is one of the helpful forms of bacteria.

Bronchitis

If your voice is so crackly and you're coughing so hard that you sound like a circus seal, you probably have bronchitis, a temporary inflammation of the mucous membranes of the bronchi, which are the main, branching airway passages of the lungs.

Acute bronchitis—which usually lasts about a week—typically follows a cold, when the virus travels from your nose to your air passages. The good news is that most cases of acute bronchitis, like most colds, disappear on their own after several miserable days. But if the bronchitis lingers, your doctor may prescribe an inhaler (the kind that's used for asthma) to help open your bronchial tubes and clear out mucus.

Bronchitis Busters

If you decide to see your doctor about your bronchitis and he or she recommends that you use an inhaler, ask about other more gentle, less

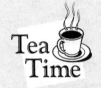

Tea Time

Soak 2 heaping tablespoons of marshmallow root in 1 quart of cold water overnight. Strain, then heat 1 cup of the tea to a boil. Add 1/2 teaspoon each of licorice root and thyme, cover, and steep for 15 minutes. Drink four cups a day. *Caution:* Avoid licorice root if you have high blood pressure or kidney disease.

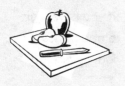
expensive ways to clear your bronchial tubes, such as the following:

- **Steam out secretions.** Warm steam soothes the lining of the bronchial tubes and loosens secretions. To make your own steam machine, first boil a pot of water. Fill a bowl with the water, then put a towel over your head and the bowl to make a "tent" to trap the steam. Lean over the bowl and inhale deeply through your nose. You can add a bit of eucalyptus or sage oil to the water to give the steam added medicinal punch. Don't try to use an electric vaporizer this way, though; its concentrated stream of steam is dangerous when used near the face.

- **Fight back with flax.** A flaxseed poultice retains heat for a long time and is ideal for soothing an irritating, spastic cough. Add ½ cup of ground flaxseed to ¾ cup of boiling water and simmer, stirring until it makes a thick paste. Spread the paste on a piece of cheesecloth, and apply it as hot as you can tolerate it to your chest. For deeper penetration, add 5 or 6 drops of thyme or eucalyptus oil to the poultice. Leave it on for 1 to 2 hours.

- **Keep the water glass full.** You need lots of fluids to keep your lungs hydrated and working at their best, so drink at least eight glasses of water a day.

- **Dump the dairy.** When you were a kid, you may have been given ice cream to soothe a tickle in your throat, but when it comes to bronchitis, that's a no-no. You want to stay away from foods that produce phlegm and those that cause inflammation. This means skipping not only dairy foods but also wheat, soy, sugar, margarine, peanut butter, preserved meats, and processed foods. What's left? Fish, legumes, and green vegetables—all of which are rich in magnesium, which helps relax the smooth muscles of your bronchial tubes so you can breathe easier.

■ **Gobble garlic.** One of garlic's key components—the volatile oil allicin—helps relax your bronchi so more air can pass through them. Garlic also stimulates the immune system and reduces phlegm.

■ **Clear congestion with a fennel chest rub.** Just combine 10 drops each of fennel oil, thyme oil, and eucalyptus oil with 4 ounces of sunflower oil, then massage the mixture gently onto your chest.

Say "Bye" to Bronchitis

When the coughing just won't stop, head for the kitchen and whip up one of these bronchitis tamers:

■ **Break up congestion.** To get mucus flowing, try this broncho-buster cracker spread: Mix small amounts of garlic, ginger, horseradish, mustard, turmeric, and chopped chile peppers

dial the DOCTOR

When Bronchitis Goes Bad

Contact your doctor immediately if your coughing keeps you awake at night, interferes with your daily activities, or lasts longer than six weeks; if the mucus you're coughing up becomes thicker, darker green, yellow, or bloody; or if you become breathless or have a fever. You could have pneumonia or asthma, both of which require immediate medical treatment.

into a paste. Spread very thinly on crackers and nibble gingerly, one tiny bite at a time. The ingredients will make everything run—your eyes, your nose, and even the thick mucus clogging your bronchial tubes.

- **Cook up a curry.** Indian curries contain turmeric, which is a great source of quercetin, a bioflavonoid-antihistamine combo that can calm reactivity in the airways. If you're not fond of Indian cuisine, simply supplement with three 200- to 300-milligram capsules of quercetin (available at health food stores) a day—one before breakfast, lunch, and dinner— for as long as your symptoms last.

MODERN MARVEL

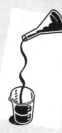

Ease into Echinacea

In one recent study, people who took echinacea twice a day for eight weeks reduced the duration of respiratory tract infections by half—possibly because the herb boosts the body's infection-fighting cells so they attack the virus with a vengeance. You can find tinctures at a health food store. Drink 1 to 1 1/2 teaspoons of echinacea tincture added to a shot glass of warm water two or three times daily for the duration of your symptoms. Disregard the slight numbness you may feel in your mouth from the herb; it will quickly pass. But don't use echinacea if you have an auto-immune disease such as lupus, rheumatoid arthritis, or multiple sclerosis, or if you are pregnant or nursing.

■ **Breathe better with onion.** Like garlic, onions contain allicin, which can open your airways by relaxing your bronchi. Coat a cast-iron skillet with olive oil and add a handful of chopped onions, a teaspoon of apple cider vinegar, and a pinch of cornstarch. Cook over low heat to make a paste. Let the paste cool and place it on a cloth. Lay the cloth on your bare chest and cover it with plastic wrap. Add another cloth, and top everything with a heating pad set on low. The onion will be absorbed into your body, and you'll know, because you'll have the onion breath to prove it.

Run Hot And Cold

You can short-circuit bronchitis by flushing out mucus with hot-and-cold wraps. Here's how: Soak a towel in water and wring it out, then heat it in the microwave for 5 to 10 minutes. Next, lay a wool blanket over your chest and cover it with a sheet. Place the steamy towel on top of the sheet, and cover it with another blanket. Let your chest soak in the moist heat for 5 minutes to bring the blood to the surface. Then repeat the process with a very cold towel, which will shunt blood away from your chest. All the while, have someone massage your legs, rubbing vigorously toward your heart for 10 minutes. The heat and cold, combined with the rubbing, create a kind of pump to flush out phlegm and draw white blood cells into circulation to kill off the virus behind your bronchitis.

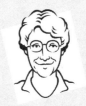

Grandma Says:

Eat your soup.
If you're coming down with a cold, whip up a batch of chicken soup. Grandma Putt knew that sipping soup made a cold-sufferer feel better—and science has proven it. New research suggests that chicken soup helps block the production of neutrophils, white blood cells that contribute to upper respiratory symptoms.

Soak Away Discomfort

Climb into a steaming tub laced with 2 drops each of eucalyptus, thyme, and rosemary oils, plus a cup or so of Epsom salts, to ease your bronchitis symptoms. The steam will increase the flow of nasal mucus; the molecules from the oils will dilate your small airways, easing your breathing; and the Epsom salts will provide bronchi-relaxing magnesium that's absorbed through your skin.

Magic Mushroom

Studies indicate that the reishi mushroom—a reddish-orange fungus that grows on the bark of withered Japanese plum trees—may be highly effective for treating bronchitis. In fact, in one study, people with bronchitis who took reishi extracts had a 60 to 90 percent improvement in their symptoms. Mix 30 drops of reishi extract (available at health food stores) in a glass of water and drink every 2 to 3 hours while your symptoms last.

Bruises

Even if you have the balance of Baryshnikov and the smooth moves of Michael Jordan, sooner or later you're going to have an abrupt encounter of the unyielding kind—such as smacking your head on a door frame or clobbering your knee on a kitchen cabinet. When that happens, your clumsiness is revealed for all the world to see in the form of an ugly, telltale bruise.

Any hard impact can damage tiny blood vessels, called capillaries, beneath your skin. Broken capillaries bleed, but you don't see blood because it's under the surface. What you do see is the dark "stain," which can range in color from slightly yellow to eggplant purple. Apart from being an unsightly mess, a bruise hurts because the same impact that damages blood vessels also injures skin and muscle. So you're left black and blue, and achy, too. Ouch!

Try Arnica

The herb arnica is a major bruise buster. Apply arnica gel, available at health food stores, gently on your bruise. Or take arnica in homeopathic form, following the package directions. Do not apply over broken skin.

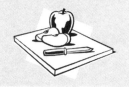
Fade Away

Most bruises aren't a big deal. Daily, your body slowly cleans up the damage by removing fluids and damaged cells. While you're healing, of course, the pain and tenderness can be a real nuisance—and you'll have to answer those endless questions about how you got that ugly blotch. There's no secret strategy for making bruises disappear like magic, but there are ways to help speed up the process.

RICE to the Rescue

The oldest treatment for bruises, and still the most effective, goes by the initials RICE: rest, ice, compression, and elevation. Performing these steps in sequence will minimize discomfort and help bruises heal much more quickly:

- **Rest.** When you've bruised an area, give it some downtime in order to let the damaged tissues start healing.

- **Ice the area immediately.** Apply an ice pack for about 20 minutes every few hours for the first day or two. The cold temperature reduces the bleeding under the skin that causes pain and discoloration.

- **Compress the area.** The best way is by wrapping it with an elastic bandage. You want the wrap to be snug, but not so tight that it cuts off circulation. You'll know you're stretching it tight enough if you can see light through the bandage while you're applying it. The pressure restricts blood flow and helps prevent swelling.

- **Elevate.** Get the bruised area above the level of your heart as often as you can. This allows excess fluid to drain away from the bruise and back into circulation where it belongs.

Change the Oil

No, not in your car—in your diet! Here are two oils you should try when you want that bruise to just go away:

- **Cure it with castor.** A powerful, traditional way to treat bruises is to apply a castor oil pack. Castor oil has excellent anti-inflammatory properties, and it penetrates the skin very well. Spread castor oil over the bruise, then wrap the area with plastic wrap. Place a heating pad (set on low) or a washcloth soaked in warm water on top of the wrap. Leave it in place for about 20 minutes, then wash off the oil. You can repeat the treatment several times a day.

- **Fix it with fish oil.** It sounds like something my Grandma Putt would recommend—and, as usual, she'd be right on the money. Fish oil is rich in omega-3 fatty acids, natural substances that make your body less prone to inflammation. As long as you're not taking aspirin or prescription blood thinners, take a tablespoon or two of fish oil daily until the bruise is gone.

Tea Time

Ginger tea is an effective treatment for bruises because it reduces inflammation and dilates, or widens, blood vessels. Wider blood vessels allow more blood to circulate, which removes pain-causing compounds and brings in more healing nutrients. You can make ginger tea by steeping 1 tablespoon of powdered ginger in a cup of boiling water for 5 to 10 minutes. Drink the tea at least three times a day until the bruise is gone.

Use Heat and Cold

After a few days of RICE, (see "RICE to the Rescue" on page 78) switch to a technique called contrast hydrotherapy, in which you alternate between hot and cold compresses. The alternating temperatures cause blood vessels to expand and contract. This creates a pumping action that brings more nutrients to the area, while pumping out waste products. Here's how it works: Soak some washcloths in hot tap water and others in cold. Apply a warm compress to the area for 3 minutes, then switch to cold for 30 seconds. Several times a day, repeat the cycle three times, always ending with the cold compress.

Pump Up Your Nutrients

Your body's need for nutrients increases dramatically when you have a bruise. Bruise beaters include zinc, vitamin A, and selenium. You'll get plenty of these and other healing vitamins and minerals by taking a multivitamin every day. Here are a few other edible cures:

- **Knock it out with nuts.** Brazil nuts are loaded with selenium, a nutrient that's essential for skin health. Eat about a cup daily while the bruise is healing.

- **Bromelain is best.** A natural substance found in the pineapple plant, bromelain helps your body break down and remove the chemical spill that causes bruises. Fresh pineapple doesn't contain

Give Bruises the Blues

Remember the girl who turned into a giant blueberry in the film *Willy Wonka and the Chocolate Factory*? It wasn't a pretty sight, but the good news is that she probably never bruised again. Blueberries are loaded with vitamin C and chemical compounds called bioflavonoids, which are essential for blood vessel repair. Eat 1/2 cup of blueberries a day. The nutrients in the berries will help bruises heal and also make your blood vessels stronger so they're better able to resist damage.

enough of the enzyme, so it's better to take it in supplement form. The recommended dose is 400 milligrams two or three times a day on an empty stomach. Don't take bromelain if you're taking prescription blood thinners.

Try the Salt Strategy

Here's a chance to use that box of Epsom salts that's been sitting in the back of your bathroom cabinet all these years. Add a cup or two of the salts to a warm bath (or a smaller amount to a basin), then soak the area for about 20 minutes. The magnesium in the salts will feel mighty soothing to bumps and bruises.

Bunions

Pass On the Pressure

Surround your burgeoning bunion with over-the-counter doughnut-shaped moleskin or a gel-filled pad to reduce pressure and friction from shoes. Check your drugstore or supermarket for protective pads that contain anti-inflammatory medicines. They'll deliver first aid to your bunion as they cushion it.

Imelda Marcos may have gotten all the headlines, but she certainly wasn't the first woman to devote more than a few yards of shelf space to fashionable shoes. Many women are into footwear, and they often choose shoes that look sharp—high heels, pointy toes, and all.

Unfortunately, buying shoes for style instead of comfort can actually change the ways your foot bones grow. Can you feel a knobby bump at the base of your big toe? If you can, that's a bunion, and it means your shoes are forcing your bones to grow in some pretty unnatural ways. Bunions really hurt when you squeeze them into tight-fitting shoes—and they can make your feet feel tired and achy at the end of a long day.

Bunion Busters

Short of surgery, there's no way to get rid of bunions once they form. Before you consider foot surgery, though—and the mortgage-size payment that comes with it—why not try some gentler ways to reduce pain and keep bunions from getting worse? Here are a few that may help:

- **Can it with cola.** Love an ice-cold soda? Your aching feet will, too. Before you pop the tab, place the can sideways on the floor, slip off your shoes, put your sore foot on the can, and roll it back and forth for several minutes. The cold will help reduce inflammation, and the motion will give your foot a good massage. Just be sure to let the can rest upright for a few minutes before you pop it open, or you'll have soda exploding in your face!

- **Heat it up.** On your tongue, the fiery capsaicin in red pepper makes you want to guzzle a gallon of water. But applying capsaicin cream (available in drugstores) to a painful bunion brings sweet relief. Capsaicin relieves pain by gradually decreasing the concentration of something called substance P, which transmits pain signals to the brain. The cream stings, so be careful not to get it in your eyes or on any area of broken skin, and wash your hands well after using it.

- **Cream it.** Head to your local health food store and look for a painkiller called Fortex. It packs aspirin-like salicylate in a peanut-oil base, and it can penetrate the skin to quickly ease bunion inflammation. Smooth the cream on your bunion several times daily, and you'll get relief.

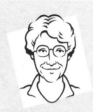

Grandma Says:

Give 'em a stretch. Grandma stretched her toes to make them strong and flexible, reducing bunion pain. Here's how to do it: Sit with your bare feet together and loop a thick rubber band around both big toes. Move your feet as far apart as they'll go, hold the stretch for 5 seconds, then relax. Repeat 10 times at least once a day.

- **Straighten 'em out.** If your big toe is starting to drift and a bunion is sprouting, a sponge-rubber toe spacer, which you can find at any drugstore, can keep it from angling outward, and relieve the pressure while you're wearing shoes. Start with a small spacer and gradually move up to wider ones until your toe feels comfortable.

Say "Aaahhh" with Herbs

The next time your bunions are barking, stop off at a health food store and get the ingredients for a soothing herbal rub or footbath. Here are two recipes that are worth a try:

- **There's the rub.** Mix 6 parts oak bark, 3 parts marshmallow root, 3 parts mullein, 2 parts wormwood, 1 part lobelia, 1 part skullcap, 6 parts comfrey root, and 3 parts walnut bark. Put the herbs in a double boiler, add olive oil to cover, and cook for 1 to 2 hours. Strain out the herbs and throw them away. Then add an equal amount of melted beeswax to the oil, and store the mixture in an ointment jar with a tight-fitting lid. Apply it daily whenever your feet hurt, and you should feel the difference within a few days.

- **Comforting comfrey.** A comfrey footbath soothes painful bunions fast. The herb contains chemical compounds that ease skin discomfort and help sore areas heal. To make a footbath, steep 1 ounce of dried comfrey leaves (available at health food stores) in a few cups of simmering water for 10 minutes. Add enough cool water to make the temperature comfortable, pour the water into a basin, and soak your feet for 20 minutes or so. If you can't find comfrey, it's okay to substitute Epsom salts.

Keep on Walkin'

Don't let bunions sideline you. Start with a foot massage, then take a walk. Here's how to do it:

- **Rub out pain.** Massage is excellent for reducing bunion pain, and you'll get even better results when you combine it with a soothing bath. The next time you're in the tub, lather your hands with soap. Slip your fingers between the toes of one foot and gently reach around to massage

If the Shoe Fits...

wear it—but make sure those shoes *really* fit your feet. Otherwise, you're just asking for more trouble. The main cause of bunion pain, and the one thing that always makes it worse, is wearing shoes that don't fit. Shoving your foot into a poorly fitting shoe literally changes the shape of your foot, so always have your feet measured when you buy new shoes. And avoid narrow styles with pointy toes. You want shoes that are wide enough for your feet to slip into comfortably, preferably with a flat or low heel.

the bottom of your foot. Bend your wrist while you rub so your foot moves in every direction. Then do the same thing with your other foot. You may be a little sore the first few times you do it, but after that, your bunions should start feeling a lot better.

- **Head to the shore.** Your feet might love a trip to the beach as much as you do. Walking barefoot in the sand is a great way to strengthen your feet and make them less sensitive to bunion pain.

Burns

You probably remember the old Saturday morning cartoons that featured Yosemite Sam. The pistol-packin' bandolero would say things like, "Now, get that flea-bitten carcass off'n my real estate!"—just before Bugs Bunny tricked him into a crackling campfire. That's life in toon town. In real life, though, there's nothing funny about burns. They're among the most painful injuries you're ever likely to get. Even a small burn damages nerves as well as the surface layers of skin, and the exposed raw tissue can take a long time to heal. Worse, it's extremely likely to become infected.

The darned thing about burns is that they happen so fast. Unlike other types of injuries—a knife cut, for example—with burns, there's virtually no time to react and save yourself from danger. By the time sensations of heat have traveled from your skin to your brain, the damage has been done.

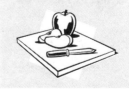

Chill the Pain

Don't Mess with Bad Burns

You can treat minor, first-degree burns at home. Second-, third-, or fourth-degree burns, which penetrate deeper into the skin, need a doctor's care—and can be life-threatening. Get to an emergency room if the burn covers an area larger than 3" in diameter, looks infected, or appears charred or white. A small burn that doesn't heal within 10 days or looks infected needs medical attention pronto!

You need immediate medical attention for serious burns or for any burn that's bigger than 2 to 3 inches around. Minor burns, however, are easy enough to treat at home. Here are some suggestions for cooling the pain and helping them heal more quickly:

- **Get the water flowing.** It's almost instinctive to throw water on something that's burning, and that's the perfect response when you've touched something that's too hot to handle. As soon as possible, flood the area with cold running water for about 10 minutes. This will stop the pain and help prevent swelling. If pain persists, repeat the cold-water treatment for 15 minutes each hour. The cold constricts the blood vessels, and taking it away opens them up again. This creates a pumping action that improves circulation and helps the burn heal more quickly.

- **Improvise if you need to.** If the closest cool liquid happens to be milk or even a soft drink, well, any port in a storm. Work with what you've got. The more quickly you cool the injury, the sooner you'll stop the damage.

- **Leave the ice in the freezer.** Even though you want to cool a burn as quickly as possible, ice will probably make things worse. It will make the area too cold, and sometimes it sticks to the skin, which can be mighty painful.

■ **Forget about butter.** Putting butter or any other oily substance on a burn is the worst thing you can do, because it will seal in the heat. After heat singes your skin, it continues to cook the tissues, so you want to try to cool the burn immediately. For that to happen, the heat has to be able to escape.

Love That Aloe!

To hasten healing and guard against infection, you can't do much better than the thick juice inside the leaves of the aloe plant. Simply cut a notch in a leaf, squeeze it until the juice appears, and apply it directly to the burn. The cooling liquid will ease pain, keep skin from blistering, stave off infection, and speed wound healing by helping fresh skin cells grow.

Herbal Soothers

Here are a handful of herbs that will help soothe the burn and aid skin healing:

■ **Ease it with oregano.** You love oregano on your pizza, and your scorched skin will love it, too. Oil of oregano contains vitamins A and C as well as minerals including calcium, phosphorus, iron, and magnesium. When rubbed on the skin, it aids in healing minor burns.

■ **Get comfort with comfrey.** The leaves and roots of the comfrey plant contain the healing agent allantoin, which stimulates healthy

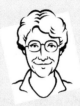

Grandma Says:

Bring out the toothpaste. To quickly ease minor burns, Grandma Putt would apply a dab of toothpaste to the site. And it worked like a charm. Turns out, most toothpastes contain menthol, which has a wonderfully cooling effect on the skin. Reapply as often as necessary to keep comfortable.

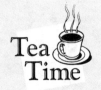

If the blisters on your burned skin burst, dab the area with plantain tea. This anti-bacterial Native American plant contains plenty of allantoin, and is sometimes called "nature's Bactine" because it's good for healing all kinds of wounds. Brew a tea (you can find packaged plantain tea at a health food store), let it cool, and apply the tea to your burn.

tissue growth. To make a cooling, cell–growth-encouraging poultice, take 1 cup of fresh leaves, or soak 1 cup of dried leaves (you can find both at health food stores) in enough water to cover them. Then mash the leaves, wrap the mash in a thin cloth, and apply it to the burn as needed.

■ **Soothe it with St. John's.** You may know this herb for its role in easing mild depression, but it also helps heal minor burns quickly and with minimal scarring. Apply the extract (available at health food stores) directly to the burn several times a day.

■ **Use an herbal mix.** Even the best herbs for burns can be made a little better by using them in combination. Pick up a cream or ointment that contains several skin-friendly herbs, such as comfrey, calendula, and goldenseal, at a health food store. Apply it according to the package directions.

Keep It Clean

One reason that burns are so dangerous is that they strip away the protective outer layers of skin—and there are plenty of germs that will jump right in. To prevent infection, wash the area with soap and water a few times each day. Just remember to wash gently: Overzealous scrubbing can easily damage burned skin. Cover the burn with a bandage if you think it's likely to get dirty, and be sure to change the bandage at least twice a day. To prevent infection, apply a thin layer of triple antibiotic ointment every time you wash the burn and change the bandage.

Clean with Calendula

This herb is an anti-inflammatory, astringent (cleanser), and antiseptic (germ killer) all rolled into one. Plus, it helps repair tissues and prevent scarring. Some physicians advise applying calendula cream directly to a burn, or you can add several drops of calendula tincture to a cup of water, dip a cloth in the mixture, and carefully dab the cloth onto the wound. Wait a day or two after the burn occurs to use this remedy, so it won't sting the tissues. You can find both calendula cream and tincture at health food stores.

Raise It High

Elevating the burned area, if it's on a part of the body that can be elevated, is definitely good. You want the area to be higher than the level of your heart so fluids that accumulate there will drain back toward the body as the normal flow of blood and other fluids mops up the damage. If you can, keep the area elevated for about 20 minutes at a time. Elevate larger burns several times during the first 24 hours.

Bursitis

Ginger is a powerful anti-inflammatory herb that can take the edge off bursitis pain. To make a healing tea, grate about an inch of fresh ginger and steep it in hot water for 10 minutes, then strain. Sip a cup of tea once or twice a day until your pain subsides.

Have you ever heard of housemaid's knee, miner's elbow, or weaver's bottom? They sound like they could be characters in Shakespeare's comedy *A Midsummer Night's Dream*. In fact, they're whimsical names for bursitis, a condition that's about as far from comedic as you can possibly get.

Bursitis occurs when small, fluid-filled sacs called bursae, which normally help joints move smoothly, get inflamed and swollen. Your body has more than 150 bursae, so you can imagine the painful possibilities. The most common sites for bursitis are joints that undergo heavy wear and tear, such as the shoulder, hip, and knee.

Be Gentle on Your Joints

If you notice that one or more of your joints hurts like the dickens, check with your doctor. Bursitis is rarely serious, but sometimes other conditions, such as arthritis, can cause similar symptoms. An X-ray will show what's causing your pain. In most cases, though, you won't have to fork over a pile of cash for expensive pain-relieving drugs. Here are a few simple tips to reduce the pain and prevent additional injury:

- **Stop the swelling.** If your joint feels hot and swollen, the first thing you should do is get some ice on it. Applying cold constricts blood vessels and reduces the flow of fluid and inflammatory chemicals to the painful area. Apply a cold pack or ice cubes wrapped in a small towel or a washcloth to the area for about 20 minutes. Repeat the treatment every hour or two until the pain goes away.

- **Raise your arm.** Or elevate your leg . . . or whatever else hurts. Raising the area higher than the level of your heart helps gravity pull out excess fluids and reduce swelling.

- **Wrap it up.** Snugly wrapping the injured area with an elastic bandage will also reduce swelling. Don't make the bandage so tight that it cuts off circulation, though. If you can just barely slip a finger under the edge, it's tight enough.

- **Add some heat.** Pain that lingers after a day or two often responds well to a heat treatment. Soak a small towel in hot water, wring it out, and place it on the area that's hurting. You can also use a heating pad set on low.

- **Swap heat and cold.** This traditional healing method uses alternating hot and cold treatments to improve circulation in an injured part of your body. It brings in more nutrients while flushing out toxins and waste products. First, soak a small towel in hot water, wring it out, and place it on the sore spot for about 3 minutes. Then soak a towel in cold water and apply it for 30 seconds. Repeat the cycle two or three times, always ending with the cold.

Pound Pain with Peppers

Call it chile pepper, call it cayenne, call it capsaicin. Just call it—this ointment is really hot stuff! Smooth it over your sore joint, and you'll begin to feel relief. The heat from capsaicin brings blood circulation to your sore bursa. You can buy capsaicin cream over the counter at your local drugstore or health food store. The best products contain 0.025 to 0.075% capsaicin. Use it up to three times a day, but keep it away from your eyes and any areas of broken skin. Wash your hands after all applications.

Soothe the Soreness

When bursitis strikes, you want quick relief from the pain and swelling. Try this plan of attack:

- **Get relief from the garden.** Two common garden plants, chickweed and comfrey, are used traditionally to relieve swelling and pain. Pick a handful of chickweed and one or two large comfrey leaves. Blanch everything in hot water and apply, using the chickweed as the first layer and holding it in place with the comfrey leaves.

- **Put bromelain to work.** This enzyme from the pineapple plant is one of nature's anti-inflammatories. To relieve bursitis, take 200 milligrams in capsule form daily on an empty stomach. Avoid bromelain if you're taking blood-thinning medications or are sensitive to pineapple.

- **Count on castor.** A castor oil pack is an old-time pain treatment that's never out of style. First, smear some castor oil over the area that hurts. Put some plastic wrap on top of the oil, then cover the whole thing with a heating pad set on low. The heat will push the oil's healing components into the aching joint. Since this is a heat-based treatment, though, don't use it if you have swelling or inflammation.

- **Get extra C.** Vitamin C is critical for repairing injured joints. You could take supplements, but a tastier solution is to add some crunch to your next salad. "Green and red peppers are good sources of vitamin C. Not a pepper fan? Then load up on oranges—but don't peel them too carefully. There's a lot of vitamin C in the white part next to the peel.

- **Pop a morning multi.** The multivitamin you take every day with breakfast is especially important when you're coping with bursitis. There are a lot of nutrients that are important for connective tissue health; a multivitamin provides them all.

Grandma Says:

Eat your berries! Once, when Grandpa Putt was felled by bursitis, Grandma baked a mixed berry pie to cheer him up. And wouldn't you know it, all dark berries, including cherries and blueberries, contain chemical compounds called bioflavonoids, which reduce inflammation and can ease bursitis pain. Eat 1/2 cup a day until you're feeling better.

■ **Oil your joints.** The omega-3 essential fatty acids found in fish are important for good health, especially when your body is coping with inflammation. Until your joints are better, plan on eating two or three servings of fish a week. The oils will tame inflammation and help you recover more quickly. If you're not a fish fan, you can get healthy amounts of omega-3's by eating ground flaxseed. Every day, add a tablespoon or two of seeds to your cereal, smoothies, yogurt, or salads.

Tame Pain with Turmeric

This pungent spice contains chemical compounds that can relieve an inflamed, irritated

Change Your Routine

Sometimes the best way to fight bursitis is to do some creative thinking. Pay close attention to what you do as you go about your daily life. Are repetitive motions putting your arms or legs in awkward or strained positions? Do you spend long periods of time with a knee or elbow pressed against the floor or a chair? Things that put pressure on a joint or tendon or restrict blood flow might cause problems down the road, so try to eliminate them from your daily routine. When you just can't avoid doing repetitive tasks that can lead to bursitis, take frequent breaks. Stretching and moving around, even for just a few minutes each hour, can make a real difference.

joint. If you're not a big fan of spicy foods, you can take supplements that contain curcumin, the active ingredient in turmeric. They're available at health food stores; just be sure to follow the label directions.

Flood Your Tissues

Your joints and bursae have a lot of water in them, so hydration is very important for joint health. Plan on drinking at least eight glasses of water throughout the day, every day.

Shape Up!

Resistance training, or exercising with weights, will help build strong muscles. And the stronger the muscles around your joints, the better they can protect you from the kinds of injuries that cause bursitis. If you've already been treated for bursitis, have your doctor prescribe an exercise program to prevent further complications.

Calluses and Corns

dial the DOCTOR

Callus Cautions

Calluses are never a medical emergency. But if you ever have a callus that hurts so much you can hardly stand it, or if it starts to ache or bleed, call your doctor for some relief.

Mother Nature must be a shoemaker at heart. If you walk barefoot a lot, you'll naturally develop calluses, thick layers of dead skin that act like the soles on a good pair of shoes. The tough skin covers the sensitive layers underneath and protects you from whatever's underfoot.

People who work hard with their hands usually form calluses that protect them from nicks and cuts. And as anyone who has ever tried to play a guitar can tell you, learning's a painful process until you develop good calluses on your fingertips. Calluses, however, sometimes have painful nerves and bursal sacs beneath them that can cause symptoms ranging from shooting pain to aches.

Callus Comfort

For the most part, you can take care of calluses with simple home care. Here's what to try:

- **Do the ol' soft shoe.** Stiff leather shoes look great, but they don't feel so good when you have corns (small calluses on the toes). The only way to get rid of corns is to get rid of friction. That means wearing shoes made from cloth or soft leather for a few weeks. Sandals are also a good choice, as long as the straps don't rub against tender skin areas.

- **Soften tough skin.** Treat yourself to one of the many creams and lotions made to soften calluses; they have ingredients such as peppermint and apple-kiwi. Also try a moisturizer like vitamin E oil, cocoa butter, or lanolin, to make calluses softer and less painful.

- **Go barefootin' at the beach.** Those gray, gritty pumice stones we use to sand down calluses are made of volcanic rock. While few of us have access to volcano slopes, sand on the beach acts like a pumice stone—only better! If you live near a beach, walk barefoot in the sand as often as you can. Your feet will feel fabulous.

- **Bring out the salts.** The next time you take a bath, treat your feet to a moisturizing salt rub. Moisten a handful of Epsom salts with a small amount of almond or olive oil, then scrub your feet until the salt's dissolved and the oil has softened your skin. Wash well and be careful not to slip.

- **Soften with citrus.** Rubbing the cut side of half a lemon on your feet, elbows, and heels will give you softer, smoother skin.

Grandma Says:

Go soak 'em. To keep your feet as soft as a baby's, follow Grandma's routine: Periodically soak your feet in a pan of warm water to which you've added a teaspoon of baking soda or soap. As the callused skin loosens, gently rub it away a bit at a time with a pumice stone or emery board. Follow up with your favorite lotion.

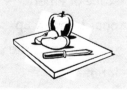
■ **File, don't cut.** Corns are just dead skin, so you'd think they'd be easy to cut away. Don't try it, though: There's a good chance that you'll damage healthy tissue and wind up with a painful sore—or even a nasty infection. It's much safer to use a nail file or a pumice stone to reduce the corn. But don't file it down all the way at one time; instead, remove just a little bit of skin each day. Most of the corn will be gone in a week or two, and you'll be less likely to hurt yourself in the meantime. (People with diabetes should see their health care provider for this procedure.)

■ **Soften before scraping.** Corns are a lot easier to remove if you soften the skin before using a file or pumice stone. First, soak your foot in warm water for 5 to 10 minutes. Once the skin is soft, gently abrade the toughened area to remove a few layers of skin, then leave it alone for the rest of the day. Repeat the soak-and-scrape routine once a day until the corn is gone.

Treat Your Feet

From foot massage to the way your shoes fit, here's a trio of treats for your tootsies:

■ **Give 'em a rub.** A foot massage is a super soother when your corns are a-poppin'. But don't put a lot of pressure directly on the corns—it hurts! Instead, work around them. Massage your entire foot, starting at the tips of your toes and working backward to your heel.

If your foot is particularly tender, you may want to use a massage technique called effleurage: long, stroking movements with a bit of pressure.

- **Redistribute the load.** Use orthotic inserts in your shoes to transfer pressure away from callused areas and absorb shock. These may help if you have calluses because of an abnormal gait, flat feet, high arches, or very bony feet. Inserts are available in most drugstores, but it's a good idea to ask a podiatrist about orthotics that can be specially made for you.

- **Size counts.** In Grandma Putt's day, clerks in shoe stores routinely measured your feet to ensure a good fit. These days, you're lucky if you can even find someone to help you find the size you *think* you need. Seek out a store where the clerks measure both of your feet. They should check the fit at the heel and the toe. After that, walk around in the shoes to make sure they're truly comfortable.

Oil Away Aches

Any oil softens the skin, but herb-infused oils stimulate circulation and help keep your feet healthy and ache-free. Try the following blend made of oils available at health food stores: Add 2 drops each of peppermint oil and carrot seed oil to an ounce of calendula oil, then mix in 5 drops each of lavender oil and geranium oil. Store the mixture in a small bottle, and massage it into your feet once a day.

Chapped Lips

Your lips are meant for more than just kissing or keeping soup from spilling out of your mouth. They're also a barometer of what's going on elsewhere in your body. If you often get chapped lips, you may have to look beyond your mouth for the solutions.

Chapped lips usually indicate nothing more serious than too much exposure to sun or wind. Chapping is especially a problem in winter, because indoor heat sucks a lot of moisture out of the air. But if your lips stay chapped for weeks at a time, or if they get better for a while, then get chapped again, you should probably see your doctor. Continually chapped lips can be a sign of chronic stress. When you're stressed out for a long time, your adrenal glands can get out of whack and disrupt your body's sodium balance. This, in turn, can make your lips dry and chapped, no matter how much water you drink.

Pucker Power

The skin on your lips is shed and replaced more rapidly than other tissues. If you aren't getting enough key nutrients in your diet, for example, the problem may start to show up on your lips before you notice other symptoms. Also, dry lips may be a signal that your body isn't retaining fluids as well as it should. So don't think of chapped lips as just a nuisance. At the very least, a lack of proper TLC can result in deep, painful cracks that are agonizingly slow to heal. Lip balm should always be the first line of defense for parched lips, but if yours still seem rough enough to scour pots, consider these additional tips:

- **Top off your tank.** Sometimes chapped lips are simply a signal that your body's water tank is too low. Try drinking several large glasses of water daily to give your lips the moisture they're craving.

- **Pump moisture into the air.** An indoor humidifier is a great way to keep your lips supple and healthy. It's especially important to use a humidifier during cold weather because heating systems, especially forced hot air systems, draw moisture out of the air.

- **Screen the sun.** Too much sun does more than just dry your lips; it can give them a ferocious burn. So use a lip balm with the highest sun protection factor (SPF) you can find. Be sure it's waterproof, and use it as often as the directions on the package recommend.

From Grandma's Kitchen

You may not see the connection, and I'm sure Grandma Putt didn't, either, but somehow she knew that eating green vegetables is a great way to keep your lips in the pink. That's because greens are rich in zinc, essential fatty acids, and riboflavin—everything your lips need to retain moisture and stay healthy.

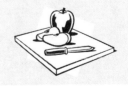

Buy Natural Balms

Herbal lip balms that contain marigold or calendula are better than synthetic goop from the cosmetics counter because they contain natural compounds that promote healing. Other lip-healing ingredients to look for in balms include lanolin, olive oil, and echinacea.

- **Bag the balm.** Avoid petroleum-based products. Rather than covering your lips with an oil slick, use protective products that contain beeswax or other natural forms of oil. (See "Buy Natural Balms" above.)

- **Lay off the licking.** If you find that your lips get severely chapped during stressful times— when visiting your in-laws at Thanksgiving, for example—you could be licking them more than usual. And licking your lips actually dries them out, so get in the habit of chewing gum or sucking on lozenges when you're nervous, and leave those lips alone!

- **Try some new makeup.** Some women get chapped lips when they use foundation makeup or lipstick. In fact, almost any cosmetic ingredient that comes near the mouth can cause reactions in some people. So if your lips are frequently chapped and you've ruled out other possible causes, try using different kinds of makeup until you find the brands that agree with you.

■ **Switch mouthwashes.** Or try a new toothpaste. As with makeup, these products may
contain ingredients that cause chapping.
Something as simple as changing brands
may make a big difference.

Load up On Bs

Chapped lips or cuts at the corners of your
mouth are classic signs of a B vitamin deficiency.
B vitamins are required for cell division and
reproduction; when the tissues in the corner of
your mouth are weak from lack of B vitamins,
cracks or splits appear. A good multivitamin that
includes all of the B vitamins should put your
lips back in working order, so be sure to take one
every morning.

Colds

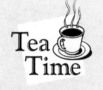
If you can't figure out why modern science hasn't found a cure for the common cold, consider the numbers. A cold is actually 1 of about 200 mild viral infections of the upper respiratory tract. Even if doctors figured out how to cure one of them, what about the other 199?

The trouble is, despite all the promises made in cold-remedy advertising, the fact remains that over-the-counter drugs just don't do much—and cost a bundle, besides. Antihistamines, for instance, will dry up a runny nose from allergies, but they won't affect the dripping and sneezing of a cold. Decongestants can leave you jittery. Aspirin and acetaminophen can suppress your immune system. And those all-in-one nighttime remedies? They come with a shot glass for good reason: The "knockout" ingredient is alcohol. It may help your head hit the pillow, but it won't do a thing to fight infection.

Feel Better Fast

Other than curling up in bed when you have a nasty cold, what's the alternative? Try some of these natural remedies. A few of them—if taken at the first sneeze—can cut your sick time by more than half:

- **Steam out infection.** Steam kills cold germs on contact if water temperatures are 110°F or more. Herbs such as eucalyptus add a penetrating scent and have disinfectant properties. Put some fresh leaves in a bowl, pour boiling water over them, and drape a towel over your head and the bowl to make a "tent." Lower your face over the bowl (carefully—you can scald yourself if the steam is too hot) and breathe in. You can also add a few drops of oregano oil to the water. It's nice—a bit like diluted Vicks.

- **Stay lubricated.** When you're in artificially controlled environments with really dry air, including offices and airplanes, your nasal membranes dry out, and tiny cracks that invite viruses may form in your nasal passages. The best defense? Drink plenty of liquids and use saline nasal spray often to hydrate the tender membranes in your nose.

- **Make a chest rub.** Using a poultice when you have a cold is a good way to make yourself rest. Make your own chest rub by adding 3 or 4 drops of herbal oil (try eucalyptus, lavender, or thyme) to 1 tablespoon of olive oil. Apply the mixture liberally to your chest, cover with a clean cloth, and settle into a comfy chair with a cozy afghan and a good book.

- **Make a Bloody Mary.** You can use booze or not, as you prefer. Start with tomato juice, add some lemon, a celery stalk, and horseradish, then drink it quickly. Tomato juice is full of vitamin C, but it's the horseradish that really does the trick. Its powerful fumes will loosen congestion, making your cold more bearable.

- **Mine some zinc.** Research indicates that zinc may cut the duration of colds by about two days. It acts as a physical barrier to prevent viruses from entering the cells that line the nose and throat. All you have to do is spritz an over-the-counter zinc nasal spray (which you can find in drugstores) in each nostril four times a day within 48 hours of the first inkling of a cold. With zinc lozenges, you have to act even more quickly—within 24 hours of your first symptom. Look for zinc gluconate tablets that aren't flavored with citric acid, tartaric acid, or sorbitol. When these ingredients mix with saliva, they cancel out zinc's benefits.

Echinacea is Excellent

Studies have shown that the herb echinacea shortens the duration of colds from nine to six days and makes them less severe—possibly because the polysaccharides it contains boost the body's infection-fighting cells. The best way to take echinacea is as a tincture (an alcohol-based extract, which is available at health food stores) because it contains more of the active constituents. At the first hint of a cold, take 30 drops of tincture every 2 hours. After a week, go to 20 drops three times a day, for a total of 10 days. Use the herb only during your cold (with continued use, it loses effectiveness), and never use it if you have an autoimmune disease such as lupus, rheumatoid arthritis, or multiple sclerosis, or if you are pregnant or nursing.

Breathe Easy with Olive

Research shows that leuropein, the active ingredient in olive leaf extract, has powerful healing properties that may beat bacteria, viruses, fungi, and even parasites. The recommended dose is one 300-milligram capsule three times a day for no more than two days. After that, gradually reduce your intake. Check with your doctor first, and never take olive leaf in any dosage for more than seven days.

Quick Cold Relief

If you can, try to take just one day off from your usual routine when your cold strikes. Stay home, get into your jammies, and try some of these cold relievers:

■ **Hooray for horseradish.** This powerful herb contains allyl isothiocyanate, which stimulates the nerve endings in your nose and makes it

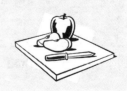

run like a faucet. Plus, horseradish has antiviral properties. Try a teaspoon of freshly grated root or a half-teaspoon of horseradish extract three times a day. The extract is available in health food stores.

■ **Soothe your cough with elm.** If you're coughing so much that your chest and back ache, try slippery elm tea. This time-honored expectorant will help break up the sticky mucus that may be clogging your bronchial tubes. Look for the tea at health food stores and follow the directions on the label.

MODERN MARVEL

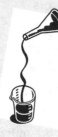

Wash Often

Hardy cold viruses can live for hours on doorknobs, faucet handles, books, money—all the things we touch every day. Frequent hand washing is the single best way to avoid catching a cold or spreading your own. Unfortunately, the habit is in decline. Researchers from the American Society of Microbiology and the Centers for Disease Control and Prevention watched 8,000 people in restrooms in several cities. Only 67 percent stopped at the sink. In a related survey, only 40 percent of women reported washing their hands after sneezing or coughing, and men were even worse—just 22 percent. (They were also asked if they washed their hands after changing a diaper or petting an animal—and believe me, you don't want to know their answers!)

- **Fight the bug with astragalus.** This Chinese herb stimulates the release of interferon in the body and thereby boosts your immune system. Unlike echinacea, you can take astragalus (available at health food stores) every day during cold and flu season to bolster your resistance. A typical regimen is eight 400- to 500-milligram capsules or 15 to 30 drops of extract daily.

- **Toss the germs.** Bacteria and viruses live on cloth towels and sponges for hours, so use paper towels, tissues, and napkins when someone in the house has a cold.

Mist Away Throat Pain

Here's a blast of natural relief for a sore throat. First, buy yourself a new plant mister. Then make a triple-strength tea by adding 3 teaspoons each of dried slippery elm, echinacea, and licorice to 3 cups of water. Bring it to a full boil, then reduce the heat and simmer for 10 to 15 minutes. Strain out the herbs, cool, and pour the brew into your new spray bottle. Open your mouth, stick out your tongue, and spray the back of your throat as needed during the day. *Ahhhh*, relief! Don't use licorice, though, if you have high blood pressure or kidney disease.

Decline Dairy

When you have a cold, stick to juices, water, and hot beverages. Avoid milk and milk products,

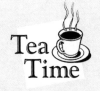

Tea Time

Garlic has long been used for its potent healing effects, and it does double duty as a cold preventive because it keeps other people at a distance! Surprisingly, garlic tea doesn't taste as bad as you'd think. Chop two medium cloves and simmer in 1 cup of water for 10 to 15 minutes. Add two to three slices of fresh ginger to improve the taste and increase the warming action of the garlic. Honey and lemon are optional. Drink two to four cups per day.

because moo juice promotes mucus formation. If you do indulge in dairy during a cold, you'll not only get a milk moustache, you're also likely to get more congestion.

M is for Mushrooms

And mushrooms are for immunity. Smoky-tasting shiitake mushrooms amp up production of interferon, a protein that girds the body to defend against viral invaders, while reishi mushrooms may help ease respiratory tract inflammation. You can either add these delicious 'shrooms to your therapeutic chicken soup, or look for them combined in extract form and follow the directions on the label.

Two to Try

Here are a pair of time-honored cold-chasers to add to your arsenal:

- **Decongest with licorice.** The steam from licorice tea speeds the flow of mucus from your nose, and the licorice itself stimulates production of interferon, a protein that not only helps the body defend against viral invaders, but also brings mucus up from the lungs and soothes a scratchy throat. You should be able to find packaged licorice tea at your local health food stores. Follow the label directions. A word of caution: Don't use this cold remedy if you have high blood pressure.

Snooze with Booze

Try a hot toddy as a cold rescue. Before hundreds of cold remedies became available at drugstores, certain home remedies were probably a lot more fun to take. And if you took enough, you absolutely felt better, because pretty soon you didn't notice the symptoms anymore. There are many variations on the hot toddy, which apparently originated in Scotland. Start with hot juice or tea and add honey and the liquor of your choice.

■ **Vinegar for vigor.** Appalachian healers make a cold remedy from common household ingredients. You may want to give this recipe a try: Mix a dash of red pepper and a pinch of salt into 1 ounce of apple cider vinegar, and drink it three or four times a day. Another remedy some folks use for colds is 1 tablespoon each of honey and lemon juice. Add them to a cup of hot water or tea, and sip it three times a day for soothing cold relief.

Cold Sores

Pain isn't always proportionate to size, as anyone who's ever had a cold sore knows. Those pesky little blisters on or near the lips are hardly bigger than a pencil eraser, but they can burn and sting like the dickens.

Despite the name, cold sores—also known as fever blisters—don't have anything to do with colds or fevers. They're caused by a virus known as herpes simplex type 1. (A close relative, herpes simplex type 2, is responsible for genital sores.) Millions of Americans are infected with the virus but never have symptoms. Others aren't so lucky.

The cold sore virus survives in the body forever, although it spends most of its life in dormancy. Periodically, it "wakes up," travels up nerves to the skin, and erupts in a painful, fluid-filled blister. The blister goes away in about a week, but that doesn't mean the virus is gone. It's just back in hiding, where it will stay dormant until the next time conditions are right for it to appear.

Healing Helpers

Most people don't get cold sores often enough to worry much about them. But they are a bother, so you'll want to do anything you can to make them go away—and help keep them from coming back. You don't have to buy a lot of fancy medicines to do it. Give these treatments a try:

- **Dab on lemon balm.** Studies show that lemon balm, also known as melissa, helps cold sores heal faster with less crusting. And since lemon balm contains at least four antiviral compounds, it's considered by some to be a first-choice herbal treatment. The key is to apply it at the first inkling of an outbreak. Make a tea by steeping 2 to 4 teaspoons of dried lemon balm leaves in a cup of hot water for 10 minutes or so, then apply the cooled solution directly to the sore. Or look for a commercial lip balm that contains lemon balm, and slather it on.

- **Excellent extracts.** At the first indication of a blister outbreak, scan the shelves of your local health food store for extracts of calendula, tea tree oil, slippery elm, and myrrh; they're all either excellent astringents or inflammation and infection fighters. Add several drops of each to a cup of hot water, let it cool, and dab the solution directly onto your cold sore for instant pain relief.

dial the DOCTOR

When It's Really Sore

While cold sores are more of a bother than a real health concern for most people, there are times when you may want to see your doctor. If you get sores every month, for example, or they're unusually large or painful, your doctor may write a prescription for a drug that can shorten the duration of outbreaks.

- **Go for the gold standard.** Goldenseal is another antiviral herb that can treat cold sores. Add ¼ teaspoon of the extract—available at health food stores—to your echinacea drink (see below) three times a day.

- **Sip echinacea.** Echinacea isn't just a plain old cold fighter; it battles cold sores, too—perhaps by boosting our natural antiviral immune fighters. Mix ¼ teaspoon of extract (available at health food stores) in water or juice, and drink it three times a day for as long as your symptoms last. *Caution:* Don't take echinacea if you have an autoimmune disease such as rheumatoid arthritis, lupus, or multiple sclerosis, or if you are pregnant or nursing.

Put Your Feet Up

The herpes simplex virus tends to awaken during times of stress, probably because tension and anxiety make your immune system work less efficiently. It's impossible, of course, to eliminate all the stress from your life, but keeping it at manageable levels reduces the risk of getting cold sores. Even if you already have an outbreak, reducing stress can prevent one sore from triggering another.

Everyone controls stress in different ways. Daily exercise is a great stress reducer. Relaxation techniques, such as meditation and deep breathing, can help, too. So can setting aside time to do things you enjoy, such as going to the movies or spending time with friends. So lighten up!

Zap Sores with Zinc

The same white ointment that lifeguards use on their noses to protect against sunburn may heal cold sores in 5 days instead of the usual 10. The catch is that you have to apply zinc oxide at least four times a day—even every hour—starting within 24 hours of the first hint of an outbreak. You can find the ointment at drugstores.

Buy the Right Balm

The herbal balms sold in health food stores reduce cold sore pain and keep the skin moisturized as the blisters dry and crust. In addition, some balms help combat the virus directly. Look for marigold and calendula balms—they're healing and have antiviral properties.

Lose Those Sores

Here are a handful of ways to short-circuit the cold sore cycle and help heal sores quickly:

- **Oil 'em.** Both lavender and St. John's wort oils, available in health food stores, inhibit the activity of herpes simplex. Once or twice a day, use a cotton swab to dab a small amount of oil on the sore. Be careful not to get the oil in your mouth, though. Even in tiny amounts, these oils should not be taken internally.

- **Flood the pain.** Even if you don't drink a lot of water most of the time, you really want to

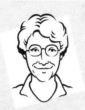

Grandma Says:

Ice it up. Grandma Putt said the best way to stop cold sores in their tracks is to apply ice at the earliest sign. Most people experience a slight tingling sensation days before cold sores erupt, and that's the time to apply an ice cube to the area. Keep it there for about 20 minutes and repeat the treatment throughout the day.

tank up when you have a cold sore. The more fluid you have in your body, the easier it is for immune cells to get where they're needed to start the healing process. So make an effort to drink 8 to 12 glasses of water a day until the sore is gone.

- **Axe the arginine.** The cold sore virus can't thrive without an amino acid called arginine, so as soon as you feel a cold sore coming on, avoid arginine-rich foods, such as chocolate.

- **Load up on lysine.** Like arginine, lysine is a naturally occurring amino acid. Unlike arginine, it actually inhibits the effects of the herpes simplex virus. Take 3,000 to 4,000 milligrams of lysine daily during outbreaks.

Try A Sheen of Vaseline

Applying petroleum jelly is an easy way to soften the skin surrounding cold sores to prevent cracks or bleeding. Smooth a generous layer on the area once or twice a day and keep applying it until the cold sore is gone.

Lick Pain with Licorice

Don't head to the candy aisle; instead, go to a health food store for natural licorice root extract. It contains chemical compounds that inhibit the virus and can help cold sores heal more quickly. As soon as a sore appears, dab it with the molasses-like extract four to six times a day.

Conjunctivitis

You've probably seen snapshots in which everyone's eyes glow a demonic shade of red. The unflattering glow—redeye, as shutterbugs call it—can make you look like an extra from the set of *Buffy the Vampire Slayer*. In real life, that redness (more of a pink hue, actually) is no less attractive—and it could mean trouble.

A condition called conjunctivitis, better known as pinkeye, occurs when the conjunctiva—the protective membrane covering the insides of your eyelids and the exposed whites of your eyes—gets infected. If your eyes are itching, burning, and discharging some sticky goop, chances are good that you've got pinkeye. It usually begins in one eye and quickly spreads to the other. Pinkeye can be caused by bacteria or an allergy, but it's most commonly the result of a virus. The good news is that you can ease the discomfort of pinkeye with some simple home remedies.

**dial the
DOCTOR**

When it Lingers

Once in a great while, a case of conjunctivitis can do some real damage. If your pinkeye doesn't clear up within a week, or if you have a fever or changes in vision along with it, call your doctor.

Ease the Irritation

While pinkeye is quite contagious, it's usually not very serious. Here's how to soothe the garden-variety types that trouble most of us:

- **Shut your eyes and chill.** Ice-cold compresses can soothe your eyes. Simply place a damp washcloth that's been chilled in the freezer or a cool, wet paper towel over your closed eyes for about 20 minutes. Stop for 30 to 60 minutes, then do it again. Reapply as often as you feel the need.

- **Relax with a berry good compress.** Strawberry tea helps soothe inflamed eyes and fight infection. Steep 1 teaspoon of leaves in 1 cup of hot water for 10 minutes, strain, and cool. Use the solution in a compress or put it in an eyecup and rinse your eyes with it once or twice daily.

- **Stay on the dry side.** Until your eyes have cleared up, don't go swimming! Not only can

The Chamomile Cure

To make a soothing eyewash from chamomile, steep 2 to 3 teaspoons of the herb (or use a tea bag) in 1 pint of boiling water for 10 minutes. Let cool and strain through a sterile cloth. Use an eyecup to rinse your eye with the solution two or three times daily until the problem is resolved. *Caution:* People with ragweed allergies may be sensitive to chamomile.

you spread conjunctivitis germs to others in the pool, but the chlorinated water can increase your eye irritation.

- **Hands off.** While your eyes are infected, avoid shaking hands; use disposable tissues; and be sure to disinfect doorknobs, countertops, and telephones. Don't share towels or pillows, and change your towels and pillowcases frequently.

The Eyes Have It

Sometimes it's the simple things you do that speed up the healing process. When conjunctivitis comes a calling, try these quick and easy eye-friendly remedies:

- **Unload your mascara.** Get rid of any mascara, eyeliner, or eye shadow that you've used since you developed pinkeye. They're harboring germs. Then, when your peepers are no longer pink, treat yourself to some new cosmetics.

- **Get out your glasses.** Don't wear contacts while you have pinkeye. Your eyes will feel worse with them in, since the lenses hold the germs against your eyeball.

- **Put on some shades.** Wear sunglasses to protect your eyes from glare and irritation. You'll look cool, and you'll feel less self-conscious about your inflamed eyes and mascara-free lashes.

- **Get all weepy.** Check your local drugstore for artificial tears and other soothing over-

Tea Time

When pinkeye is recurrent or particularly severe, support your whole body with infection-fighting herbs. Combine equal parts of echinacea, eyebright, calendula, and cleavers. Steep 1 teaspoon of the mixture in 1 cup of hot water for 10 minutes, then strain and drink two or three cups daily.

the-counter eye remedies. According to the American Academy of Family Physicians, these lubricating eyedrops are especially helpful if your pinkeye is due to allergies, but they can also help reduce swelling of the conjunctiva.

- **Stop allergy attacks.** If your conjunctivitis is allergy related, ask your doctor if you should take an over-the-counter antihistamine such as diphenhydramine (Benadryl), which can help reduce itching, swelling, and discomfort. If an oral medication doesn't do the job, ask if prescription antihistamine eyedrops are right for you.

Constipation

Sometimes constipation, like beauty, exists only in the eye of the beholder. Most of us grow up thinking that a daily bowel movement is necessary for good health, but everyone experiences constipation in different ways. For someone who's accustomed to having a bowel movement every day, a reduction to three or four a week could be a sign of constipation. For others, having three bowel movements a week is normal, but having fewer than that is a problem.

There are literally hundreds of things that can cause constipation. Sometimes it's a side effect of medications. Lack of exercise can cause it, or drinking too little water, or not eating enough fiber. The list goes on and on.

And since regularity varies so much between people, doctors offer this advice: If there's been any change in your usual bathroom habits, get help.

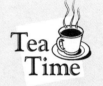

Tea Time

This old-time remedy really seems to loosen things up. Any time you boil potatoes, save the cooking water. The next morning, mix 2 tablespoons of potato water and 2 tablespoons of honey into a mug of hot water, and drink it before breakfast.

Start Things Moving Again

Fortunately, you don't have to put up with constipation—and you definitely shouldn't fork over your hard-earned cash for over-the-counter laxatives. There are a lot of less expensive—and safer—treatments to try first. Here are the best:

- **Fill 'er up.** All experts agree that the simplest way to wake up your colon is to drink water—lots and lots of it. Try to down 10 glasses (a total of 80 ounces) within 24 hours. Need to get things moving right now? Drink a large glass of water every 10 minutes for 1 hour to soften your stools and spur elimination.

- **Praise the plants.** The best diet for beating constipation is the same one that doctors recommend for preventing heart disease, cancer, and dozens of other serious health problems: a lot of plant foods and very little, if any, junk food. In other words, eat as though processed foods had never been invented. Aim for a diet that's high in fiber and complex carbohydrates. That means lots of fruits and vegetables, whole grains, and legumes every day, as well as high-fiber cereals such as oatmeal and oat bran.

- **Have another slice of pie.** Just make sure it's rhubarb—one of the yummiest natural laxatives around. Rhubarb stimulates mucus production in the large intestine to ease elimination, which typically occurs within 6 to 10 hours. You can also eat it stewed, or try this lip-smacking smoothie: Juice 3 cups of raw rhubarb stalks and

1 cup of fresh or frozen strawberries. Add ¼ cup of water and ¼ cup of honey, then sip and go!

- **Heed the call.** If you're reluctant to use a public restroom no matter how urgent the need, you're setting yourself up for trouble. Resisting the urge to have a bowel movement—whether you're in a restaurant or at home—can make it difficult to go later on. In fact, delaying bowel movements can make your large intestine lazy. Essentially, you're teaching your body to resist its natural urges. You'll be a lot more regular if you go as soon as possible when you feel the need.

Get-Regular Roundup

When constipation lingers, try some of these solutions to get yourself going:

- **Rub in regularity.** To encourage movement in sluggish bowels, try a simple belly-button rub. Use your favorite massage oil and lightly massage your stomach with the tips of your fingers, starting at your belly button and moving in small, clockwise circles. Gradually expand the circles until you're massaging your whole abdomen. If you do this for 10 to 15 minutes every morning, you may find that your daily routine will be a bit more regular.

- **Move often.** Any kind of physical activity—walking, lifting weights, riding a bicycle—helps the intestine work more efficiently. In fact, it's not uncommon for people who have been con-

dial the DOCTOR

Watch for Changes

If feelings of discomfort or bloating linger after a bowel movement, or if constipation persists after you've tried to treat it, call your doctor. Persistent abdominal pain or fever, a change in the color or consistency of stool, or blood in the stool could be signs of obstruction or disease. If constipation goes on too long, stools can get so hard and impacted that they won't budge without medical help.

From Grandma's Kitchen

Grandma Putt always encouraged me to eat my oatmeal. She said it would keep me regular—and she was right! Oatmeal has lots of mucilage, a gummy fiber that soaks up water, softening stools and making them easier to pass. That's the reason it's often recommended as an excellent breakfast choice to jump-start your system. Just don't top your bowl with bananas, which can be binding.

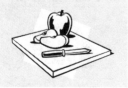

stipated for years to get completely better once they start exercising for 20 to 30 minutes daily.

- **Regulate with supplements.** The mineral magnesium helps soften stools and make bowel movements easier. Talk to your doctor about starting the day with 500 milligrams of supplemental magnesium. Another option: As long as you don't have stomach or kidney problems, take 1,000 to 2,000 milligrams of vitamin C a day, split into two or three doses. If either supplement causes diarrhea, reduce the dose.

- **Dig some dandelions.** To make a dandy drink that'll relieve constipation, puree some young dandelion leaves in a blender with water, then pour the juice into a glass. Drink up to three times a day. Or add fresh dandelion greens to a salad. Just be sure your dandelion comes from a lawn that hasn't been blasted with chemicals. And don't use dandelion if you're taking diuretics or potassium tablets.

Mind Your Medicines

Constipation is among the most common side effects of medications. Antacids are typical culprits, as are pain medications. It's worth making a list of all the drugs you're taking to review with your pharmacist. If it turns out that one of them may be responsible for your constipation, your doctor shouldn't have any trouble finding an acceptable alternative.

Just Say "Ahhh..."

Open wide and down these remedies. They're all but guaranteed to get you back on the regularity track:

- **Multiply by three.** In hospitals, prunes, bran, and applesauce are frequently mixed together and offered to patients to get things going. To make your own cocktail, mix 4 to 6 chopped prunes with 1 tablespoon of bran and ½ cup of applesauce. Try it just before bed.

- **Give psyllium a try.** Check your local health food store or drugstore for powdered laxatives that contain psyllium seeds. Once a day, add 2 tablespoons to a large glass of water or juice and drink it immediately, before it thickens. To avoid an intestinal blockage, be sure to drink lots of water throughout the day—at least six extra glasses—while you're taking psyllium. And don't use it within 2 hours of taking any other supplements or medications, since it could delay their absorption into your bloodstream.

Sit and Soothe

The abdominal cramps that often accompany constipation can be excruciatingly painful. A fast way to get relief is to soak in a warm bath for 15 to 20 minutes. The warm water will relax your muscles and help reduce painful pressure and spasms.

■**Pop some prunes.** Ounce for ounce, prunes are packed with more fiber than almost any other fruit or vegetable—including dried beans. What's more, they contain dihydroxyphenyl isatin, a natural laxative. Down a glass of prune juice before bed to encourage a morning movement, then nibble on dried prunes (or figs and raisins, which also contain isatin) during the day. For a tasty, high-fiber dessert, try baked apples stuffed with prunes, figs, or raisins.

Say Yes to Yoga

Perform this yoga exercise, and you could have a bowel movement within 10 minutes. First, stand with your hands at your sides, inhale deeply through your nose, and exhale through your mouth. Lift your arms over your head, while inhaling deeply again through your nose. Next, exhale while lowering yourself into a squat, bringing your hands to your knees, and lowering your head. As you finish the exhalation, still squatting, pump your abdomen in and out 20 times. Stand up and repeat three times.

Kick Back After Meals

It's the best way to encourage your digestive tract to shift into gear. If you're the type who likes to eat and run, you're diverting blood to other parts of your body and leaving your intestine short-changed. The old adage 'rest and digest' is just as true today as it ever was.

Coughs

Coughing is your body's equivalent of a bouncer. It's rough, and it tosses out all the potential troublemakers in the exclusive night-club of your respiratory system. Unfortunately, there are a lot of troublemakers out there: dust, pollen, viruses, and the smoke from your spouse's cigar, to name just a few. Coughing does its job pretty well, and for the most part, you want to encourage it. But you also want to soothe the irritated tissues in your throat and airways until the cough goes away, as well as boost your immune system so any germs will disappear as quickly as possible.

Breathe, Sip, and Sleep

A simple cough often responds to simple solutions. Here's what may help:

- **The poultice that pleases.** Traditional healers swear by herbal oil poultices for easing coughs. To make one, add a few drops of thyme or

dial the DOCTOR

Count the Days

If your cough really hurts, is accompanied by fever, or gets worse after a week or so, see your doctor. You may have an infection that needs antibiotics. Coughing can even be a symptom of heart disease, so don't wait.

Coughs 129

eucalyptus oil to a teaspoon of olive oil. Rub the mixture on your chest and the outside of your throat, then cover the area with an old towel or a piece of flannel so you don't stain your clothes. Leave the poultice on for about 20 minutes. The vapors will soothe your irritated airways, and reduce the urge to cough.

- **Hang out with hyssop.** A good way to eliminate mucus—and the coughing that goes with it—is to drink hyssop tea. A traditional herb for treating coughs, hyssop makes mucus thinner and easier to cough up. Buy dried hyssop at a health food store and add 1 teaspoon to a cup of freshly boiled water. Steep for about 10 min-

A Honey of a Cure

Honey mixed with onion juice was widely used for coughs during the Great Depression, when few folks could afford drugstore remedies. To this day, people still use it. Honey or sugar is used to draw the juice from an onion, forming an effective cough syrup. The onion, it's said, stimulates saliva flow, which clears the throat and may reduce inflammation.

Here's what to do: Slice an onion into rings, and place them in a deep bowl. Cover them with honey and let stand for 10 to 12 hours. Strain out the onion, and take 1 tablespoon of the syrup four or five times a day. Or you can finely chop an onion, mix with 1/2 cup of granulated sugar, and let stand overnight. Take 1 tablespoon of the resulting syrup every 4 to 5 hours.
Caution: Never give raw honey to children under one year of age.

utes, then strain out the herb. Drink it warm throughout the day.

- **Heat some wine.** A traditional Belgian remedy for coughs is to combine hot red wine with lemon, cinnamon, and sugar. At the very least, it will put you right to sleep, so you won't know if you're coughing (and probably won't care). Alcohol is a component of many cough medicines, but use it cautiously—too much will weaken your immune response, which you need to fight infection.

- **Sleep on a slant.** When your chest is congested and you're coughing up a lot of mucus, pile on several pillows or sleep on a foam wedge. Sleeping with your head raised 6 to 8 inches will prevent the mucus from pooling in your bronchial passages, thus easing your coughing and promoting more peaceful sleep.

Cough Busters

Your kitchen cabinets hold an array of cough suppressants. Here are a few you'll want to try to tame that hack:

- **Keep fluids flowing.** Any time is the right time to drink lots of fluids, but especially when you've got a cough. Enjoy a cup of hot tea with honey—it's good at loosening mucus.

- **Add extra nourishment.** Even if you get all of the essential nutrients in your diet, your body needs extra vitamins and minerals when you're fighting an upper respiratory infection. Taking

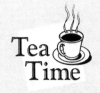

Tea Time

Thyme is great for fighting off a nagging cough. It inhibits bacteria and reduces inflammation in your throat. This familiar kitchen spice is also an expectorant: It thins mucus, so you don't have to cough as hard to get rid of it. Make a tea by steeping 1 teaspoon of dried thyme in a cup of hot water for 10 to 15 minutes, then straining out the herb. Or visit a health food store, pick up a bottle of thyme tincture, and take 10 to 20 drops up to four times daily.

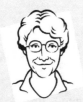

Grandma Says:

Take a break. If you ever came down with a cough around Grandma Putt, the first thing she'd have you do is put up your feet. After all, since most coughs are caused by upper respiratory infections, your first approach should be to help your body heal. The best way to do that is to kick back and take it easy.

a daily multivitamin is an easy way to ensure that you get all the nutrients you need to heal.

■**Forget the fruit juices.** While vegetable juices are great when you have a cold or the flu, fruit juices can hurt more than they help. They're loaded with sugar, and all that sweetness is just what germs need to flourish. Also, the acids in citrus juices can irritate your throat and make a cough worse. Stick with vegetable juice until you're well again.

■**Pop extra C.** This all-purpose nutrient is essential when you're sick because it strengthens your immune system and can help reduce cold symptoms, including coughs, in a hurry. Unless you have kidney or stomach problems, take 500 milligrams of vitamin C every few hours until you're feeling better. If you start having diarrhea, reduce the dose to a level you can tolerate.

Tame a Cough with Herbs

These cough cures have been around for ages, and there's a good reason why—they work!

■**Ask for anise.** The herb anise, which has a pleasant licorice flavor and fragrance, is a traditional cough remedy. You can buy anise tea bags at health food stores. Or raid your spice cabinet, and steep a teaspoon of anise in a cup of hot water. It's also fine to use as a tincture. The recommended dose for quelling a cough is about 20 drops up to four times daily.

- **Gulp down some gum plant.** Also known as grindelia, this common herb is a top-flight cough remedy. It's great when you have a dry, raw kind of cough. Take about 20 drops of grindelia tincture two to four times daily. You can find the tincture at health food stores.

- **Soften with marshmallow.** When mixed with hot water, the herb marshmallow (which was used to make the candy in the days before high-tech laboratories) forms a slippery liquid that coats and moisturizes a dry, raspy throat. Slippery elm has similar effects. You can buy both herbs in powdered form at most health food stores. Add a tablespoon of either to a cup of hot water, and sip it slowly several times a day.

Drink Your Veggies

Fresh vegetable juice is packed with nutrients that will feed your immune system. The advantage of juices over solid foods when you're sick is that your body is able to absorb the nutrients quickly and easily. So unpack that juicer someone gave you for your birthday five years ago, and crank it up. Green leafy vegetables are the best choices for juicing. Be sure to use organic veggies so you don't ingest any pesticides.

Cuts and Scrapes

dial the DOCTOR

When the Blood Keeps Flowing

Cuts that bleed a lot or continue bleeding for more than a few minutes may be too much for you to handle. If you can see deep inside the cut—say, more than 1/4 inch into the tissue—see a doctor right away.

How many times have you been sorting papers on your desk when "Yee-ow!"—all of a sudden you're bleeding from a nasty paper cut? Most of the cuts and scrapes we endure in the course of our busy lives are caused by the smallest things: trimming gnarly tree branches, say, or moving a little too fast with the paring knife. When you get a cut or scrape, your body almost immediately mobilizes specialized cells in your skin and blood vessels. They secrete a host of chemical compounds, including gluelike substances that stop bleeding and seal the cut.

Fast First Aid

Cuts are painful because some parts of your body, especially your fingertips, are jammed with sensitive nerves. Even shallow cuts on your hands or fingers can deliver a surprising amount of pain, and the risk of infection is very real. Obviously, you need to see a doctor if you're bleeding a lot or have a deep puncture wound.

In most cases, though, all you need is some simple first aid:

- **Clean and clean again.** Hold your wound under running water or pour cool water over it from a cup. Using mild soap and a soft washcloth, thoroughly clean the edges of the wound and the surrounding area, being careful not to let any soap stray into the open skin. If dirt is embedded in the wound, dip some tweezers in rubbing alcohol, then pick out the particles. Or use a very soft, clean nailbrush to remove any tiny, deeply embedded bits of debris.

- **Put on some pressure.** Once the wound is clean, press a clean cloth or tissue on it for 15 minutes (that's about how long it takes to stanch the flow of blood), especially if the cut is on your scalp, hand, or foot, where blood vessels are close to the surface. If blood seeps through the cloth, add another layer, and reapply the pressure gently, but firmly. If the cut is on your arm or leg, you can raise it above the level of your heart to help slow the bleeding. *Note:* If your cut bleeds in spurts or blood drenches the bandage after 10 minutes of firm, direct pressure, go to the emergency room immediately.

- **Cover it.** Once the injury is clean, cover it with a bandage. It should be snug enough to keep out dirt, but not tight enough to hinder circulation.

- **Do it all again.** Even if you wash and cover a wound promptly, bacteria can still get inside and cause trouble. To prevent infection, it's

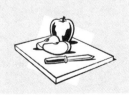

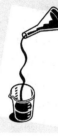

Modern Marvel

Cream the Pain

One of the quickest ways to ease the pain of abrasions is to apply a thick coat of triple antibiotic ointment. The cool cream feels good going on, it protects the wound from infection, and it can even help prevent scars.

important to change the adhesive bandage every day. Wash the wound with soap and running water, dry the area with a clean towel, and apply a fresh bandage. Most cuts don't require any more attention than that. And don't bother dousing it with hydrogen peroxide—in some cases, it can actually damage the tissue.

Cures for Cuts

Cuts, especially on your fingers, are a real pain. You want them to heal pronto so you can get back to using your hands without saying "ouch". Here are some ways to get cuts closing fast:

- **Knock out the germs.** Calendula fights a broad range of bugs, including bacteria and fungi. You can use it as a poultice to clean out debris. To prepare one, saturate a piece of sterile gauze or cloth with calendula tea (available at health food stores), place the soaked material on your injury, and leave it there for about an hour to help soften the skin and make any debris easier to remove. Afterward, pour a drop or two of extract directly onto the wound to keep it germ-free and minimize scarring.

- **Put rosemary to work.** To reduce the risk of infection, wash the wound with rosemary tea, available at health food stores. This herb is a mild antiseptic that appears to penetrate the skin and may allow the wound to dry out better than antibiotic creams and ointments, which can smother the skin and seal in germs.

- **Yell for yarrow.** Yarrow acts as both an astringent to stem the flow of blood and as an anti-inflammatory to calm the pain. Simply rinse some fresh yarrow leaves, chew them into a paste, and spit out the mashed poultice directly onto your wound. The fresher the leaves, the more quickly the bleeding will stop.

- **Heal faster with comfrey.** The leaves and roots of the comfrey plant contain the healing agent allantoin, which stimulates healthy tissue growth, speeding healing and reducing scar formation. You can find comfrey cream at a health food store, or you can crush fresh, clean leaves to apply to your wound. Comfrey encourages scab formation, so use it only on shallow cuts that you've cleaned thoroughly. Otherwise, you may seal in germs.

- **Stop scars with gotu kola.** This versatile Indian herb contains three compounds that simulate collagen, which is the connective tissue at the heart of skin repair and scar reduction. In fact, studies indicate that gotu kola can help prevent keloid scars—those large, bulging scars that come about when more tissue grows than needed to repair the wound. Simply pour a drop or two of extract (available at health food stores) directly onto the wound daily as it heals.

- **Clobber pain with cloves.** Raid your spice rack for whole cloves, which contain the chemical eugenol—an excellent antiseptic and painkiller. Crush the cloves into a powder, then sprinkle it directly onto your wound to speed healing.

Nature's Germ Fighter

Echinacea, a natural immune booster, will help bring white blood cells to a wound to fight infection. Take two capsules three times a day for a week.

Don't Mess with Infection

Even minor abrasions sometimes become infected. When you change the bandage, look for redness, swelling, pus, or increased tenderness. These are all signs that bacteria are winning the battle, and you may need antibiotics to turn the tide. Another risk to be wary of is tetanus, especially if there was wood or rusted metal in the injury. Tetanus is a life-threatening condition, so be sure you're protected. If you haven't had a tetanus vaccination in the past 10 years, go to your doctor and get the shot.

Dandruff

If aliens (that is, assuming that there are any) could somehow manage to tap into our television signals during commercial breaks, what would they think of us? They'd naturally assume that we're obsessed with cars, clean floors, and—oh, dear!—the horrors of dandruff. Shampoo manufacturers have somehow convinced us that dandruff is a serious social faux pas, if not exactly life-threatening.

The truth is, we all shed dandruff flakes now and then, especially in winter, when our scalps tend to become dry due to indoor heating. Usually the flakes are so few and far between that we're not even aware of them. It's only when the dandruff multiplies that we begin to notice little specks in our hair or on the shoulders of dark jackets or shirts. That's when it's time to reach for some tried-and-true home remedies like the ones you'll read about here.

dial the DOCTOR

If the Itch Spreads

You should see a doctor if you're losing hair, your scalp seems inflamed, or you have itchy, scaly skin on other parts of your body. These symptoms may indicate a more serious problem, such as psoriasis.

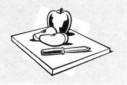
High-Speed Turnover

Most dandruff occurs when tiny oil glands at the base of the hair roots run amok. The scalp's skin normally replaces itself once a month, but if you have dandruff, somehow this shedding process is accelerated. Your hair becomes greasy, and those telltale crusty, yellowish flakes sprinkle onto your shoulders. Chances are, they're not your favorite fashion accessories.

More men than women have dandruff, so doctors suspect that the male hormone testosterone may have something to do with it. Other factors that can give you a case of the flakes include family history, food allergies, excessive sweating, alkaline soaps, and yeast infections. And although no one knows exactly what causes dandruff, stress does provoke it.

Banish the Flakes

In most cases, you can control dandruff with a few basic steps—without spending a fortune on expensive hair-care products. Here are some healthy-hair options:

- **Get a shampoo with fire power.** A good dandruff-fighting shampoo reduces scaling of the scalp, and allows medication to penetrate. Look for shampoos that list coal tar or salicylic acid among the ingredients. Although there are many over-the-counter dandruff shampoos, the FDA has approved only five active ingredients as safe and effective against dandruff: coal tar, pyrithione zinc, salicylic acid, selenium sulfide, and sulfur. The FDA also recognizes a combination of salicylic acid and sulfur as effective.

- **Wash your hair daily.** This breaks up larger flakes of dandruff, making them less noticeable. It also prevents the buildup of hair spray, gels, and other hair preparations, some of which can look a lot like dandruff as they wear off the hair. Massage the shampoo into your scalp and let it sit for 3 to 5 minutes—longer if your dandruff is severe. Rinse thoroughly.

- **Steam it out.** Steam your scalp with nutritive herbs for a deep-cleansing dandruff treatment. Mix together equal parts of fresh or dried leaves of rosemary, nettle, and peppermint. (If you use fresh nettle, be sure to wear gloves while preparing the mixture to avoid being stung by the prickly leaves.) Steep 2 tablespoons of dried herb mixture or ½ cup of fresh herbs in 2 cups of hot water in a covered container for 10 minutes. Strain the infusion, let it cool slightly, and apply it carefully to your scalp. Cover your hair

---

Beat It with Bs

The B vitamins, particularly biotin, are essential to a healthy scalp, so make sure you get a multivitamin that contains biotin. Or take a B-complex supplement that includes 300 micrograms of biotin to keep dandruff at bay.

with a shower cap and wrap your head in a hot, wet towel. Leave the treatment on for 30 minutes, then use an herbal rinse (see "Herbal Itch Relief" below).

Herbal Itch Relief

There are a number of herbs that are time-honored dandruff fighters. Give some of these a try:

- **Soothe with an herbal rinse.** Herbal rinses add sheen to the hair shaft and relieve scalp irritation at the same time. Traditional herbs include rosemary and sage for dark hair, chamomile and marigold for blondes, and cloves for auburn or red hair. Make a strong tea using 4 tablespoons of herb to 1 quart of boiling water. Steep for 15 minutes, then add ¼ cup of apple cider vinegar to restore the scalp's normal pH. Use as a final rinse after shampooing.

- **Tame it with thyme.** Another herbal approach to dandruff control is to dab some thyme oil diluted with olive oil (4 drops of thyme oil per teaspoon of olive oil) on your scalp 1 hour before washing your hair. Then, after shampooing, it's thyme for an anti-dandruff rinse. To make it, boil a handful of dried thyme in a quart of water, strain, and cool.

Styling Solutions

You can fight dandruff even when you're styling your hair. Follow these two hair care rules for flake-free tresses:

- **Turn off the power.** Whenever you can, let your hair dry naturally rather than blowing it dry. When you must have extra volume for a special occasion, be sure to use a lower heat setting. That hot wind really dries out the scalp, making you more vulnerable to dandruff.

- **Brush it out.** Using a natural-bristle brush, brush your hair from the scalp outward with steady, firm strokes. This carries excess oil away from your scalp, where it can cause dandruff, to the hair strands, where it gives your hair a healthy shine.

Hops Is Tops

It flavors beer—that's how most of us know about hops. Yet the wild hops plant is found all over the world, and Native Americans use it as a cure for dandruff, among other things. But you don't need to comb the fields for hops—just rinse your hair with beer or add a good squirt of the "suds" to your regular shampoo.

Denture Pain

dial the
DOCTOR

Hidden Heart Trouble

If you wear dentures, the last thing you would expect is to have a "toothache" in your lower jaw. Don't ignore it—you could be having a heart attack. If you have what seems to be tooth pain in your lower jaw, call 911.

Dentures have sure come a long way since George Washington wore his famous artificial teeth. Today, it's hard to distinguish dentures from natural teeth, at least by the way they look. Wearing them, on the other hand, does take some getting used to. If the fit isn't perfect, dentures can feel clumsy or uncomfortable. And even if they fit perfectly, they simply don't feel like real teeth. There's always an adjustment period—and the adjustment, in some cases, can be downright painful.

Your own teeth come properly fitted, and even the best dentist can't compete with Mother Nature. When you get dentures, your dentist will do everything possible to ensure proper fit, and to minimize pressure points on your gums. But for various reasons—changes during adjustments, for example, or even changes in your own mouth—the way dentures fit can vary over time. You'll know there's a problem if you develop a sore spot somewhere along your gum line. It's similar to the blisters you get when your shoes don't fit well, and the pain increases every time the area is rubbed the wrong way.

Take a Bite Out of Pain

Denture pain is incredibly common, but that doesn't mean it's normal. Pain always means that something's wrong. If your dentures start hurting, you need to visit your dentist. You most likely only have to have them adjusted, and won't be shelling out big bucks for a whole new set. In the meantime, here are a few ways to reduce the pain and help the sore spots heal properly:

- **Eat softly.** New dentures are always uncomfortable at first. As a matter of fact, during the first two months, most patients will probably need to have their dentures adjusted two or three times. During that time, you can keep soreness to a minimum by sticking to foods that are soft and easy to chew, such as pasta or steamed vegetables.

- **Give your gums a break.** Once you get a sore spot on your gums, your best bet is to wear your dentures as little as possible until it heals. Otherwise, they will continue to irritate the area. Most sores heal completely within 10 to 14 days, although you'll probably be able to wear your dentures comfortably before then.

The Clove Cure

A traditional remedy for tooth pain is to dab on some clove oil, which you can buy at a health food store. This remedy works just as well for gum sores, too, and it takes effect almost instantly. Simply dip a cotton swab in the oil, and apply it directly to the sore for soothing relief.

- **Heal faster with gargles.** Antibacterial mouth-washes can help gum sores heal more quickly because they prevent bacteria from irritating the open wound. Be sure you choose a brand that's formulated to kill germs, not just freshen your breath.

- **Get plenty of vitamin C.** It's an essential nutrient for gum health. If your dentures have rubbed you the wrong way, take 2,000 to 3,000 milligrams of vitamin C daily to help the sore heal more quickly. Don't take this amount of C, however, if you have stomach or kidney problems. And since high doses can cause stomach upset or diarrhea in some people, take it in two or three smaller doses during the day. It also helps to take it with food.

MODERN MARVEL

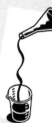

Count on Q10

Available in health food stores, drugstores, and supermarkets, coenzyme Q10 is a supplemental nutrient that promotes gum healing by increasing the amount of oxygen that's available to tissues in the mouth. Check with your doctor first, but it should be okay to take anywhere from 30 to 200 milligrams daily until the sore spots heal. Keep your mouth properly lubricated by drinking at least eight full glasses of water daily. You don't have to drink it all at once; just sip it throughout the day to keep your tissues moist.

Check Your Belt Size

Have you lost or gained weight recently? If so, you may have found the reason for your denture pain. Believe it or not, your gums can actually shrink with weight loss, and swell with weight gain. And even these small changes in the size or shape of your gums can throw your denture fit out of whack. If you aren't able to maintain a stable weight, stay in touch with your dentist, who will adjust your dentures to compensate for your weight changes.

Brush Often

Plaque and tartar, the same nasty substances that promote tooth and gum disease, can adhere to dentures just as easily as they cling to natural teeth. Once plaque and tartar build up, they can push your dentures out of alignment. Brush your dentures at least twice a day—before you put them in, and again after you take them out. It's a good idea to use a toothbrush that's specially made for dentures and designed to get into all the cracks and crevices.

Feel Better With Folic Acid

This B vitamin is another nutrient that's good for your gums. It helps your body replace cells that were damaged by poorly fitting dentures. If you have a gum sore, take at least 400 micrograms of folic acid daily until the sore heals.

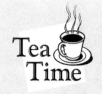

Tea Time

Here's a quick (and tasty) way to ease denture-related gum pain. Drop a teaspoon of dried chamomile (available at health food stores) into a cup of hot water, steep for 10 to 20 minutes, and strain. When it's cool, take a mouthful of tea, swish it around for 30 seconds or so, and spit it out. Keep rinsing with the tea until it's all gone. *Caution:* You shouldn't use chamomile if you're allergic to ragweed.

Depression

dial the DOCTOR

Know the Signs

Untreated depression can lead to suicide. If you have any thoughts of suicide, are depressed for more than two weeks, can't concentrate, can't sleep or sleep too much, or have a noticeable change in weight, get help right away.

Think depression is just about the blues? Think again. Serious, clinical depression can last for months or even years, and it has a profound impact on both physical and mental health. Researchers at Johns Hopkins University found that depressed people were four times more likely to have heart attacks than those who said they were not depressed. A study of middle-aged women found that those who had depressive symptoms (sleeping problems, lack of energy, frequent boredom, and crying), and who felt unsupported by their friends and families, had low levels of high-density lipoprotein (HDL)—the "good" cholesterol that helps prevent heart disease.

What's Behind It?

Genes, which help determine the levels of various brain chemicals that affect mood, may be partially to blame, but depression is usually a one-two punch. Genes set the stage, and then a stressful event tips your brain chemistry into the abyss. And chronic stress—the kind that arises from constantly trying to meet too many daily obligations—floods the body with the hormones cortisol and prolactin, which can lower levels of the mood-stabilizing brain chemical serotonin.

There are other causes of depression as well. The spikes and dips in hormones that normally occur during the menstrual cycle (giving rise to the irritability and general moodiness of premenstrual syndrome, or PMS), after giving birth (triggering postpartum depression), and before menopause can affect brain chemistry and dampen your mood. Abnormalities in the thyroid, pituitary, and adrenal glands can do the same. Even the gloomy days of winter, or simply being cooped up in a dark house or win-dowless office, can add to your doldrums, since inadequate exposure to sunlight can inhibit the release of serotonin. This sleepy, moody type of low is called seasonal affective disorder (SAD) and usually lifts during the sunny spring and summer months. If you're underexposed to light in general, however, it can contribute to general depression year-round.

Natural Mood Lifters

Depression needs to be diagnosed by a doctor. People with moderate or serious depression need to be under a doctor's care and should seriously consider taking medication if it's recommended;

Don't wait until the holidays to get your dose of tryptophan, an amino acid that's converted into serotonin in the body. In one study, when women ate turkey, fish, dairy products, nuts, and other foods high in tryptophan, their depression eased.

When you're eating a tryptophan-rich food, pair it with a lower-fat carbohydrate, such as whole grain bread, brown rice, or mashed potatoes. Carbs trigger the release of insulin, which allows tryptophan to enter your brain so that serotonin levels rise.

in some cases, antidepressant drugs can be life-savers. But if your depression is mild, you might not have to start out with antidepressants—or spend the rest of your life (not to mention your life savings) in therapy. At least in the beginning, ask your doctor if you can try some of these gentle (and less expensive) treatments. Just one caveat: If you're already taking prescription antidepressants or have bipolar disorder (also called manic depression), avoid the herbal anti-depressants recommended in this section:

- **Build up your Bs.** Nearly 80 percent of people with depression are deficient in vitamin B_6. Check with your doctor first, but to get B_6 plus the rest of the Bs (all of which your body needs to deliver oxygen to the brain, turn blood sugar into energy, and keep feel-good brain chemicals in circulation), take a B-complex supplement that supplies 20 to 100 milligrams of B_6, 500 micrograms of B_{12}, and 400 micrograms of folic acid. Take it with food.

- **Feel better with fish.** Cold-water fish, such as salmon and tuna, are packed with omega-3 essential fatty acids, which help the brain receive serotonin. But they also contain eicosa-pentaenoic acid (EPA), one of the components in fish oil that has been shown to help reduce feelings of worthlessness. Since you'd have to eat a boatload of fish to get the antidepres-sant effects of EPA, your best bet is to eat fish several times a week and take 1 gram (1,000 milligrams) of fish-oil supplements (available at health food stores) twice a day. Just be sure your supplements contain at least half EPA and half docosahexaenoic acid (DHA). Fish oil can thin your blood, so avoid it if you take aspirin or prescription blood thinners.

■ **Breathe hard.** A study at Duke University Medical Center revealed that people with major depression who exercised aerobically for 30 minutes three times a week experienced the same relief from depression as people who took antidepressants. There are several reasons for this effect. First, aerobic exercise forces oxygen into your cells, increasing energy production. Second, it signals the brain to release "feel-good" brain chemicals called endorphins,

MODERN MARVEL

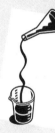

Swallow SAM-e

SAM-e (short for S-adenosylmethionine)—a compound that helps regulate the breakdown of feel-good hormones—may be an effective mood booster for people with mild to moderate depression. You get results from SAM-e within six weeks with no major side effects. Check with your doctor first, then look for quality brands such as Nature Made coated tablets (to reduce the risk of stomach upset) at health food stores. If you don't see results in a few days, gradually increase your dose, but never take more than 400 milligrams four times a day. Once your mood stabilizes, gradually reduce the dose to 400 milligrams twice a day.

which boost mood. Finally, it enhances sleep and curbs weight gain, both of which can increase energy.

Battling the Blues

Try some of these feel-better suggestions to help take the blues away:

- **Hit the switch.** If seasonal affective disorder (SAD) is a problem, try what's called a dawn simulator—essentially a bedside lamp whose glow increases gradually from dim to more intense light, mimicking a natural sunrise in mid-May. All you do is program the fake dawn to start 1 to 3 hours before you awaken, and your body detects the changing light through your closed eyelids. Look for 250-lux models on the Internet and in catalogs and stores that sell personal health care products.

- **Get a helping hand.** Preliminary studies indicate that massage may help reduce symptoms of depression, perhaps by combating a buildup of the stress hormone cortisol. To enhance the effect, use some mood-boosting herbal oils, such as bergamot, geranium, jasmine, neroli, or ylang-ylang, all available at health food stores.

- **March forward.** When you feel yourself beginning to slip into darkness, don't panic—and don't even think about it. Just act. As quickly as you can, slip on your sneakers and head outside for a brisk 10-minute walk, literally counting

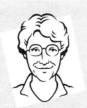

Grandma Says:

Plan a girls' night out. When you're feeling blue, spend time with friends. Studies indicate that when a woman spends time with another woman, her body releases a brain chemical called oxytocin that counters the kind of stress that can contribute to depression. So get together with a buddy and you'll feel better.

your steps in a 1–2, 1–2 military fashion. This simple, focused, almost meditative activity will not only crowd out negative thoughts, it will also encourage your brain to release endorphins to help lift your mood.

- **Get the point.** One university study found that three months of twice-weekly acupuncture treatments reduced depression in more than half of the women tested, although researchers aren't sure why. It's possible that insertion of the thread-thin needles stimulates the release of mood-lifting endorphins or corrects a chemical imbalance involved in depression. Ask your doctor to recommend a reputable practitioner in your area.

Healing Rays

If you exercise outdoors, you may enhance the natural antidepressant effect of your workout. Exposure to sunlight—even on dim, overcast days—helps boost levels of vitamin D, which then helps the body maintain higher levels of serotonin. In fact, even in a downpour, there is 30 times more light outside than in.

Act Happy, Feel Happy

Remember the famous restaurant scene in the movie *When Harry Met Sally*, when Meg Ryan noisily shows Billy Crystal how she can fake an orgasm? "I'll have what she's having," says a

Tea Time

Flowers do more than make our world a more beautiful place: Their fragrance, color, and chemical makeup can also lift our mood. Passionflower, lavender, vervain, borage, rosemary, and skullcap can be just the things for chasing the blues away. Try making a tea with one of these herbs, or use two or three in combination. Steep 1 teaspoon of either a single dried herb or mixed herbs in 1 cup of boiling water for 10 minutes, then strain. Drink two or three cups per day.

nearby patron. You can "fake yourself out" to lift your mood, too. Put on your favorite music, dress in your best clothes, stand up straight, and go about your day as if it were the best day of your life. If your depression is severe, however, be realistic—and get help. Putting a happy face on a serious problem is denial, and that's unhealthy.

Improve Your Mood with St. John's

A slew of studies since the 1970s have shown that St. John's wort can ease mild (but not severe) depression. Check with your doctor first, then look in your local health food store for a high-quality brand such as Kira or Nature Made and take 300 milligrams three times a day. You may not feel the effect of St. John's wort for up to two months, and in some people, it can cause stomach upset, allergic reactions, and heightened sensitivity to the sun. *Caution:* Never take herbal antidepressants with any antidepressants that your doctor prescribes.

Diarrhea

In the world of physics, as Isaac Newton discovered under the apple tree, what goes up will always come down. In the world of digestion, what goes in will eventually come out. All too often, however, it comes out way too quickly—in the form of watery diarrhea.

Don't blame the flu, at least not right away. Viral infections that settle in the intestine are a common cause of diarrhea, but so are dozens of other things, including bacteria, stress, or simple overindulgences, such as eating a giant bowl of cherries.

Stem the Tide

It's easy enough to "dry up" diarrhea with an over-the-counter drug that contains loperamide hydrochloride, such as Imodium, but doctors don't recommend this approach very often. For one thing, diarrhea is your body's way of giving harmful substances the boot. More important,

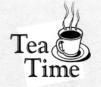

Tea Time

The tannins in blackberry root dry the mucous membranes in your intestine and bind up the bowel. Check in your local health food store for blackberry tea (the real McCoy, not simply tea flavored with blackberry) and follow the package directions. Drink several cups a day.

you can almost always control it with drug-free approaches. Here's a bunch of inexpensive alternatives:

- **Spoon up some yogurt.** It's brimming with healthful bacteria cultures that restore balance in the intestine and help tame the trots. If you're not a yogurt fan, take a probiotic supplement that contains lactobacillus GG (LGG). One study found that LGG could shorten the normal course of diarrhea from eight days to a more tolerable two. If you can't find LGG, any probiotic supplement that contains lactobacillus will help.

- **Spit out the gum.** Many chewing gums are made with the artificial sweetener Sorbitol, which can cause diarrhea. If you want to chew gum, read labels to find a Sorbitol-free brand.

- **Dump the dairy.** You'll need to give up milk and other dairy products until you're feeling better. When you have diarrhea, your intestines' ability to digest milk and other dairy products is impaired. Likewise, you'll want to avoid citrus and vegetable juices, alcohol, and caffeine, which also make things worse.

- **Bind with bananas.** Along with rice, apples, and toast, bananas and other bland foods will help you recover from diarrhea. Another option is eating chicken-rice soup to replenish the sodium and potassium you've lost.

- **Make nice with rice.** The next time you prepare a batch of rice, add an extra 1½ cups of water to the pot. When the rice is cooked to the texture you want, drain off the extra water, chill it if you like, and drink it for a hydrating, binding tonic. If you need a sweetener, use a small amount of sugar or honey.

- **Tame your sweet tooth.** For some people, sugar in any form—whether it's the fructose in fruit or the lactose in milk—is simply not well digested and can cause intestinal distress. So cut back on your sugar intake to see if it curbs your diarrhea.

- **Get on the sauce.** When nothing else seems to work, let carob and applesauce come to the rescue. Mix 1 teaspoon of carob powder in ¼ cup of applesauce and eat it slowly. You may need two or three doses throughout the day.

Tame the Runs

Cut down on those mad dashes to the bathroom with some natural remedies:

- **Relax your intestines.** Valerian, an herbal sedative long recommended as a sleep tonic, can settle intestinal spasms and is especially helpful if you're doubled over with crampy diarrhea. Take 100 to 300 milligrams a day for as long as you have symptoms. Since valerian is a sleep aid, it can cause drowsiness, so it's best to take it before bedtime, and don't take it if you're using any other kind of medication, particularly anti-depressants or anti-anxiety drugs.

dial the DOCTOR

The Three-Day Rule

Diarrhea usually takes care of itself, but sometimes it signals serious problems, such as food poisoning, a digestive disorder, or even thyroid disease. Call your doctor if it lasts more than 72 hours—or immediately if you have bloody diarrhea, pain, or a fever.

Bland though it may be, barley has long been known to slow intestinal motion and curb diarrhea. Grandma Putt gave it some pizzazz by adding 1 cup of beef broth to prepared pearl barley. This mixture will replace your lost fluids and electrolytes in addition to calming your innards.

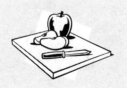

- **Soothe with slippery elm.** This herb soothes the mucous membranes of the bowel with few or no side effects. Stir ¼ teaspoon of slippery elm powder into a cup of applesauce, and eat it three or four times a day. Or add 30 to 40 drops of tincture to a glass of water, and drink it every 2 hours until your diarrhea stops. Both forms of the herb are available at health food stores.

- **Go for garlic.** Garlic is one of the best ways to fight infection internally—whether your diarrhea is caused by a flu virus or bacteria that you picked up from food. Since cooking garlic neutralizes its healing properties, pick up some garlic capsules at a health food store or drugstore, and take 200 to 400 milligrams three times a day until your diarrhea subsides.

Take Away The Burn

If you have burning diarrhea, marshmallow tea can minimize the irritation by attracting moisture to your intestinal walls. Look for the tea or powder at a health food store. Make the tea according to the package directions, and drink a cup several times a day. To use the powder, add a teaspoon to a flavored gelatin product and snack on it throughout the day.

Rest Easy with GSE

Made from the pulp or seeds of grapefruit, grapefruit seed extract (GSE), which you can find in health food stores, can knock out any bacterium, parasite, or virus that may be behind your diarrhea. Add two drops to a glass of water, and take it twice a day until you've killed whatever you picked up. Never take GSE straight, or it may wipe out the beneficial bacteria along with the troublemakers, and don't use it if you're taking cholesterol-lowering medication.

Pamper with Peppermint

Peppermint is a natural menthol and antispasmodic. Try a cup of calming peppermint tea to relax the muscles of your digestive tract and relieve the spasms that trigger diarrhea. Just stir 1 teaspoon of leaves (fresh or dried) into 1 cup of boiling water and simmer for 10 minutes. Strain out the leaves and enjoy. Drink as many as three cups a day after meals until your symptoms clear up.

Dry Eyes

When your eyes are so dry that simply blinking feels like the rasp of sandpaper, and you can watch *Old Yeller* without shedding a tear, you can be pretty sure that you're heading for trouble. Your eyes should naturally be a little misty. Tears are constantly flowing across their surface, washing away grit and keeping the tender tissues lubricated. But as we age, tear production decreases (even if you cry more than ever at weepy movies). The result: Hot, dry, sore eyes that feel as parched as the Sahara.

Contact lenses are a common cause of dry eyes. Some medications, especially decongestants, antihistamines, blood pressure medications, and tranquilizers, can cause it. So can living in a dry, dusty climate.

Soothe and Lubricate

Since dry eyes can be a sign of serious illnesses, including lupus and rheumatoid arthritis, check with your doctor just to be safe. In most cases, though, you can get fast relief at home without hauling out your credit card. Here's some eye-opening advice:

- **Warm them up.** Heat opens clogged oil glands in the eyelids, so placing a warm compress over your eyes may help increase moisture flow. Just run some hot—but not too hot—water over a small towel, wring it out, and lay it over your closed eyes.

- **Splash and rinse.** When you are in a dry, dusty climate, rinse your face and eyes often with cool, clean water. This will ease irritation, and add some moisture to offset the arid atmosphere.

- **Brighten up.** Eyebright is a favorite for almost any eye ailment, and a warm compress of eyebright and fennel seeds can be very refreshing. Make a tea by adding 1 teaspoon of eyebright and 1 teaspoon of fennel seeds to 1 cup of hot water. Add a clean cloth, and steep for 10 minutes. Wring out the cloth, and apply it to your eyes for 20 minutes once or twice daily.

- **Don some shades.** If you have a fan blowing near you, wear regular glasses or sunglasses, even indoors. Breezes can evaporate moisture on the surface of your eyes. Any glasses will help, but wraparound shades will offer the best defense.

- **Wear eye protection.** Ever notice how red people's eyes look when they've been in the

MODERN MARVEL

Bottled Tears

Using "artificial tears" eyedrops regularly will restore the film of moisture over your eyes, but ask your doctor which products are best and how often you should use them. Some eyedrops can blur vision, so choose those made with saline (salt) or synthetic cellulose. Some contain vasoconstrictors that help relieve bloodshot eyes, but these products can dry your eyes further, and even increase redness and soreness when used for more than three days.

pool too long? That's because chlorine can irritate the eyes and dry them out. So wear goggles when you swim, especially in chlorinated pools.

- **Humidify the air.** Use a humidifier if you live in a dry climate or work in a place that's very dry. Adding moisture to the air will help combat the effects of the dryness. Just be sure to keep the humidifier clean so you don't add other eye irritants, such as mold spores, to the air.

- **Think like a fish.** Drink lots of water to keep your body well hydrated, especially if you live in a dry place where your body moisture evaporates quickly. This will help keep your own natural tear supply flowing freely.

Dry Skin

Your skin is the one part of your body that's constantly exposed to air. Unless you spend your entire life in a sauna, the air is continually sucking moisture from your skin's surface. And if you happen to live in a dry climate or are exposed to drying indoor heat in winter, your skin probably feels as dry and crackly as an old paper bag.

Doctors have a fancy name for dry skin. They call it xerosis, which simply means that so much water has evaporated from the top layer of the skin (the stratum corneum) that it feels like a shriveled autumn leaf. As we get older, the uppermost layer of our skin naturally loses some of its ability to hold water. In fact, by age 65, more than half of us have xerosis.

While natural aging isn't within our control, many other factors that contribute to dry skin are, such as: dry indoor heat; prolonged sun exposure; long, leisurely baths; frequent air

From Grandma's Kitchen

Oats aren't only for eating. Do what my Grandma Putt often did and treat yourself to a whole-body oat mask. Make a big pot of oatmeal, let it cool a bit, and slather it on your lightly oiled skin from head to toe. When it's dry, soak it off in a warm tub.

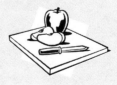

travel (the air on planes is always very dry); and the overuse of citrus-, alcohol-, or menthol-based skin care products.

From Dry to Dewy

You can almost always treat dry skin without spending a fortune on fancy skin care products. The equation is simple: Add things that seal in moisture and take away things that encourage evaporation. Here are the top picks:

- **Select the right soap.** Look in your local health food store for oil-based bars that contain super-moisturizing olive oil or coconut oil, are not labeled as soap (which is drying), and are scented with palmarosa, rosewood, and/or sandalwood. All of these can help stimulate oil production.

- **Change the oil.** After bathing, pat your skin to remove most of the water. Then, while your skin's still damp, slather on almond or sun-flower oil (the same oil you use for cooking). Both are brimming with vitamin F, which pro-vides plenty of unsaturated fatty acids that may help regulate the oil glands. If you'd rather not smell like a Caesar salad, simply add a few drops of lavender oil.

- **Take your time.** We are often so rushed that we barely have time to apply moisturizer after a shower when our bodies are damp. So do your skin a favor and give yourself a few more minutes for a mini-massage, and rub a moisturizer all over your body. Take your time. The massage will stimulate blood flow to your skin, which makes the moisturizer more effective.

■ **Bathe in an oil slick.** Add a fragrant bath oil to your bathwater, soak, pat yourself dry, and moisturize (but be careful not to slip in the tub). Experiment with bath oils to find the ones that feel best to you. In places where your skin is extremely dry, such as your feet, rub on some additional moisturizer, then wear socks to bed so you won't get your sheets greasy.

Honey, Pass the Milk

A milk-and-honey massage is one way to start your day off on the right foot. Mix equal parts of honey and milk and, starting at your feet, massage the lotion into your thirsty skin. This is best done in the shower, where you can simply rinse off when you're done.

Get on the A-List

Vital for proper skin growth and repair, vitamin A is one of a family of natural and synthetic derivatives known as retinoids, which are the primary ingredients in many prescription anti-aging drugs such as tretinoin (Retin-A). You can get pretty much the same protection (at a fraction of the cost) simply by filling your plate with foods rich in beta-carotene (which converts to vitamin A in the body), such as cantaloupe, carrots, and apricots.

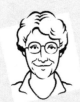

Grandma Says:

Eat your fish. Grandma urged us to eat lots of cold-water fish, such as tuna and salmon, to keep our skin moist. Nowadays, you can also take 2 tablespoons of flaxseed oil (available at health food stores) daily. Both provide omega-3 essential fatty acids, which help your skin retain water to keep it plump, supple, and smooth.

Run for the Roses

EPO, or evening primrose oil, contains the essential fatty acids linoleic acid and gamma-linolenic acid, both of which may alleviate skin dryness and reduce the potential for future water loss. Check your health food store for EPO, and take 1,000 milligrams (about a tablespoon) of the oil three times a day, or get gel-caps and follow the directions on the label.

Rosehip oil also has a high linoleic acid content, which studies show can both tone and moisturize skin. Look for rosehip oil at a health food store, douse a cotton ball, and dab the oil all over your face, neck, and upper chest.

Soothe and Smooth

Water is an important part of the equation for conquering dry skin. Here's the lowdown:

- **Fill your internal rain barrel.** You need lots of water to keep your entire body working well, including your skin. It's really quite simple: The more water you drink, the more water is available to pump up and out to your epidermis. So don't be stingy with the water—drink a minimum of 8 to 10 glasses a day.

- **Enjoy an herbal steam.** An herbal facial steam can deep-six dryness—especially if you use a type of oil that encourages oil production in your skin. Simply bring 3 cups of water to a boil, then remove the pot from the stove. Add 1 drop each of rose, geranium, rosemary, fennel, and peppermint herbal oils to the water. Drape a towel over your head and tuck the ends around the pot so the steam is captured inside a "mini-sauna." Be careful not to get close enough for the steam to burn your face, and limit your steam sessions to about 5 minutes once a week.

- **Smooth your skin with E.** As an ingredient in lotions or as an oil, topical vitamin E—particularly the form known as alpha tocopherol—reduces skin roughness, the length of facial lines, and wrinkle depth. When it's combined with topical vitamin C in the form of ascorbic acid (which seems to help promote the growth of collagen, the skin's underlying support), the effects may be enhanced. Check your health food store for skin care products that include both of these skin-friendly vitamins.

- **Pass up the petroleum.** For years, dermatologists have lauded petroleum jelly as the thickest emollient and therefore the best treatment for very dry skin. Now there's evidence that moisturizers with large amounts of glycerin (which has a less greasy feel) may work just as well, if not better. Glycerin appears to increase space between cells in the stratum corneum, creating a reservoir of moisture-holding ability that makes the skin more resistant to drying. Look for glycerin in commercial moisturizers or simply make your own—buy pure glycerin from a health food store and combine 1 part glycerin with 2 parts rosewater.

Brush Up Oil Production

Starting at the soles of your feet and moving up your legs toward your heart, gently rub your body in a circular motion with a super-soft, dry-bristle brush. Then do the same with your hands and arms. Brushing will help stimulate your sebaceous glands to produce more sebum, and will also remove dead skin that makes your skin look dry, dull, and old.

When Paste Ain't Safe

If your lips always seem to be dry, check out the ingredients in your toothpaste. If it contains cinnamate—a flavoring agent that can be drying—you've nailed the culprit. Simply switch to a brand that's cinnamate-free. Also avoid tartar-control toothpastes, which, like long-lasting lipsticks and mouthwashes that contain alcohol, can be drying.

Slather on Shea

Made from the shea nut of the karite tree, shea butter is loaded with vitamins A and E and may even protect your skin from oxidative damage. Perhaps its best quality, though, is that it's a thick emollient that sinks into the skin and feels smooth, not greasy like petroleum jelly. Check at health food stores for shea butter sold alone or combined with other skin care ingredients.

Soften with Sesame

Indian women have long used sesame oil, which is rich in both vitamin E and linoleic acid, to moisten and soften dry, cracked hands and feet. Pour ½ cup of sesame seeds and ¼ cup of warm water into a blender, and process for 3 minutes. Strain the lotion, apply it to your skin, and leave it on for as long as possible. Rinse first with warm water, then with cool water, and blot dry. You can also buy sesame oil at a health food store—but making it yourself will save you big bucks.

Earaches

From Grandma's Kitchen

Here's an old-time remedy that soothes an earache with warm, moist heat. Grandma Putt used to boil an onion (but you can heat it in the microwave), let it cool slightly, then put it in a clean cotton sock for me to hold against my aching ear.

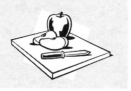

Adults sometimes get ear infections, but they're a lot more common in kids. And if you really want to get, well, an earful of complaints, talk to almost any parent. You'll hear a long litany about missed school days, last-minute visits to the doctor, and the difficulty of giving eardrops to pain-racked children.

Most ear infections occur when cold germs settle in the eustachian tubes, the narrow passageways between the throat and eardrums. In kids, the tubes are nearly horizontal, which means that it's hard for mucus to drain out. As mucus accumulates, internal pressure rises, which is why ear infections are so painful. The good news is that ear infections gradually taper off as children get older because their heads and necks get longer, causing the eustachian tubes to assume a more vertical position. The more easily the mucus drains out, the less likely it is that infections will occur.

Improve the Flow

In the majority of cases, ear pain is caused by simple infections—often triggered by a cold, allergies, a sinus infection, or simply moisture. You'll almost certainly need to see a doctor, but you won't have to sell the family car to afford a bunch of visits to a specialist. There's a lot you can do at home to reduce irritation and even eliminate the germs. Here's how to get started:

- **Heat away the pain.** Gentle heat is probably the most soothing home treatment for aching ears. For adults, the easiest approach is to use a heating pad. Set it on low, cover it with a towel or pillowcase, and lie down for a while with your ear against the pad. As long as the pad doesn't get too hot, it's fine to lie there for 20 to 30 minutes, or until the pain subsides. Set a timer so you don't fall asleep. If you don't have a heating pad, or if it's your child who's hurting, you can gently heat the ear with a hair dryer set on low. Hold the dryer at least 6 inches away from your ear, which should feel comfortably warm but not hot. If your ear starts getting too warm, it's time to stop the treatment. To check the temperature for a child, put one hand over her ear when you turn on the dryer. Gradually move the dryer away until the airflow on your hand feels warm but not hot.

- **Count on analgesics.** Aspirin, ibuprofen, and acetaminophen aren't just for headaches. They quickly ease ear pain and help control the fever that often accompanies infections. These medi-

**dial the
DOCTOR**

Protection from Infection

Ear infections are hardly ever serious, but if the infection isn't eliminated quickly, there could be scarring or other damage that can result in hearing loss. As long as the pain is mild, it's okay to wait a day or two before seeing a doctor. But if the pain is severe or comes on very suddenly, go to an emergency room right away.

A natural way to reduce pain-causing congestion is to massage the outer part of your ear. It helps the eustachian tubes drain normally, which reduces pressure on the eardrum. Simply put your index finger behind your ear and your middle finger right in front of the little triangular flap (the tragus) that covers the opening of your ear canal. Stroke with both fingers down toward the outer corner of your jaw, squeezing your fingers together as you pull.

cations are very safe as long as you follow the directions on the label. There is one exception, however: Don't give aspirin or ibuprofen to children, because these drugs can increase the risk of Reye's syndrome, a serious neurological illness. Acetaminophen, however, is safe for children of all ages.

- **Add potato punch.** The next time you have an earache, reach for a simple spud. Cut the potato in half, microwave it until it's soft, and let it cool to a comfortable temperature. Then hold the cut end against your ear for 10 to 15 minutes. The heat is very soothing.

Fight Back with Vinegar

Anytime you're going to swim in a body of unchlorinated water, such as a lake, a river, or the ocean, take along a mixture of half vinegar and half rubbing alcohol (a drying agent). Dry your ears well, then dribble 2 drops of the solution into each ear after your dip.

Beat It with an Oil Blend

Rubbing oil behind your ear (where your lymph glands are located) or placing a cotton ball saturated with oil inside your ear may soothe the ache and help stimulate the lymph glands to remove infectious agents. Many people find that something called sweet oil—which is really olive oil with other oils such as lavender, tea tree, chamomile, and hops mixed in—works really well. Check your health food store for sweet oil, or simply make your own by combining the oils in equal amounts.

Ease Ear Woes

We all know that you can get swimmer's ear if you spend a lot of time in the water, but what many people don't realize is that sometimes water isn't just a culprit—it can be part of the cure for ear pain, too:

- **Snort some saltwater.** Dissolve as much table salt as you can in a glass of warm water without the water becoming cloudy (it should taste like tears), then pour a little of the saltwater into the cup of your hand and sniff the mixture into one nostril, then the other. Repeat several times. This nasal wash acts as a natural decongestant to shrink swollen tissues, and unplug the eustachian tubes.

- **Do some steam cleaning.** Eucalyptus is an herbal decongestant that may help ease the pressure in your eustachian tubes and nudge drainage of fluid that has been dammed up in the middle ear—especially if you combine it with steam, which also encourages the flow of mucus. Fill a bowl with boiling water, add several—as many as 10—drops of eucalyptus oil (available in health food stores), and drape a towel over your head and the bowl to capture the steam. Lean over the bowl, being careful not to scald your skin, and inhale the mist for at least 5 minutes. You can also place a few drops of eucalyptus oil in your bathwater, but don't put it directly into your ears.

Try The Garlic Cure

Take advantage of garlic's natural antibiotic properties. Simply mash a garlic clove with a fork, and saturate it with several drops of olive oil. Let the mash sit overnight, strain out the garlic, and warm the oil so it's pleasantly tepid, but not hot. Tilt your head so your sore ear faces up, and plop two or three drops of the warm oil into your ear. Lie down—again, with your sore ear up—and let the oil settle for 2 or 3 minutes before you raise your head. Do this a few times a day, and your discomfort should disappear within a day or two.

Prevent Pain with Boric Acid

If you're prone to ear infections, ask your pharmacist to mix up a solution of 3 percent boric acid, 70 percent alcohol. Squeeze a few drops into your ears every day to keep yourself infection-free. The boric acid will acidify the ear canal, discouraging any bacterial or fungal invaders from venturing down that path, while the alcohol will dry it up.

Flu

The only way to confuse a cold with the flu is to be one of the lucky ones who have never had the flu. A cold isn't exactly pleasant, but the flu is in a whole different category—the virus really hits with a vengeance. Your symptoms may start with a mild cough, a headache, or a few sniffles, but that's just the beginning. Before long, you'll know that this is no ordinary cold. The flu can knock you right off your feet with a fever, chills, aches, and a racking cough, along with a sore throat and congestion.

The flu usually hits from late fall into winter, although it can occur at any time of year. The virus is easily passed from one person to another, and it tends to last for a week or more.

Fight the Viral Villain

If you act quickly, you can almost stop the flu in its tracks by getting antiviral medications from your doctor. The problem is, most people don't

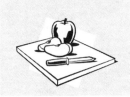

even know they have the flu until a few days have passed, and by then the drugs won't work. For most people, the best remedies are also the oldest—get lots of rest and try to stay comfortable while your body takes care of the viral invader. Here are some other super suggestions for reducing your discomfort and healing more quickly:

- **Welcome a fever.** Nobody enjoys having a fever, but that high temperature is doing you a favor. An increase in temperature is one of the most potent defenses your body has against viruses. In other words, lowering fever with aspirin or other drugs may actually prolong your illness. Unless you're just too uncomfortable or the fever's very high (above 102°F), it's best to leave it alone.

- **Sip some slippery elm.** This herb forms a slick coating that can soothe a sore throat faster than you can shout "Relief!" You can buy the powdered form at a health food store and make a slightly sticky tea by adding 1 teaspoon of the powder to a cup of hot water. Or take slippery elm lozenges, also sold at health food stores. Sucking on a lozenge will keep your throat coated and comfortable for hours.

- **Enjoy a salty soak.** The flu is almost always accompanied by muscle aches and pains. A quick way to get relief is to soak in a bath spiked with Epsom salts. They contain magnesium, which is good for relieving muscle tension. Pour about a cup of the salts into the bathtub while the water's running.

- **Cool and soothe.** It won't affect the underlying fever, but applying a cold compress to your skin will make you feel a lot more comfortable. Soak a washcloth in cool water, wring it out, and put it on your forehead or neck. When it warms up, soak it again and repeat the process.

Feel Better With Menthol

Slathering a menthol rub over your chest is a traditional remedy for flu, and it seems to help with aches and pains as well as congestion. The active ingredient is eucalyptus, and it works very well. You can make your own herbal rub by adding 6 to 12 drops of oil of menthol, eucalyptus, or camphor (available at health food stores) to an ounce of olive or almond oil.

Foil the Flu

When the flu strikes, the last thing you'll be thinking of is what to eat or drink. But you must—keeping hydrated and eating right will go a long way toward making you feel better faster. So prepare yourself now by noting these four flu dietary rules:

- **Suck down the fluids.** Lots of liquids are in order when you're battling the flu. When you're not adequately hydrated, your symptoms feel worse, and your immune system won't function

dial the
DOCTOR

When You Need to Worry

Anyone with heart disease, immune system problems, lung disease, or other serious health conditions should call a doctor at the first sign of flu symptoms. Even if you're in great shape, talk to your doctor if you don't start feeling better within a week. It's not uncommon for viral flu to lead to a secondary bacterial infection. You may need antibiotics in order to recover.

If flu has your
nose stuffed to
the rafters, har-
ness the power
of the humble
onion. The same
vapors that make
cooks weep can
help clear up your
congestion, so
start peeling and
let them work
their magic. Once
you're breathing
easier, chop the
onion and toss
some pieces into a
salad: Onions con-
tain compounds
that strengthen
your immune
system and thin
mucus.

as well as it should. Water is the best choice; try to drink at least eight glasses a day.

- **Eat light.** Big, heavy meals aren't a good idea when you're sick, because your body will put more energy into digestion than into stomping the virus. Nor do you want to go hungry, because your body needs nutrients in order to recover. A good compromise is to plan your menu around soups, vegetable juices, and other easy-to-digest foods.

- **Hold the milk.** Milk, cheese, and other dairy products tend to make mucus thicker, which increases congestion and other symptoms.

- **Tank up on nutrients.** Some of the vitamins and minerals you should be getting every day—including vitamins A, C, and E and the minerals zinc and selenium—are especially important when you're contending with the flu, because they strengthen your immune system. You can't count on the amounts of vitamins in foods when you're sick, so be sure to have on hand a multivitamin/mineral supplement that provides 100 percent of the recommended daily amount of each of these important nutrients.

Get Steamed

Inhaling steam is a great way to open up your congested airways and soothe irritated tissues. Just heat a pot of water on the stove, carefully move it to a table or counter, then lean over and breathe in the steam. Drape a towel around your head and shoulders to trap as much steam as possible.

To get even more relief, add a few drops of eucalyptus oil, available at health food stores, to the water.

Heal with Echinacea

This flu-fighting herb contains polysaccharides, which boost your body's infection-fighting cells. Echinacea is most effective when taken as a tincture (available at health food stores) because it contains more of the active constituents. Take 30 drops of tincture every 2 hours for a week, then switch to 20 drops three times a day, for a total of 10 days. *Caution:* Don't use echinacea if you have an autoimmune disease such as lupus, rheumatoid arthritis, or multiple sclerosis, or if you are pregnant or nursing.

MODERN MARVEL

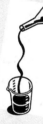

Get the Vaccine

If you're at high risk for getting the flu—you're elderly, work in a health care setting, or have chronic health problems—you should get the flu vaccine annually. The vaccine isn't 100 percent effective at preventing the flu, but if you get the shot and practice good preventive measures—such as washing your hands frequently and supporting your immune system with a good diet—you'll dramatically improve your odds of getting through flu season unscathed.

Gallstones

It's hard to imagine that something smaller than a grain of sand could trigger pain that rivals that of childbirth, but that's what a lot of people say about gallstones. The tiny granules cause such intense pain that they've been known to make even tough men cry.

On the Move

Bile, a digestive fluid that your body uses to digest fats, is stored in a small pouch called the gallbladder. Bile usually stays in liquid form, but sometimes one of the substances it contains, such as cholesterol, forms a hard little crystal, or gallstone, that floats around in your gallbladder. Most gallstones don't cause symptoms; you can have them all your life without ever knowing it. Sometimes, however, a stone lodges in one of the ducts leading out of the gallbladder. When that happens, *ouch!*

The crazy thing about gallbladder attacks is that they're totally unpredictable. You may be in agonizing pain for a few minutes or a few hours. You may have three attacks a day for three weeks, then never have another. There's just no way to tell.

No More Stones

There's both good news and bad news about gallstones. The good news is that as long as you're not having symptoms, you don't have to worry. The bad news is that the main—and by far the best—treatment for symptomatic stones is to have your gallbladder removed. It's a fairly simple "band-aid" procedure, and most people are back on their feet in a day or two. But who wants surgery if it can possibly be avoided?

If you've had gallstones in the past, your doctor may give you a medication that helps dissolve any new ones in the gallbladder. Another approach involves using painless sound waves to break up the stones. Yet another option is to make some simple lifestyle changes that can help prevent stones from recurring, like these:

- **Trim the fat.** The more fat in your diet, the more bile your liver will generate to digest it— and the greater your risk for gallstones. Studies have shown that people who get no more than 30 percent of calories from fat are less likely to get gallstones than those who eat more fat. Look for foods that have less than 5 grams of fat per serving.

- **Divide your meals.** Most of us were raised on three square meals a day. If you divide the same

From Grandma's Kitchen

Because the liver and gallbladder are intimately involved with digestion, it makes sense that food therapies can give them a little boost. A traditional way to help the gallbladder work more efficiently is to drink vegetable-juice cocktails that include celery, parsley, beets, carrots, radishes, and lemon. (Grandma Putt would mix and match ingredients to suit her taste.) Drink two cups a day.

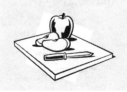

A gallbladder attack can be mistaken for a heart attack. Gallstone pain begins in the lower right abdomen and shoots upward to the shoulder and around the back to the right shoulder blade. If you have any abdominal pain that won't go away, fever, sweating, chills, yellowish skin, yellowing of the whites of your eyes, or clay-colored stools, see your doctor immediately.

amount of food into smaller, more frequent meals, though, you'll be less vulnerable to gallstones because the gallbladder won't secrete as much bile at once. You should eat something every 3 to 4 hours. For instance, instead of eating a sandwich, a bowl of soup, and a piece of fruit for lunch, you might have a cup of soup and half a sandwich, then eat the rest later on.

■ **Diet smart.** We've all seen those ads for diet plans that promise to change us from Titanic to Twiggy in a few weeks. But crash diets are bad news for the gallstone prone. In fact, rapid weight loss increases the risk of gallstones. So if you're planning a weight-loss program, it's a good idea to contact a health care provider for advice on how to lose weight gradually.

Tame It with Turmeric

The spice turmeric, commonly used in Indian cooking, is a traditional gallstone remedy. If you don't care for the taste of turmeric but still want the benefits, you can take 50 to 100 milligrams in capsule form three times a day, with meals.

Sensible Stone Busters

These simple steps can make quick work of gallstones and get you feeling like yourself again:

■ **Count on castor oil.** A fast way to help ease the pain of gallstone attacks is to relax with a castor oil pack. First, rub castor oil over the painful part of your abdomen. Cover it with a layer of plastic wrap, then put a heating pad set on low on top of the wrap. Relax for an hour or two, then remove the pack and wash off the oil. The soothing warmth will make the pain easier to live with until you can see your doctor.

■ **Eat naturally.** Studies suggest that processed foods, especially refined sugars, may be associated with an increased risk of gallstones. So replace processed foods in your diet with fresh fruits, vegetables, whole grains, and other natural foods.

■ **Get moving.** Since research shows that the more active you are, the less likely you'll be to develop gallstones, it pays to increase the time you spend exercising to 2 to 3 hours a week. Need more motivation? Think about 20/20 (not the TV show). Walk briskly for 20 minutes a day, five to seven days a week, and you'll reduce your chances of developing gallstones by 20 percent, according to studies.

■ **Manage your meds.** If you're taking cholesterol-lowering drugs, you may be on the gallstone A-list. These drugs cause the gallbladder to excrete excess cholesterol, which can raise the risk of stones. Don't stop taking the medicine, of course, but talk to your doctor about lowering your cholesterol without medications.

Don't Ignore the Pain

Even if you've had gallstone attacks in the past, don't assume that everything's going to be fine when you have your next one. Extreme pain may be a sign that your gallbladder is infected, which can be life-threatening without immediate medical treatment.

Gas

dial the DOCTOR

Gas Shouldn't Last

If you've suddenly noticed increased gas, or it seems more painful than it should be, talk to your doctor as soon as possible. While flatulence itself isn't a disease, it may be a symptom of more serious digestive problems.

Now, don't blame the dog. Intestinal gas may be embarrassing, and it's certainly unpleasant when the windows are closed, but it's a natural part of digestion—for people as well as our four-legged friends. Pointing the finger at Rover might get you off the hook, but what will you say—or do—the next time?

Flatus, as gas is known among doctors, is a result of swallowed air and the fermentation process triggered by intestinal bacteria. Food that enters your digestive tract provides nourishment for enormous colonies of them, and they, in turn, emit clouds of smelly chemicals. Basically, their gas becomes your gas. Excess gas isn't only a social problem, it's also uncomfortable because it puts pressure on your intestine.

Fight the Flatulence

Of course, there are times when we all generate more gas than we would like. While you can't get rid of it altogether, there are a number of strategies for keeping it at manageable levels. Here are a few tips you may want to try:

- **Enjoy leisurely meals.** Believe it or not, most people release about 2 pints of gas a day. And half of that is swallowed air. There would be a lot less swallowed air—and expelled gas—in the world if everyone would eat the way their mothers told them: Take small bites, don't talk while you're eating, and eat slowly. Why? Because hurried eating increases the amount of air you swallow.

- **Dump the antacids.** Low stomach acid can cause gas problems because it may interfere with normal digestion.

- **Be bitter.** Bitter herbs have been used for thousands of years to improve the digestive process, but you don't have to eat pounds of arugula

MODERN MARVEL

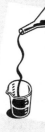

Rely on Beano

This over-the-counter product is made from a plant enzyme that breaks down the sugars in food. Put a few drops of liquid Beano on your first bite of food, or take a Beano tablet before eating. You'll enjoy your meal without that bloated feeling. There are also activated charcoal products that will absorb gas, but because they could also absorb any medications you take, you should check with your doctor before using this alternative.

Tea Time

For centuries, people of many cultures have used natural gas-fighting, (carminative) herbs to tame the effects of poor digestion. You can take advantage of these herbal gas busters by whipping up an after-meal tummy-taming tea. Just mix equal amounts of caraway seeds, fennel seeds, and aniseed. Crush 1 teaspoon of the mixture and add it to a cup of freshly boiled water. Steep for about 20 minutes, strain out the seeds, and sip.

or dandelion to get the benefits. Instead, sip a little Angostura bitters. This classic after-dinner drink is available in most supermarkets.

- **Cultivate culture.** The live cultures (called acidophilus) in some yogurts break down milk sugars and keep a balance of healthy bacteria in the digestive channels. Read labels to be sure the yogurt you buy contains acidophilus, and eat it often for better digestive health.

- **Stroll after meals.** Regular exercise promotes bowel function and helps your body digest food. Flopping your butt down on the couch after dinner encourages food to ferment, creating gas, so get moving!

Pass on the Gas

It's a safe bet to say that a lot of the gas your body is producing comes from what you're putting in your mouth. So chew on these tips:

- **De-gas strong foods.** Add anise, fennel, or ginger to "gassy" vegetables such as brussels sprouts, broccoli, and cabbage. Along with enhancing flavor, the herbs offset the gas-producing effects of these healthy foods.

- **Bubbles are trouble.** We all have gas to spare, so the last thing you want to do is pump more gas into your system by drinking carbonated beverages. It's fine to enjoy a soft drink or soda water now and then, but the more you drink, the gassier you're going to be.

■ **Take the gas out of beans.** On the scale of gas-producing foods, beans, along with broccoli, cauliflower, and other high-fiber foods, are almost off the chart. What you may not know is that these foods cause trouble mainly for people who don't eat them very often. Adding beans and their high-fiber cousins to your menu more frequently will often cut down on the excess emissions. And that's good news for everyone!

Rub Away Cramps

Relieve gas pains with a simple rubbing solution containing antispasmodic herbs. Add 4 to 6 drops each of lobelia and catnip tincture to 2 tablespoons of olive oil, then gently massage it into your abdomen in a clockwise pattern.

Lemon-and-Spice Relief

Lemon and cinnamon both have gas-relieving properties. Choose your favorite:

■ **Digest with lemon.** Lemon water slips your stomach into gear, and helps your digestive system work more efficiently. When you're having trouble with gas, squeeze the juice from a slice of lemon into a glass of water, and drink it before and after meals.

■ **Sweeten with cinnamon.** To make a sweetly spiced, gas-busting after-dinner drink, steep a stick of cinnamon in boiling water for about 10 minutes, then let the tea cool slightly. Discard the cinnamon and sip the tea.

Intestine Protection

Basil makes a sweet drink that can reduce painful and embarrassing gas. Make a tea by steeping 2 tablespoons of chopped fresh basil (or 2 teaspoons of dried basil) in 1 cup of freshly boiled water for about 15 minutes. Strain and sip.

Gingivitis

It's not just a figure of speech when dentists say that gum disease can sneak up you. They mean it literally because the stuff that causes gingivitis—gum inflammation—is invisible. It can lurk on your teeth for days, months, or even years, releasing acids that slip beneath the gums. If the process isn't stopped, your gums may shrink and pull away from your teeth. Eventually, your teeth loosen and fall out.

The clingy film that causes all this trouble, called plaque, is constantly produced by bacteria that live in the mouth. Redness, bleeding, and soreness are the first signs that plaque is out of control. So, by the time you notice something's wrong, you already have gum disease.

Put Your Gums in the Pink

Here's the good news. Gingivitis is entirely reversible—and you probably won't have to write a fat check to your dentist. All you have to do

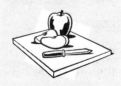

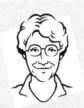

Grandma Says:

Make your own paste. If you want to clear up a persistent case of gingivitis, try Grandma Putt's homemade gum paste. Shake 1 teaspoon of baking soda into a small dish, and drizzle in enough hydrogen peroxide to make a paste. Work it gently under your gum line with your toothbrush. Leave it on for a few minutes, then rinse well.

is be more diligent about flossing and brushing. Severe gum disease always requires a dentist's care, but there is no reason at all to let things go that far. If you follow these tips, you'll keep your gums in the pink—and totally free of pain:

- **Swish with salt.** Plain salt is a wonderful gum healer. Add ¼ teaspoon to ¼ cup of warm water. Stir until the salt dissolves, then use as a mouthwash two or three times daily.

- **Brush 'round and 'round.** Don't make the mistake of using too much elbow grease when you brush. You're not trying to sandblast the sides of a building, just break up the thin layers of plaque that may have formed. To be sure you get it all, move the brush in little circles rather than up and down. If you've only recently started having problems, a week or two of gentle brushing should erase the pain.

- **Bag the old brush.** Don't forget to change your toothbrush a few times a year. Old brushes are often full of bacteria, which means you could actually be causing more problems. You can also clean your brush periodically—soak it in hydrogen peroxide overnight to kill bacteria.

- **Go electric.** You're supposed to brush your teeth for 2 minutes or more, but it's easy to cut the time short when you're in a hurry. Some electric toothbrushes are a great help with this because they have a built-in signal mechanism that reminds you to work on all four areas of your mouth for 30 seconds each.

- **Water your mouth.** Water stimulates the production of saliva that you need to fight excess mouth bacteria. Drink 8 to 10 glasses a day.

That's a Mouthful!

Fight gingivitis with these tried-and-true routines:

- **Fix it with folic acid.** This B vitamin helps repair and replenish gum cells that have been damaged by gingivitis. Take a daily multivitamin to get enough folic acid (the recommended amount is 400 micrograms a day).

- **Paint on some goldenseal.** This herb helps protect against infection while strengthening the tissues of your gums and mouth. Use a small, unused paintbrush to apply goldenseal tincture (available at health food stores) to your gums once or twice daily. Goldenseal can be irritating, so test it first by dabbing just one spot on your gums with the brush. If no irritation shows up by the next day, paint away.

- **Follow this sage advice.** Myrrh, sage, and calendula tone tissues and protect them against infection. Two or three times a day, add 5 drops of each tincture to a small amount of warm water, swish it around in your mouth for several minutes, then spit it out.

- **Rinse with chamomile.** A swish of chamomile tea will bring soothing relief to sore gums. Steep a tea bag in hot water for 10 to 20 minutes, then let the tea cool. Take a mouth-

dial the DOCTOR

Save Your Choppers

Periodontal disease, or periodontitis, occurs when a buildup of plaque causes irritation and inflammation. Unless it's stopped, periodontitis weakens your gums and supporting bones so much that you may lose your teeth. If your gums have pulled away from your teeth, or you have discharge between your teeth and gums, see a dentist immediately.

ful, swirl it around for about 30 seconds, then swallow it or spit it out. Continue the process until you've used all the tea. *Caution:* Don't use chamomile if you are allergic to ragweed.

- **Bark up the right tree.** Two herbal tinctures, prickly ash bark and Jamaican dogwood, are traditional favorites for reducing gum pain. Moisten a cotton ball or swab with one of the tinctures, and apply it to the painful spots two or three times a day.

Clobber Pain with Cloves

Clove oil is a natural painkiller that works well for just about any kind of oral pain. Dip a cotton swab in the oil, which you can find at health food stores, and dab a little on the sore areas of your gums. Don't have clove oil? Open the spice rack, take out a whole clove, and tuck it between your cheek and gum. It's not as effective as the concentrated oil, but it will turn the throbbing down a notch.

Join the Queue for Q

Talk to your doctor about taking coenzyme Q10 (CoQ10). This supplement increases the amount of oxygen that's available to cells inside your mouth. The extra oxygen helps gum cells grow and reproduce, and it kills gum-damaging bacteria. Until your gums are better, consider taking 30 to 200 milligrams of CoQ10 daily.

Hay Fever

The next time you're sneezy, you might want to take a moment to blame Grandpa Kerchooey for giving you his genes. Sure, hay fever usually gets worse in spring and summer, but pollen's only part of the reason. It's a fact that a lot of the pesky symptoms—congestion, coughing, and those watery, red-rimmed eyes that you make resemble a white rabbit—crop up more often in folks with a family history of allergies.

Of course, every season does give us something to sneeze at. Airborne pollens pounce in the spring, grasses make us gasp in the summer, and leaf molds float merrily through the brisk fall breezes. Unfortunately, lots of other things are blowin' in the wind, such as increasing air pollution from industry and automobiles. Add to all that the global warming that's confusing the seasonal clock, and those hereditary tendencies, and it's Allergies 'R Us!

Scrub with Eucalyptus

Some folks swear that they can clear a stuffy nose with eucalyptus soap, just by using it in their daily shower. It may be that the scent permeates the nasal passages along with the hot steam. Pick up a bar at your favorite bath shop, and give it a try.

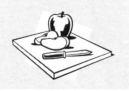
Chemistry Gone Awry

Hay fever is nothing more than an extreme immune reaction. Inhale a simple speck of pollen, for example, and your immune system may react as though your body were fighting off a pack of wolves. Racing to the rescue (when there's no real threat), your immune system cranks out quantities of a disease-fighting protein called immunoglobulin E (IgE). The IgE charges through your bloodstream like Paul Revere, signaling the release of chemicals such as histamine and alerting special cells in the linings of the throat, nose, and lungs to pump up their production of mucus. This is why your eyes and nose run or you're plugged up with congestion.

Dry Up the Drips

Drugstore shelves practically collapse under the weight of all the hay fever drugs out there. Medications can do only so much, though. Anti-inflammatory nasal sprays usually work, but only if you begin using them weeks before allergy season starts. Decongestants clear your sinuses and shrink swollen nasal membranes, but taking them for too long causes rebound congestion. The other problem with over-the-counter drugs, as hay fever sufferers know all too well, is that they cost a bundle. Fortunately, as long as you don't have asthma, there are better solutions—home remedies with no side effects that also won't break the bank! Here's a sampling:

- **Dig into blackberries.** They're loaded with quercetin, a natural chemical that halts the production of histamine, the substance that makes people with allergies sneeze, wheeze, and generally feel miserable. Isn't it wonderful that blackberries ripen just as hay fever season starts?

- **Breathe better with ginkgo.** Ginkgo is best known for improving memory, but its leaves contain ginkgolides, a medicinal component that helps fight allergies. Try a tea made of ginkgo leaves to clear up your runny nose and itchy eyes. Steep 1 teaspoon of dried leaves in a cup of boiling water, then strain out the herb. Let the tea cool, add some honey, and you're good to go. *Caution:* If you're taking any kind of blood-thinning medication—even aspirin—don't use ginkgo without checking with your doctor first.

Soothe Your Sinuses

When those headachy, runny-nose, sneezy allergies hit, you really need to have a plan of action. Start here:

- **Seal out the culprits.** During pollen season, keep the windows of your car and house closed, and stay in air-conditioned spaces whenever possible. Be especially cautious during early-morning hours—pollen counts are at their highest between 5 and 10 a.m. Never hang your clothes to dry outside, where they can collect pollen, and wash your hair every night to keep from contaminating your pillowcase.

Tea Time

It's not surprising that nature provides its own remedies just when allergy season hits. Spring greens and flowers often make the best potions for allergy relief. Look in your neighborhood for nettle, eyebright, cleavers, and elderflowers. Pick them fresh and steep 1/4 cup of these herbs in 1 quart of water overnight. Strain out the herbs, then drink the liquid, hot or cold, throughout the day.

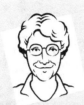

Grandma Says:

Steam your sniffer. Grandma Putt's favorite hay fever treatment still works wonders for me. Soak a washcloth in the hottest water you can stand, wring it out, and lay it across your nose and sinuses. If you keep the cloth as hot as you can, it seems to work on the same principle as hot soup or spicy food: It loosens and liquefies mucus.

■ **Cut the collecting.** Swear off eBay and stop filling your house with tchotchkes. The dust they collect is just an extra trigger for your hay fever. The culprits include books, drapes, figurines, blinds, carpets, dried flowers—nearly every object in the house. Instead, go for a lean decor.

■ **Fire up the washer.** Dust mites are major allergens, and even the cleanest households are full of these microscopic critters. They love to sleep in your bed, which is full of cozy places for them to accumulate, so wash your bedding often. Mites live in any bedding material, but you can wash synthetics to drown the little buggers. So, unless you can find a down comforter that's washable, buy synthetics for your bed.

Soothe with Salve

Try placing a dab of soothing salve on your temples to ease allergy symptoms. Choose one that contains an herbal oil, such as lavender, eucalyptus, or peppermint. The scent will soothe and relax you while the oil opens your respiratory passages and eases congestion.

Hooray for Horseradish!

Horseradish clears air passages from the nose right up into the sinuses. This powerful root is best taken raw. Grate some into a glass of tomato juice, or mix it up with your favorite salsa, or, if you're very brave, eat it right off a celery stalk.

Headaches

You overslept. The kids shrieked and fought for the TV remote. You can't find your purse. In the middle of all this craziness, you might notice that your head is starting to throb—and you know from painful experience that within a few minutes, this minor headache could escalate into a major-league skull banger.

Tension headaches are the most common type of head pain, and they're aptly named. Whenever you're tense, muscles in your scalp, neck, and shoulders contract and tighten up. Tight muscles have to pull against something, and it's often your head that feels the squeeze.

Take Away the Tension

Nearly everyone gets headaches sometimes. It's worth checking with your doctor if you get them all the time or if the pain interferes with your daily activities, but you'll probably be able to manage most headaches on your own. The

dial the DOCTOR

The Sledgehammer

If your headache is so intense that it feels as if you've been hit with a sledgehammer, or if a bad headache won't go away, see your doctor. Strokes, high blood pressure, and adverse reactions to medications can be the cause.

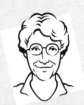

Grandma Says:

Can the coffee.
When it came to java, Grandma just said "No". She knew that caffeine is addictive, and can give you withdrawal headaches as soon as two hours after having a cup of coffee. If you can't give it up entirely, at least cut back to a cup or two of joe a day. You'll still get the lift, but without the headaches later.

vast majority of headaches (about 95 percent) are "primary" headaches, which means that they aren't caused by some underlying illness.

It's fine to take aspirin, ibuprofen, acetaminophen, or any other over-the-counter headache medications as long as you're not sensitive to them. Keep in mind, however, that these drugs don't eliminate the underlying problems, and they may cause side effects that are more uncomfortable than the headaches themselves. It's best to start with gentler approaches, like these:

- **Rub in some lavender.** A drop or two of lavender oil massaged into the temples can help relieve a headache. If you have sensitive skin, apply a thin layer of lotion before using the oil. Or, massage the lavender into the pad of muscle between your thumb and index finger—an acupuncture point for headaches.

- **Willow works wonders.** Willow bark contains salicin, which metabolizes in the body like aspirin, its synthetic cousin. Chew some fresh willow twigs to ease headache pain. If there isn't a willow tree nearby, head to the health food store for a tea or a tincture (30 drops of tincture every 4 to 6 hours). If you are sensitive to aspirin, choose another remedy.

- **Discover the sole solution.** It's hard to imagine that foot problems could cause head pain, but it happens sometimes, especially in women. Wearing high heels or shoes without good support can lead to muscle strain that in turn causes headaches. Always buy shoes with plenty of padding. And if you wear high heels, slip out of them now and then to give the muscles in your legs and feet—and your scalp—a chance to relax.

■ **Heat the upstairs.** You've probably seen movies or television shows that portray headache sufferers holding huge ice bags on their heads. Ice is good for pounding headaches, but heat is usually better for tension headaches because it causes muscles to relax instead of contract. Put a heating pad or a washcloth soaked in warm water on the areas that hurt, or hang out in a steamy bath or shower for 10 to 15 minutes.

Head for Relief

When you have a headache, or feel one coming on, you definitely want fast relief. Here's how to short-circuit the pain:

■ **Put your fingers to work.** A quick way to ease tension headaches is to press your fingers firmly where it hurts while flexing those muscles against the pressure. Doing this a few times helps tense muscles relax. Suppose that your shoulder muscles are unusually tight, and you're feeling the pain in your scalp. Press your fingers into the muscles and shrug your shoulders at the same time to increase the pressure. Next, while maintaining the finger pressure, relax your shoulders for a few seconds, then shrug them again. The combination of pressure and relaxation knocks out tension in a hurry.

- **Try high-speed C.** Vitamin C has powerful anti-inflammatory properties, which is important because inflammation plays a role in some tension headaches. You can try taking 1,000 to 2,000 milligrams of vitamin C at the first sign of a tension headache. If it's going to work, you should feel the benefits within an hour or two. If you have stomach or kidney problems, though, you shouldn't take high amounts of vitamin C. Also, to avoid diarrhea or stomach upset, take it in two or three smaller doses throughout the day.

- **Sit straight.** If you spend a lot of time slumped in a chair or hunched over a keyboard, your head will pay the price. Poor posture is among the most common causes of tension headaches. When you're sitting, your legs should be at a 90-degree angle to your hips. Keep your shoulders back, and don't let your head hang backward or forward; keep it in line with your spine.

- **Kick the salt.** A lot of women get tension headaches during the week to 10 days before their menstrual periods. Eating salt during this time can make things worse because it promotes fluid retention and sometimes raises blood pressure. You may find that cutting back on salt—not only when you're premenstrual but throughout the month—will prevent a lot of headaches. Don't focus just on the saltshaker, though. Only a small percentage of the salt we eat is added at the table. Most is found in processed foods—canned soups, for example, or those lunches at fast-food restaurants. If you eat plenty of natural foods like fruits, vegetables, and whole grains, you'll almost automatically reduce your salt intake to healthier levels.

- **Flex and stretch.** A good way to prevent tension headaches is to do some stretching exercises. Focus on your neck, because that's where these headaches often originate. Several times a day, gently turn your head from left to right as far as you comfortably can in each direction. Then lower your chin toward your chest, hold for a moment, and tilt your head all the way back until you're looking at the ceiling. This stretching exercise is especially helpful on those days when you've been chained to the computer or stuck in rush-hour traffic, and your muscles are tighter than usual.

Sleep Tight

You may not realize it, but the way you sleep can result in an aching head. Keep these in mind:

- **Stare at the ceiling.** Sleeping on your back is the best position for supporting your head and neck muscles. Sleeping on your stomach, on the other hand, means that your head is turned to the side for hours at a time. This can be a real strain on the neck—and a pain in the head.

- **Pop for a new pillow.** Some pillows do an excellent job of supporting your head and neck, while others are so soft that you might as well be sleeping on air. Firm pillows are usually best for preventing tension headaches, but you'll have to experiment to find the pillow that works best for you.

Relax with Magnesium

This common mineral appears to promote muscle relaxation. The next time you have a tension headache, take anywhere from 250 to 750 milligrams of magnesium, and see if it helps. Start by taking the lower amount, and increase the dose only if you don't get relief. Taking more than 400 to 500 milligrams of magnesium a day can cause diarrhea in some people. If this occurs, reduce the dose.

Move Stress Away

You don't want a heavy-duty workout when your head is hurting, but gentle exercise, such as walking or yoga, will relieve tension headaches fast. Exercise helps eliminate muscle-tensing stress hormones from your body and stimulates the release of painkilling chemicals called endorphins.

You may also want to try this acupressure technique from traditional Chinese medicine: Grip the skin between your thumb and index finger and give it a firm pinch. Pressing that area often takes headache pain away.

Heartburn

You probably already know that heartburn has nothing to do with the heart, but it's easy to understand how it got the name. When that miserable, burning feeling flares, usually at night or after meals, it can literally feel as though your heart's on fire. The source of the burning is stomach acid that surges upward into your esophagus, the tube that carries food from your mouth to your stomach. There's a valve at the bottom of your esophagus that's supposed to prevent this upsurge, but sometimes it doesn't work very well. When this happens, you'll know it. UGH—it hurts!

Rapid Relief

If you get heartburn only once in a while, don't give it a second thought. If you have it more often—say, at least once a week over a period of months—you need to check with your doctor. For one thing, heartburn is too painful to live

Tea Time

Chamomile tea is an excellent heartburn remedy because it contains anti-inflammatory substances that soothe irritation. It also settles your stomach after heavy meals. Look for it and other soothing herbal teas, such as slippery elm, marshmallow, and plantain, at health food stores.

Grandma Putt always knew that cabbage eased heartburn. But what she didn't know is that this veggie is loaded with glutamine, an amino acid that appears to promote healing in the digestive tract. People who eat cabbage several times a week may be less likely to experience heartburn than those who never eat it.

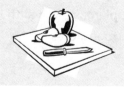

with every day. For another, the constant irritation can lead to all sorts of health problems. In most cases, though, you can manage heartburn yourself—without spending all of your cash on over-the-counter products. Here's how:

■ **Suck down some fluid.** Water is one of the best remedies for heartburn because it dilutes the burning acid and flushes it back into your stomach. Chug it every chance you get.

■ **Moo-ve away from milk.** Milk has a reputation as a stomach soother, but it can actually make heartburn worse by increasing acid production, so avoid it like the plague.

■ **Stand up to it.** Everything that goes up has to come down. It was true for Isaac Newton's apple, and it's equally true for stomach acid that splashes upstream. To help gravity do its job, stand up at the first pangs of heartburn. You'll feel much better when the acid drains back into your stomach.

■ **A heavenly healer.** The herb angelica has the power to cool your heartburn. You can make a tea (it tastes a bit like celery) by putting 1 teaspoon of dried herb or 3 teaspoons of crushed fresh leaves in 1 cup of boiling water. Steep for about 10 minutes, strain out the herb, and enjoy a cup after meals.

■ **Try meadowsweet.** It's a digestive herb that protects and soothes the stomach lining while reducing excess acidity. Sip a cup of meadowsweet tea between meals. To prepare it, steep

1 heaping teaspoon of dried herb (available at health food stores) in 1 cup of hot water for 15 minutes, then strain and drink.

Cool the Burn

Head heartburn off at the pass with these tried-and-true relievers:

- **Loosen up.** Tight clothing presses on the stomach and literally pushes acid uphill. So get comfortable: Loosen your belt a few notches, untuck your shirt, or undo a few buttons. Less pressure means less heartburn.

- **Get your jaws moving.** It may not be polite at formal gatherings, but chewing on a stick of gum is a great way to stop heartburn fast. Chewing increases the flow of saliva, which acts as a natural acid neutralizer.

- **Trim the squares.** Eating gargantuan meals almost guarantees heartburn because all of that food in your stomach requires enormous quantities of digestive acids. You'll be much less likely to get heartburn if you eat five or six small meals a day instead of gorging yourself on two or three large ones.

- **Tip your bed.** A lot of people get heartburn after going to bed because lying prone puts the stomach at the same level as the vulnerable esophagus. An easy solution is to raise the head of your bed a few inches by putting boards or sturdy, wide blocks under the legs.

dial the DOCTOR

Don't Get Burned

People who have frequent heartburn are at risk for cancer of the esophagus. Chronic heartburn that's accompanied by weight loss, trouble swallowing, or visible blood when you cough or have a bowel movement can indicate that acid has already caused serious damage. If you have chronic heartburn, play it safe and see your doctor right away.

- **Pick up licorice.** Licorice root soothes stomach fires and increases circulation to help healing at the same time. Look for chewable tablets of de-glycyrrhizinated (DGL) licorice, which do not contain glycyrrhizin, a component of licorice root that may cause spikes in blood pressure. Chew two to four tablets before meals.

Play it Safe

Emergency room doctors see a lot of people with heartburn who think they're having heart attacks. Don't laugh, though—even doctors can't always tell the difference right away. The bottom line: Go to the emergency room immediately when you have chest pain, especially if you have a history of heart problems, if you smoke, or if you have other risk factors for heart disease.

Mind Your Meals

Of course, heartburn flares up after meals, so you need to watch what—and when—you eat. Follow these guidelines:

- **Catch the culprits.** Caffeine, alcohol, and chocolate are notorious for causing and aggravating heartburn. You don't necessarily have to give them up, but a little moderation may bring blessed relief.

- **Eat lean.** Fatty foods stay in the stomach for a long time and trigger the release of more acid. Drop the fat and switch to leaner meals.

Modern Marvel

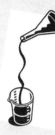

Tame the Acid

Over-the-counter antacids will do the trick. There are dozens of brands, and they all work equally well at stopping heartburn. Liquid antacids work better than tablets because they neutralize more acid.

- **Give up the mints.** Peppermint, spearmint, and other mints may freshen your breath, but they also trigger heartburn by relaxing the muscle in the esophagus that's supposed to keep acid out. So just say "no" to those after–dinner mints.

- **Eat early.** As you'd expect, the production of stomach acid peaks soon after meals. You're a lot more likely to get heartburn when you eat late and go to bed within an hour or two. If you can, eat earlier in the evening so that most of your food is digested by the time you hit the sack.

Hemorrhoids

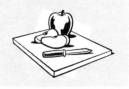
Hemorrhoids are a real pain-in-the-you-know-what. But forget the fancy name for a moment; they're really nothing more than the anal equivalent of varicose veins—blood vessels that are swollen or inflamed. Of course, that little explanation won't make you feel one bit better when the pain is so intense that you can't sit down, or when the itching keeps getting worse—and you can't even scratch in public!

No More Vein Pain

The main cause of hemorrhoids is straining during bowel movements. Sitting for a long time can also contribute to them, as can lack of exercise or not getting enough fiber or water in your diet. In most cases, you can take away the pain of hemorrhoids—and keep them from coming back—without contributing to your doctor's retirement fund. Here are a few things to try:

■ **Soak away pain.** A soak in the bathtub is just the ticket for hemorrhoid pain, and it doesn't have to be lengthy. A 10-minute bath will relax the muscles surrounding the hemorrhoids and reduce irritation and discomfort. And it feels so good, no one will blame you if you soak a bit longer.

■ **Ease the ouch with okra.** Even if you're not a big fan of okra, it's one of the best foods for soothing as well as preventing hemorrhoids. For one thing, it's loaded with fiber. It also has a naturally slimy texture that augments the natural coating of mucus in the intestine. It's a good excuse to eat lots of gumbo.

■ **Say *ahh* with aloe.** Aloe gel is one of the most soothing treatments for hemorrhoid pain. Apply a little to your finger and dab it directly on the tender spots. It may help the tissue heal more quickly, and it will lubricate the area so there's less irritation. You can buy the gel at a health food store or simply squeeze some from a freshly cut aloe leaf.

■ **Keep a regular schedule.** Having regular bowel movements is among the best ways to prevent constipation, which in turn prevents vein-damaging straining. For starters, get in the habit of having bowel movements at the same time every day. For most people, nature's call comes early, usually after breakfast or a cup of coffee. Don't ignore your body's signals. If you wait until later to go, your intestines will have to work harder than they should.

dial the DOCTOR

Seeing Red

For the most part, hemorrhoids aren't serious. They almost always go away on their own in a few days. But there are a few things you need to be aware of. While it's common for hemorrhoids to bleed a bit, it's impossible to know for sure if blood in the toilet bowl is from a hemorrhoid or something serious, such as colon cancer. Never ignore blood in the stool—see your doctor right away.

Sittin' Pretty

Here are some more ways to ease the pain of hemorrhoids and get back to feeling like your old self:

- **Don't force things.** Since straining to have bowel movements aggravates hemorrhoids, don't try to force the issue. Your body knows when it's time to go. If you miss your regular time, let your body decide when it's ready. If you don't get results within 10 minutes, it's time to get off the throne. There's no prize for success, and there's certainly no penalty for coming back later to try again.

- **Reduce your reading time.** That's right, get those *National Geographics* out of the bathroom. They only encourage you to spend too much time on the toilet.

- **Tank up.** Getting enough water throughout the day will go a long way toward making stools softer and easier to pass. Everyone needs different amounts of water, but a good goal is at least 5 full glasses daily; 8 to 10 may be even better.

- **Cool the pain.** Soak a washcloth in cold water, wring it out, and hold it against the affected area until the cloth warms. Don't rub. Rinse the washcloth out, douse it in cold water again, and reapply. Repeat until the pain and itching stop.

- **Baby yourself.** The discomfort of hemorrhoids can make a baby out of anybody, so even if you're a big bruiser, be bold and venture into the baby goods aisle of the grocery store for some baby wipes. They're softer than any toilet paper and they'll help you avoid irritating an already uncomfortable area.

Get off the Couch

People who exercise regularly are less likely to get hemorrhoids than those who spend most of their time lounging. Twenty minutes of exercise a day, even if it's no more than a slow walk, helps your intestines work more efficiently and with less straining.

Heal from the Inside Out

Available in health food stores, mild-tasting aloe juice is a traditional remedy for digestive problems because it soothes your system right where it counts. Drink a glass a day until your hemorrhoids are gone.

Catch the Clots

It's not uncommon for little blood clots to form inside hemorrhoids. While they aren't serious health threats, they can be excruciatingly painful. If your hemorrhoids are making you miserable, your doctor may recommend having any clots removed. It's a simple office procedure that takes just a few minutes and eliminates the pain immediately.

Wash with the Witch

One of the fastest ways to ease itchy hemorrhoids is to apply a little witch hazel. Pour some on a washcloth or tissue, then gently apply it to the tender area. Witch hazel evaporates quickly and leaves a cool, soothing sensation.

Eat More Fiber

The indigestible fiber in fruit, vegetables, legumes, and whole grains soaks up water in the intestine like a sponge. A high-fiber diet makes stools softer and easier to pass, so you strain less and put less pressure on tender hemorrhoids.

Doctors advise getting 30 to 35 grams of fiber daily, but you don't have to put your produce on a scale to be sure you get the right amount. When you fill your plate, salads or vegetables should take up about a quarter of the space. Also, snack on vegetables or fresh or dried fruit during the day.

High Blood Pressure

In the deadly realm of health threats, high blood pressure is like the stealthy cat burglar. It doesn't make a sound, and you don't know you have it until long after the dirty deeds are done. In fact, doctors often call high blood pressure, or hypertension, a silent disease because it usually causes no symptoms until it has already wreaked havoc in your body.

To understand high blood pressure, imagine a nice, new garden hose, all smooth and flexible, warm from the sun. It coils and uncoils easily; it does its job. But what happens if you neglect it and leave it out year-round through all kinds of weather? Yep, after a season or two, it hardens, stiffens, doesn't work very well—and may eventually spring a leak. In a way, your arteries are like that. The "tension" in hypertension is about them. Your arteries must continually contract and relax to accommodate the powerful force of blood pumping

Shake the Salt

Reducing sodium intake definitely helps people with hypertension, and not just those especially sensitive to it. That's why doctors suggest you consume less than 1,500 milligrams of sodium a day. Keep in mind that just 1 teaspoon of salt contains 2,400 milligrams.

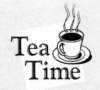

Tea Time

Hawthorn berries are widely used to help lower blood pressure. Combining them with other herbs and relaxants can increase their effect. Combine equal parts of dried hawthorn, motherwort, passionflower, and skullcap, then steep 1 heaping teaspoon of the mixture in 1 cup of hot water for 15 minutes. Strain and drink two or three cups daily.

into your heart—60 to 70 times a minute, and that's while you're resting. When the blood is moving at too high a pressure, it literally wears out the arteries. Down the line, untreated hypertension can also damage your heart, which gets bigger as it works harder to pump. Eventually, it can become more inefficient. Your kidneys and eyes take a beating, too, and a stroke can damage your brain.

A Lifetime of Care

Although it's dangerous, high blood pressure is also highly treatable. Because it sneaks up without symptoms, though, once your doctor says you have it, you have to make a commitment not to go into denial. Just do what's necessary to keep it under control.

If you have high blood pressure, you need to be under a doctor's care, and you may need a variety of prescription drugs to control it. But doctors have also learned that lifestyle factors can be just as important as drugs—and they're a whole lot cheaper. Here's what you need to do:

- **Stop the stress.** If you are easily stressed, your body repeatedly pumps adrenaline into your bloodstream, causing a rise in blood pressure. Take an honest look at your stress level, and take control. You can commit yourself to reducing the stress in your life. Regular exercise, yoga, and meditation are good places to begin.

- **Lower pressure with lime.** Lime blossoms may be effective when your high blood pressure is associated with tension and stress. Toss 1 heaping teaspoon of blossoms into 1 cup of hot water, steep for 15 minutes, then strain. Drink one to three cups per day.

- **Lay off the licorice.** Here's an instance where the artificial is better than the real thing. Natural licorice can raise blood pressure and wash potassium from the body. It's found in some herbal teas, dark beers, and candy. So, if your blood pressure is a little iffy, read labels and buy only licorice made with artificial flavoring.

Know the Numbers

The first step toward controlling your blood pressure is to understand the numbers used to define it. Pressure is expressed as two numbers, one over the other. The upper number (systolic pressure) is a measurement of the pressure during the contraction of the heart as it pumps blood into arteries. The lower number (diastolic pressure) indicates the pressure as the heart relaxes between beats. Blood pressure varies within a normal range during waking hours and should be around 120/80 millimeters of mercury (mm Hg). When it stays above 140/90 for a period of time, it is considered high, can damage the surface of blood vessels, and can lead to cholesterol being deposited on artery walls. Many doctors suggest you start trying to lower your pressure well before it gets to that level.

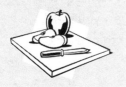
■ **Watch out for stowaways.** Many packaged, prepared, and junk foods are loaded with sodium—some are as much as 85 percent sodium! Always read the labels before you buy lunch meats, soups, canned foods, packaged meals, frozen dinners, and other prepared foods. There are healthy, low-sodium alternatives to these foods, but avoid fast foods altogether, except for an occasional salad (be prepared, and tote your own bottle of low-sodium dressing).

Get it Down

There are a number of do-it-yourself techniques for lowering your blood pressure. Here are a few to check out:

■ **Pump up the produce.** A diet low in salt but high in fruits, vegetables, and low-fat dairy products can lower blood pressure as much as medication can, according to research. Load up your shopping cart and stock your fridge with a variety of these products. Fruit is especially good because its fiber apparently works even better than the fiber from vegetables and grains to lower systolic blood pressure (the top reading). Strawberries, blueberries, and peaches are especially good examples. And in some studies, strawberries lowered diastolic pressure (the bottom reading), too. So top your morning oatmeal or cold cereal with these fruits and reach for a fruit snack later in the day—every day.

- **Get moving now!** We're not naming names here, but many people with high blood pressure are couch potatoes. Even moderate exercise will help—as long as you do it for 30 minutes four or five times a week. Check with your doctor before you start, then pick a regular exercise program you will enjoy and stick with it. (Even if you don't like it at first, you'll soon grow to love feeling fit.)

- **Drink lightly.** Limit daily alcohol consumption to one 12-ounce beer, one 4-ounce glass of wine, or one drink made with 1.5 ounces of hard liquor. More than that can send your blood pressure moving up the scale.

- **Pamper yourself with pets.** Some studies have shown that having pets to care for and love lowers high blood pressure. A cat purrs, and you purr. A dog looks into your eyes, and you melt. If you don't already have a pet, visit a humane society or other shelter and choose a four-legged creature to share your life.

Read This

Both aggressive, let-it-all-hang-out folks and the quiet types who repress their anger are likely to send their blood pressure soaring. If you tend to respond to negative events by acting like either Clara Clam or Rick the Raging Bull, pick up a copy of *LifeSkills*, by Duke University psychiatrist Redford Williams, M.D. By following his simple anger-management techniques, you'll not only lower your blood pressure, you'll also change your life.

De-stress with Passionflower

This herb is one of Mother Nature's best tranquilizers. When you need to be rescued from anxiety or stress—and the high blood pressure that can result—try a cup of passionflower tea. Simply steep 1 or 2 teaspoons of the dried herb in 1 cup of boiling water for 20 minutes, strain, and drink.

Forgive and Forget

Forgiveness is good not only for your soul, but also for your body. A study tracked blood pressure and heart rate as people talked about betrayals in their lives. When some participants reported forgiving a grievance, their readings returned to normal, while the readings of those who held a grudge remained high. Across the board, men were more likely to forgive than women.

If you find it hard to forgive, remind yourself that the word does not mean excuse, forget, or condone. It simply means that you release yourself from the anger and resentment you've been holding—literally—in your heart.

High Cholesterol

With all of the scary headlines about cholesterol, you probably think that the waxy goo sloshing around in your blood is all bad. The truth is, you can't live without it. Cholesterol is a key ingredient in fat-digesting bile. It's used to fortify brain and nerve cells. And the body uses it to manufacture important hormones.

Cholesterol itself isn't the problem. It's the amount. When there's an excess of the fatty stuff in your blood, it clings to artery walls like sludge in a drainpipe. And—no surprise—it's hard for the heart to pump life-giving blood when the main channels are clogged. We talk about cholesterol as if it were a single substance, but there are actually several different forms. Low-density lipoprotein (LDL) is the nasty stuff that hangs onto artery walls. High-density lipoprotein (HDL) is the good stuff that grabs excess LDL from the blood and carts it to the liver for disposal. Thus, the key to con-

From Grandma's Kitchen

Grandma Putt ate oatmeal for breakfast nearly every day—because she liked it. Now we know that this fiber-filled grain helps lower cholesterol. So eat your oats!

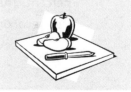

trolling cholesterol—and lowering your risk of heart disease and stroke—is to do everything you can to lower levels of harmful LDL while boosting levels of beneficial HDL.

Look to Your Diet

The new generations of cholesterol-lowering drugs are very helpful, but some of them cause muscle pain or other side effects. They also cost a bundle. In most cases, before your doctor advises you to take drugs to lower cholesterol, he or she will give you detailed advice about natural strategies. They often work—and are a lot less expensive than heart surgery! Here are the best ones to try:

- **Change your bread spread.** We already know that the saturated fat in meats and dairy prod–

Magic Margarines

Even though traditional margarines raise cholesterol more than just about anything else, some new brands, including Benecol and Take Control, actually lower it. They contain a cholesterol-like plant fat that blocks the absorption of cholesterol in the small intestine. As a result, the level of harmful LDL cholesterol drops by 7 to 10 percent. The American Heart Association says 2 tablespoons of Benecol or 3 tablespoons of Take Control daily is enough to have significant cholesterol-lowering effects.

ucts damages arteries, so too much of those foods can sabotage a heart-healthy diet. Even worse are the hydrogenated oils and trans fats used in margarine. Research has shown that people who load up on margarine can see rises in cholesterol of 14 points—which translates to a 10 percent increase in heart attack risk. Give up margarine now, or look for trans fat-free products when you shop. (See "Magic Margarines" at left.)

- **Bet on barley.** Researchers at Texas A&M University tested the effect of barley bran flour, barley oil capsules, and wheat flour on men and women with high cholesterol levels. All the participants followed a low-fat diet for about a month. The result: Those who used either kind of barley significantly lowered their cholesterol levels and their blood pressures. What's the magic ingredient in barley? It's beta-glucan, a type of fiber that study after study has shown lowers cholesterol. (By the way, it's also what gives barley its creamy texture.) Barley also boasts tocotrienol, a substance that deactivates an enzyme that tells the liver to produce artery-clogging LDL cholesterol.

- **Eat lean.** In a study of 145 men and women with mild to moderately high cholesterol, researchers at three major medical centers compared the effects of eating lean white meat with those of eating lean red meat on the partici-pants' cholesterol levels. For about nine months, one group ate a diet in which 80 percent of the meat was lean red meat. The other group ate lean white meat. After a four-week break, the groups switched the types of meat they were eating. During the entire study, the participants were instructed to follow a healthy eating plan recommended by the American Heart Association. The result: Whether the participants ate red or white meat, they lowered their levels of LDL and improved their levels of beneficial HDL. A heart-healthy diet containing up to 6 ounces of lean red or white meat daily can positively impact blood cholesterol levels.

Food Do's and Don'ts

When you're trying to combat high cholesterol, you've got to watch what you eat. Here's what's good for you, and what you should avoid:

■ **Mind the Mediterraneans.** Scores of studies and many doctors agree that the heart-healthiest diet is the one Mediterranean populations enjoy. Consisting mostly of vegetables and fruit, beans, fish, nuts, and plenty of olive oil, Mediterranean meals have a positive effect on both cholesterol levels and blood pressure. Add generous amounts of these foods to your low-fat diet, and you'll lower both your total and LDL cholesterol levels by twice as much as people who eat ordinary low-fat meals, according to study results.

■ **Eat less—but more often.** It may seem surprising, but the more often you eat, the lower your cholesterol may be. In a study of men and women between the ages of 50 and 89, those who ate four or more meals a day lowered their cholesterol by 2.5 percent compared with participants who ate only once or twice a day.

- **Forgo the fast food.** Hydrogenated oils and trans fats are widely used in fast food (especially French fries) and most commercially prepared snacks (like cookies). Forget the fries on your next lunch break, and get into the habit of reading labels on cookies and other snack foods.

Sweet and Sour

You can help lower your cholesterol by including a variety of fruits and vegetables in your diet. Here's the lowdown:

- **The power of pectin.** It binds up cholesterol, preventing its absorption in the blood. Good sources include apples, grapefruit, carrots, prunes, and cabbage.

- **Lower it with lemon.** Living in a toxic world, as we do, can compromise the liver's ability to metabolize fats and cholesterol. Perk it up a bit by squeezing a lemon into your daily water ration. The lemon juice helps prod your digestive system, including your liver, and encourages it to go to work.

- **Know your beans.** They contain soluble fiber that not only lowers cholesterol but may also make your arteries more flexible.

Grandma Says:

Go nuts. Every evening, Grandma Putt would munch on the same snack—a handful of walnuts. Maybe she knew they were great for her heart. According to some studies, 8 to 11 walnuts a day can lower cholesterol even more than olive oil. The nuts lowered the risk of coronary heart disease by 11 percent.

Ditch the Sticks

Along with all of its other terrible consequences to your health, smoking raises cholesterol levels by increasing the stickiness of blood platelets, which makes clotting in narrowed arteries more likely. It also reduces the blood's capacity to carry oxygen and damages the lining of coronary arteries, most likely by contributing to the formation of plaque. Consider this for motivation: When you quit, your risk of heart disease drops rapidly, as does your cholesterol. If you haven't tried in a while, see your doctor for help.

'Chokes Clobber Cholesterol

Ever since Roman times, globe artichokes have been used in traditional European medicine

MODERN MARVEL

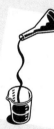

Filter out Trouble

Apparently, the rumors about coffee raising cholesterol levels are not true. The cholesterol connection actually comes from the brewing method, not the coffee itself. When coffee's unfiltered, as it is when it's made with a French press, it can add as many as 20 points to your cholesterol tally. Scientists believe that two compounds in coffee—cafestol and kahweol—are to blame. Brewing through paper or gold-plated filters is said to remove these troublemakers, so if you prefer the French press method, just strain the brewed coffee through a filter before you drink it.

for liver complaints. With its liver-protective, cholesterol-reducing, and appetite-stimulating actions, the artichoke is an excellent all-around digestive herb—especially if you have trouble digesting fat and often feel bloated or nauseated after rich meals. Simply add the plant to your diet (skip the buttery dipping sauce!) or take it as a dried extract (2 grams three times a day). *Caution:* If you have gallbladder disease, talk to your doctor before eating artichokes, and if you're allergic to them, skip this remedy (even the extract) altogether.

The Garlic Cure

It's the real deal for lowering cholesterol, with the ability to drop levels by up to 15 percent, according to many scientific studies. To keep your arteries free and clear, try a glass of garlic tea or juice once a day. Follow it up by chewing a big sprig of fresh parsley, so you don't asphyxiate all your friends!

Another idea: Peel and chop a clove or two, let it rest on the cutting board for at least 10 minutes, then slip it into anything from soups and stews to salads and poultry dishes. Letting the clove rest allows the cholesterol-lowering compounds to form.

Hives

Okay, we all know that beauty is skin deep, but beauty isn't the first word that comes to mind when you're dealing with an outbreak of hives. Those nasty little bumps can make you look as though you fell into a vat of polka dots. On the other hand, you'll probably be too busy scratching the itch to stare in the mirror anyway!

Hives are usually an allergic reaction to food or medication and should be checked by a doctor. They can also pop up after you touch a plant like stinging nettle, or are stung by an insect. Hives can erupt on any part of your body—even in your mouth—but they're usually on your skin, and, boy, are they visible! In some cases, the red wheals may be as large as 1 inch in diameter. Most hives develop within hours of contact with a trigger substance, but sometimes they appear days later, particularly if you're reacting to a medication.

Ditch the Itch

Hives usually don't stick around very long, but why put up with them longer than you have to? Here's what you can do to soothe and save your irritated skin:

- **Attack with antihistamines.** Hives can fade within minutes, or last for days or even weeks. But you can fight back. Your first line of defense is to take an over-the-counter antihistamine such as diphenhydramine (Benadryl). In most cases, it will ease the reaction. A topical anesthetic ointment or lotion may also provide relief. If the problem persists, ask your doctor whether a prescription antihistamine might prevent additional eruptions.

- **Screen for tartrazine.** It's the technical name for a food dye known as Yellow Number 5. Reading food labels can help you avoid this common cause of hives. This not-so-mellow yellow is found in cheeses, artificial fruit drinks, and in the coatings of vitamins and candies.

- **Search for the source.** When hives first hit, try to remember everything you've recently eaten. If you can identify the trigger early, you can avoid a more serious recurrence. Drawing a blank? Keep a daily food diary until you're sure whether or not something in your diet is triggering the hives.

- **Axe the aspirin.** This common analgesic is a frequent cause of hives. If you're allergic to aspirin, also try eliminating foods that con-

Grandma Says...

Soothe with oats. To reduce the itchiness of hives, Grandma Putt would have me soak for 10 to 15 minutes in a bathtub full of warm water to which she'd added finely ground colloidal oatmeal. This over-the-counter bath powder stays suspended in water and won't clog your drain—but it will sure fix your itch.

tain salicylate, the active ingredient in aspirin. These include apricots, berries, grapes, raisins and other dried fruit, and tea.

- **Don't be a sourpuss.** Foods that are processed with vinegar, such as pickles, may cause hives in some people. Give up the sour stuff for a while and see if it helps.

- **Chill the chick.** Chickweed salve soothes itching, burning hives in no time. For extra relief, keep the salve in the fridge and dab it on cold. Or make an infusion by steeping a handful of fresh chickweed in 2 cups of hot water for 15 minutes. Strain the liquid into a spray bottle, chill, and spritz it on your hives.

Nix the Niacin

Eating foods high in niacin increases the chance of hives. The most common foods that cause this reaction are niacin-rich shellfish, nuts, and berries, but you may also be sensitive to poultry, seeds, cereals, and breads. Boycott these foods for a week to see whether niacin could be the trigger for your hives.

Mend with Mint

You may find some temporary relief from those hot, itchy hives by dabbing them with cool mint tea. Stir 1 teaspoon of fresh or dried leaves into 1 cup of boiling water, and simmer for 10 minutes, then strain. Rub the cooled tea on your skin.

Ingrown Hairs

It's hard to believe that something the size of a hair could cause so much, well, hair-raising pain. But an ingrown hair, which curls downward instead of growing out straight, is like a sharp needle that digs deeper and deeper into the skin—not all at once, but over days or weeks. You don't feel it at first, but once bacteria take advantage of the tiny wound, you get an inkling of what pain is all about. At the very least, you develop a tender little bump.

Help for Wayward Hairs

In most cases, you can take care of an ingrown hair—and prevent a recurrence—without medical intervention. Here are a few things to try:

■ **Wipe out the germs.** It's not necessary to pull an ingrown hair out of your skin; your body will eventually expel it. But you should gently clean the affected area twice a day with soap and water, and definitely keep an eye out for

dial the
DOCTOR

When it Really Hurts

If an ingrown hair bump becomes large and very painful and/or if the infection spreads and causes fever, dizziness, or other symptoms, you should see your doctor right away.

infection. Warning signs include increasing heat, redness, swelling, pain, or pus. If an infection doesn't clear up on its own in a day or two, see your doctor.

- **Hit it with heat and cold.** To ease painful or infected ingrown hairs, alternate hot and cold compresses. Soak a washcloth in hot water, wring it out, and drape it on the sore area. Keep it there for 3 minutes, then replace it with a cold cloth for 30 seconds. Repeat the cycle two more times, ending with the cold compress. This technique, called contrast hydrotherapy, improves skin circulation and speeds healing.

- **Cream it with calendula.** A quick way to take the sting out of irritated skin is to apply a cream that contains the herb calendula. Ready-made creams are available in health food stores, or you can make your own version. Just add 6 to 12 drops of calendula oil to an ounce of almond or olive oil. Rub it on the irritated area once a day until the problem is gone.

- **Stay wet.** Shave in the shower—it keeps your skin clean and the pores open. It also reduces the chances that your skin will be irritated and allows for a closer shave, which can keep hairs from growing inward.

- **Wash before and after.** It's important to wash with soap and water before, as well as after, shaving. Thorough cleansing reduces the risk that bacteria will survive long enough to colonize tiny shaving nicks or ingrown hair follicles.

Forget the Antibiotics

A lot of people insist on using antibiotic soaps and creams, but they shouldn't. These products tend to irritate your skin, including areas where hairs may be growing inward.

Turn Off the Juice

Electric shavers may allow you to shave without using lather or water, but they're more likely to irritate your skin. If you're having problems, go back to blades.

For some men with extremely curly facial hair, not shaving may be the only solution to persistent ingrown hairs. Give it a try and see how well the bearded look suits you—or at least go a few days between shaves to give your skin a much-needed break.

Shave, Don't Save

You're less likely to get ingrown hairs if you shave just once with a disposable razor, then throw it out. I know it's wasteful in this day and age, but if you continue to reuse a razor, it makes it easier for yesterday's bacteria to get into today's shaving cut or ingrown hair follicle. And that turns into tomorrow's painful bump.

Ingrown Toenails

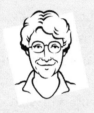

Grandma Says…

Take your vitamins. Grandma always took a daily multivitamin to help ensure that her body had the right nutrition for proper nail growth. Healthy nails are less likely to become ingrown or infected.

Mother Nature isn't all sweetness and light. She has her own form of torture—one that can reduce you to tears if you don't take care of it quickly. The "nail" in toenail isn't just a figure of speech. Humans don't have the daggerlike claws that cats do, but if you've ever had an ingrown toenail, you know that your nails are still plenty sharp. An ingrown nail starts out like any other nail, but sometimes its sharp edge curves into the side of your toe instead of growing out straight. The more the nail grows, the deeper it digs into your skin.

Prevent the Pain

Some people are simply prone to ingrown toenails—and the infection that sometimes comes along for the ride. Others get ingrown nails when they wear too-tight shoes or trim their nails in the wrong direction. You'll have to see your doctor once a toenail starts penetrating the skin. But before that happens, here are a few tips to try:

- **Start with a salt soak.** An Epsom salts bath will help draw out pain and infection. Fill a basin with warm water, add a cup of Epsom salts, and soak your foot for 20 to 30 minutes.

- **Pack it in clay.** A clay pack, available at health food stores, will help keep swelling and infection under control. Look for French green clay, or ask a pharmacist for pharmaceutical-grade kaolin clay. Apply the clay to the affected toe and leave it on until it dries, which usually takes 30 minutes to an hour. Then rinse away the clay and dry your foot thoroughly. Repeat the treatment once or twice a day.

- **Rub out infection.** An herbal foot massage can soothe the pain of an ingrown nail and protect the area from a potentially serious infection. Start with a trip to the health food store for infused calendula oil and oregano, thyme, and lavender oils. Then combine 1 ounce of the calendula oil with 10 drops of each of the others, and slather the mixture all over your foot. The hands-on attention will make the area feel a lot better, and the oils will help reduce swelling and pressure around the sore nail.

- **Change your socks.** To reduce the risk of infection, put on clean socks two or three times a day. For additional protection, add a few drops of lavender, oregano, or thyme oil (available at health food stores) to a basin of water

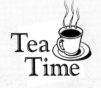

Tea Time

Here's a tea treatment that's taken by foot, not by mouth. Put a quart of water in a saucepan, then add 1 cup of dried calendula flowers, 1 tablespoon of dried thyme, and 1/2 cup of dried lavender flowers (all available at health food stores). Simmer the mixture for 5 minutes, then let it cool to room temperature. Put it in a basin and soak your foot for about 5 minutes.

and soak your socks in the solution overnight. The germ-killing action of the oils will help ensure that your socks don't allow infection-causing bacteria to thrive.

Let the Sun Shine In

Germs are never happier than when they're in a dark, tight space. To keep them under control, expose the toe with the ingrown nail to the air as often as possible, and try these:

- **Bare it all.** Take off your shoes and socks when you're lounging around the house.

- **Don some sandals.** They're a wonderful option for airing out an ingrown toenail. Footwear made of natural materials, such as leather and cork, will probably be the most comfortable and least aggravating to your toe.

- **Be foot-loose.** Shoes that don't leave enough room for toenails to grow naturally can force them to grow into your tender toes. Take the time to try on a lot of shoes until you find the ones that fit well and feel good.

Groom 'Em Right

Your best defense against ingrown toenails is to learn how to care for your nails. Try these pedicure tricks:

- **Cut it straight.** If you know that one of your nails is prone to becoming ingrown, check it every week so you can cut it before it gets too long. Then trim straight across the top of the nail. Don't try to round the edges so the nail follows the shape of your toe; this just makes it more likely to curve into the flesh.

- **Don't dig.** It's fine to snip away a toenail that has just started to grow in the wrong direction, but you don't want to mess with a nail that's already embedded in the skin. Trying to trim it at that point is likely to damage the tissue and increase the risk of infection. To play it safe, see your doctor.

- **Train your nails.** Here's a safe, painless way to encourage an ingrown nail to head in the right direction before it can cause real trouble. Take a small piece of cotton and roll it into a tight cylinder. Slip the cylinder under the nail right where it's touching (or almost touching) the skin. The cotton will relieve the pressure and may make the nail grow out rather than in.

Insomnia

Whoever came up with the idea of counting sheep obviously never had insomnia. If anything, your brain is too active when the lights go out, and the last thing you need is some kind of woolly math problem.

We all have sleepless nights now and then. Doctors estimate that about a third of Americans spend at least a few nights watching the clock s-l-o-w-l-y advance. In most cases, there's no mystery about what causes it. Stress is a big factor. So are lack of exercise, depression, and miscellaneous aches and pains.

Nighty-Night

Most people with insomnia don't need a pricey prescription or over-the-counter drugs. In fact, these simple tips from top sleep experts will do the trick:

- **Wear yourself out.** Physical activity during the day will help you sleep better at night. Exercise reduces stress and induces sleep by promoting deep relaxation. Exercise also helps you fall asleep faster and sleep longer. Even a brisk walk before dinner can make a big difference.

- **Take a hint from kitty.** Catnip may turn your lazy feline into a rowdy cat, but it has the opposite effect on us humans. A little catnip tea after dinner may be just the ticket for winding down after a long day. Steep 1 teaspoon of the herb in 1 cup of hot water for 10 minutes, then strain and enjoy. *Note:* Stash your catnip out of the reach of all cats!

- **Sleep by your brain clock.** Sleep, much like a muscle, can be trained and refined. The key is to repeat the same sleep pattern every day to set your brain clock to a good schedule. Your body will adapt to the regularity, restoring normal hormonal sleep-wake cycles and easing you

Modern Marvel

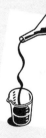

Meddling Meds

If you're wondering what's keeping you up at night, it just might be your medications. Drugs that interfere with sleep include beta-blockers for high blood pressure, thyroid medications, bronchodilators and corticosteroids for asthma, sinus and nasal decongestants, and antidepressants. If you're taking any of these, ask your pharmacist whether a change in medication may help ease your insomnia.

into more restful sleep. If you stay as regular as you can and don't skimp on sleep, you will feel great in the morning.

- **Soak up sunshine.** If you fall asleep at 8 p.m. instead of 10 p.m. and wake up at 4 a.m. instead of 6 a.m., your sleep cycle is off. Spend more time outdoors during the day. That way, daylight can help your internal clock counteract its tendency to put you to sleep earlier in the evening and wake you up earlier in the morning.

Don't Blame it On Age

Many older folks toss and turn and barely get five hours of sleep a night. So the assumption has long been that as we age, we actually need less sleep. But what researchers have discovered is that losing sleep has nothing to do with aging itself—it's the aches and pains that often

Snooze with Valerian

Valerian, an herb also known as heliotrope, is a mild sedative that smells like stinky socks and is reputed to help you sleep. Research shows that valerian root depresses the central nervous system and relaxes smooth muscle tissue. It can be used as a tea or taken in pill or tincture form. Valerian isn't recommended if you have asthma or use sleeping pills, alcohol, antidepressants, or anti-anxiety medication.

accompany aging that are the real culprits. Older people tend to have more medical conditions, such as arthritis or bladder problems, that keep them awake. If you think this may be what's causing you to lose sleep, don't be a stiff-upper-lipper when it comes to pain or discomfort. Talk to your doctor about relief.

A.M. or P.M.?

A morning person goes to sleep relatively early in the evening, wakes up early, and is most effective at doing complex tasks in the morning rather than in the evening. A night person goes to bed later, gets up later, is slower to reach full horsepower, and does better at complex tasks in the evening. If insomnia is a major part of your life, the odds are good that you're fighting your natural sleep type. Just decide which type you are and try to readjust your daily priorities so that complex tasks are scheduled for the proper time. Sleep will soon follow.

The Sleep Zone

Making a few changes to your sleep arrangements can help you get to the land of Nod quickly and keep you asleep. Here's what to do:

■ **Follow the same routine.** The best way to get to sleep quickly is to establish and follow bedtime routines. These rituals have a big influence on your ability to get to sleep and

Travel to Dreamland

Native American healers invented a sleep-enhancing "dream spirits" pillow to ease insomniacs into dreamland. To make your own, put equal amounts of dried leaves of catnip, rabbit tobacco, mint, and sage into a small calico or plain cotton pillowcase and sew it shut. This aromatic, sedative pillow is said to make dreams more memorable, and its effects are even more noticeable in hot, humid weather.

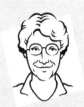

Grandma Says...

Cut back on caffeine. When I was a young man, I had a terrible time with sleepless nights, until Grandma Putt told me to keep the caffeinated coffee for the morning, and switch to decaf in the afternoon or evening. It sure made a difference. After a while, gradually wean yourself from full-caffeinated coffee by mixing half decaf and half regular in the pot.

wake up on a regular basis. Try reading a book, breathing deeply, or sipping a cup of herbal tea. They all can work in the same way that shaving, washing your face, and having a cup of coffee help you accelerate when you get up in the morning.

■**Snooze in comfort.** Be as comfortable as possible for the third of your life that you spend in bed. A good mattress and bedding help you enjoy your stay. There are many kinds of mattresses out there, from foam to air to pillow-tops and more. The best way to get a mattress that's right for you is to actually go out and test it by lying on it for several minutes in your usual sleep position. And treat yourself to high-quality, smooth sheets and covers that will caress you rather than make you itch or sneeze.

■**Pull the shades.** Your body needs darkness to trigger its sleep cycle. If you have a big streetlight shining in the window, or you have to sleep during the day because you're on night shift, close the blinds or pull opaque drapes across your windows so the light won't get through. Another alternative: wear a comfortable sleep mask.

■**Stop trying so hard.** Striving to sleep only makes the problem worse, so if you haven't fallen asleep after a little while, get up and distract yourself. Sit in another room to read or listen to soft music.

Pillow Talk

Your pillow may be the culprit behind all that tossing and turning you do each night. When was the last time you bought a bed pillow? If you're like most folks, it's been a while. So ditch that lumpy, bumpy old one and buy yourself a new model. You'll find ones made specifically for back sleepers and for side sleepers, stuffed with everything from feathers to fiber to foam.

Welcome Some Whoopee

If you can't sleep, have sex. After getting worked up sexually, your body goes quite naturally into a state of total relaxation. If your significant other is sound asleep, make some romantic moves. Turn on the sexual vibrations, and you'll turn off any others that may be keeping you awake.

You're Getting Sleepy...

Use guided imagery, a form of self-hypnosis, to help yourself get to sleep. Listen to a meditation tape or use a progressive muscle relaxation exercise to become deeply relaxed, then picture yourself comfortably asleep. While you're at it, imagine that you're in a more comfortable bed, in a luxury hotel, on a mountaintop, or in a gently rocking sailboat. Visualize every possible detail of the scene to increase the suggestion's power. Do this nightly for several weeks, and you'll soon be able to fall asleep more easily.

Irritable Bowel Syndrome

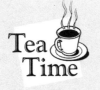

Tea Time

Peppermint is a powerful antispasmodic and pain reliever. Use peppermint leaves to make a soothing tea. Put 1 heaping teaspoon of leaves in 1 cup of hot water, cover and let steep for 10 to 15 minutes, then strain. Drink three cups daily between meals.

Even though irritable bowel syndrome, better known as IBS, is among the most common conditions treated by doctors, they still don't know what causes it. They don't always agree on what to call it. And they sure don't know how to cure it. With all of this confusion, IBS might as well stand for Incredibly Baffling Syndrome.

For some reason, people with IBS have intestines that are, well...irritable. They seem to have abnormal electrical activity that causes frequent, uncomfortable muscle contractions, or spasms. Everyone with IBS has a slightly different pattern of problems. Some people have mainly cramps, some have episodes of diarrhea and/or constipation, and others are afflicted with gas and bloating. The symptoms may occur daily for years, or they may disappear for a while, then come roaring back with no warning.

Calm the Chaos

If your intestinal symptoms are so severe that they interfere with your day-to-day life, you should see a doctor right away. If it turns out that you have IBS, lifestyle changes may be just as important as medical care. Here's what many doctors advise:

- **Sweet isn't neat.** If you have IBS, sweets are a one-way ticket to disasterville. Sugary foods appear to interfere with the normal muscle contractions that propel food through the intestine, so nix the sweets.

- **Slip and slide.** When mixed with water, slippery elm powder makes a drink that will soothe your irritated gut from end to end. This is a good remedy to take first thing in the morning and last thing at night to help your tissues heal 24 hours a day. Pour 1 cup of warm water over 1 teaspoon of powder, stir briskly, and drink immediately.

- **Say no to joe.** Either eliminate or strictly limit the amount of caffeine you consume. Whether it comes in coffee or your favorite soda, caffeine is a bowel stimulant.

- **Bubbles mean trouble.** Reach for noncarbonated drinks, such as fruit juice or water. The fizz in carbonated drinks can cause problems for people with IBS.

- **Feast less, graze more.** Many people with IBS find that it helps to split their day's calories

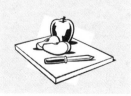

among five or six small meals rather than following the traditional breakfast–lunch–dinner schedule. Eating less food at one time puts less strain on the large intestine.

- **Fish for relief.** Some foods can help quell the intestinal inflammation that contributes to IBS symptoms. For example, salmon and other cold-water fish, as well as ground flaxseed, contain omega-3 fatty acids that help your body suppress inflammation.

Take a Deep Breath

Studies show that meditation (which involves controlled breathing) can lower the levels of stress hormones in your body and reduce anxiety and pain. But deep breathing can be soothing on its own. Instead of breathing shallowly from your chest, inhale deeply until you feel your abdomen expand, then slowly exhale. Repeat three more times. This is an effective technique because when your diaphragm moves, it lowers your body's stress response.

Rub Your Tummy

Chronic conditions like IBS can create a vicious cycle when flare-ups are greeted with increased stress, tension, and anger toward a body that isn't behaving the way it's supposed to. A good exercise for breaking this pattern and focusing on healing your gut is to give yourself a 10- to 15-

minute abdominal massage every day. To make a massage oil, mix ¼ teaspoon of lobelia oil or catnip tincture per 1 tablespoon of vegetable oil (any kind will do). Then begin at your belly button and massage in small, gentle, clockwise circles until you've covered your entire abdomen. Visualize your intestines relaxing and returning to their normal, healthy state.

Spoon Up Some Culture

Not all germs are bad germs. In fact, we couldn't get along without certain types of bacteria that live in our intestines and aid digestion. To help your digestive system, eat live-culture yogurt. It contains beneficial Lactobacillus acidophilus organisms, which appear to reduce IBS symptoms. Check labels when you shop to be sure the yogurt you buy contains live cultures, and plan on having at least a few servings a week.

The Castor Cure

A castor oil pack provides relief from abdominal pain and cramps. To make one, moisten a washcloth with the oil, drape it over your abdomen, and cover it with plastic wrap. Put a heating pad set on low on top of the plastic and leave it on for 20 minutes. The combination of oil and plastic traps the heat and helps reduce spasms and cramping.

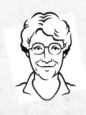

Grandma Says…

Get moving. Grandma Putt always said that exercise works wonders for your digestive system. Now, you may not be up to it when your symptoms are in high gear, but 15 to 20 minutes of exercise every day is an important IBS-stopping strategy. Physical activity reduces levels of emotional stress, and it helps your bowel work more regularly.

Kidney Stones

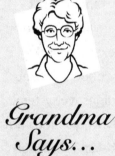

Grandma Says...

Peel a banana. Grandma Putt never had kidney stones. Maybe that's because she ate so many bananas. They're packed with potassium, the mineral that can help prevent some types of stones from forming.

If you were experiencing kidney stone pain right now, you wouldn't be reading this book. You'd be on the floor, curled up in agony. Even though most kidney stones aren't much bigger than a grain of sand, every now and then one gets stuck in the narrow tubes, called ureters, that connect your kidneys and bladder. Or they irritate the urethra, the tube that carries urine out of the body. In either case, the pain can be excruciating.

Chemicals and minerals that are normally present in urine sometimes solidify and form hard little crystals, or stones. Most are so tiny that they pass harmlessly through your body without making you aware of their existence. Larger stones that get stuck, on the other hand, usually cause pain in the lower back or groin. Some people also experience nausea, blood in the urine, or an increased urge to urinate.

Roll 'Em Out

A kidney stone obviously isn't something to handle on your own; you need to see a doctor immediately. You'll probably need X-rays or other tests to determine exactly where the stone is. Once your doctor knows its location and size, there are a number of treatment options. He or she may recommend "watchful waiting"—giving the stone a little time to exit your body on its own—or give you medication to dissolve it. If the problem is severe, however, you'll probably need surgery to remove the stone.

Crush Stone Pain

Fortunately, your body is pretty good at getting rid of kidney stones. If you get them frequently, though, you need to find ways to minimize the pain—and more important, to keep them from coming back. Don't keep throwing money at specialists if you don't have to. Instead, try these tips and see if they help:

- **Drink up.** Staying well hydrated should be a top priority for those who are stone-prone. Keeping enough water flowing through your system reduces the concentration of stone-forming minerals. Water can also help flush out small stones that have already formed.

- **Heat up—or cool down.** During a kidney stone attack, one of the best things you can do is apply an ice pack or a heating pad to your

dial the DOCTOR

Symptoms to Heed

Don't assume that everything's going to be fine if you've been diagnosed with kidney stones. While pain is normal, you shouldn't have fever, nausea, or vomiting, nor should the pain get significantly worse. If you experience any of these symptoms, call your doctor immediately. There's a good chance that the stone has caused an infection, and you may need antibiotics right away to keep it from getting worse.

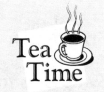
abdomen, lower back, or wherever you're feeling the pain. Either will take the edge off until you can get professional help.

- **Squeeze an orange.** If you're concerned about kidney stones, start your day with an orange or a tall glass of juice, then continue to eat oranges or quaff OJ throughout the day. The citrus fruit raises your body's level of citrates, natural chemicals that keep new stones from forming and existing stones from getting worse. Discuss this with your doctor first, though—not all types of stones are affected by citrates.

- **Calm them with corn.** Herbalists have traditionally recommended the herb cornsilk for kidney stones, and there's good evidence that it works. Cornsilk coats and soothes irritated tissues in the body, including tissues in the urinary tract. Drink one or two cups of corn-silk tea daily when you're coping with kidney stones. To make it, steep 1 teaspoon of herb in a cup of hot water for about 10 minutes, then strain and sip.

Take The Produce Express

You'll do yourself a big favor by adding more fiber to your diet. Why? Because people who have high-fiber diets are less likely to get stones. You can get loads of fiber by filling up on fresh fruit and vegetables as well as legumes, whole grains, and high-fiber cereals. You want to get at least 20 grams of fiber a day.

Cork the Bottle

Avoid alcohol when you're coping with a kidney stone. Its dehydrating effects will interfere with your body's ability to dissolve and flush the stone. The same goes for caffeine—it increases activity in the nervous system, which can aggravate the pain.

Supplements to the Rescue

Make sure you're getting enough magnesium and B_6 in your diet. Both can help reduce your kidney stone symptoms. The mineral magnesium relaxes muscles throughout your body, which can reduce pain during kidney stone attacks. Take 600 milligrams a day. This amount may cause diarrhea, so if it occurs, reduce the dose.

While it hasn't been proven yet, there is some evidence that people who don't get enough vitamin B_6 in their diets are more likely to get kidney stones. If you've had stones in the past, an easy preventive strategy is to take a daily multivitamin that contains 100 percent of the Daily Value of B_6.

Got Milk?

Some types of kidney stones are composed mainly of calcium. In the past, people who got these kinds of stones were advised to cut back on the mineral. Doctors now believe that the calcium you get from foods actually helps prevent kidney stones, although the calcium in supplements may make you more prone to them.

When you talk to your doctor, find out if your stones are the calcium variety. If they are, ask whether you should increase or cut back on calcium in your diet.

Ease Them Out

The herb cramp bark (*viburnum opulus*) is a muscle relaxant that makes it easier for stones to move through your body. It's available at health food stores in many forms, including capsules, tinctures, and teas. Each product contains different amounts of the active ingredient, so follow the label directions to be sure you're taking the proper amount.

Soak That Stone

Your doctor will probably advise you to take an over-the-counter or prescription painkiller during kidney stone attacks. While you're waiting for it to work, add a cup or two of Epsom salts to a warm bath and soak for a while. The warmth of the water will ease your stress as well as the discomfort. In addition, the magnesium in Epsom salts may help relax your muscles and further reduce the pain.

Lactose Intolerance

Most American diets are filled with dairy products, from the milk we put on our breakfast cereal, to the butter we slather on toast, to the cheese we load into sandwiches and casseroles. But many folks (particularly African Americans, Native Americans, Asians, and Hispanics) have a hard time digesting dairy. In fact, most people begin to lose their ability to digest milk and milk products at about age 2, although they may not have symptoms until much later. It turns out that once our ancestors were weaned, they never got milk again, so the enzyme necessary to digest it—lactase—got programmed out of existence. And without lactase, milk can't be digested without the discomfort of gas and cramps.

Soothe Your Gut

If you haven't been diagnosed with lactose intolerance, but you suddenly start experiencing

Replace the Calcium

Because milk is such a rich source of calcium and vitamin D—major dietary bone builders—you need to find those nutrients elsewhere if you're avoiding dairy foods. So eat plenty of dark green, leafy vegetables and almonds, and fatty fish like salmon and herring. And ask your doctor if you should take calcium supplements.

Grandma Putt
would often drink
hot cocoa when
she was feeling
bloated. While she
didn't have lactose
intolerance, she
knew the cocoa
would soothe
her gassy tummy.
Now a study from
the University of
Rhode Island has
shown that cocoa
may stimulate
an enzyme that
breaks down the
lactose in milk
that's responsible
for bloating and
gas. So if you have
trouble digesting
milk, stirring in a
few teaspoons of
cocoa may help.

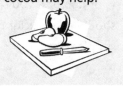

digestive discomfort, check with your doctor. The symptoms are nearly identical to those caused by many other conditions, including irritable bowel syndrome and colitis. But if you know from experience that dairy puts you in the dumps, try these:

- **Heal with marshmallow.** Marshmallow tea soothes inflamed tissues and helps the lining of the gut heal. Make a cold infusion by soaking 2 tablespoons of marshmallow root in 1 quart of cold water overnight. Strain and drink it throughout the day.

- **Ferment and feel better.** Traditional nomadic peoples, who continued to use dairy products as a food source beyond infancy, cultured their milk products to make them more easily digestible. If you are lactose intolerant, you may be able to handle fermented dairy products (such as yogurt and kefir) and perhaps even goat's- or sheep's-milk cheeses. If your lactose intolerance is severe, however, it's best to omit milk from your diet completely.

- **Look for hidden lactose.** Many foods contain milk solids as filler. If you're especially sensitive to lactose, these can cause you discomfort if you ingest enough, so read food labels carefully and search out lactose-free products instead.

- **Have cookies with your milk.** Studies have found that eating other foods with a dairy product increases the odds that the lactose can enter your body without bothering your gut.

MODERN MARVEL

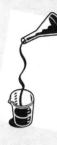

An Excellent Enzyme

Lactaid, along with several other over-the-counter products, does the work of natural lactase. Just drop a caplet in a glass of milk, then guzzle the moo juice. Follow the package directions to take it before eating cheese, sour cream, and other high-lactose foods. Your bones will benefit from the calcium, and you can enjoy your favorite Ben & Jerry's without uncomfortable after-effects.

Shop for Substitutes

Look around until you find as many lactose-free products as you can—or products that are supplemented with extra lactase. There is now a brand of yogurt with added lactase, for instance. You can also buy lactose-free cheese that melts just like real American cheese. Pop it under the broiler, and you can have a melted cheese sandwich, a tuna-cheese melt, or a baked potato topped with cheese.

Recipe Relief

Check out the Internet for Websites such as www.lactaid.com, to find recipes and menu ideas to help you enjoy dairy-free living.

Laryngitis

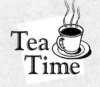

Tea Time

A red sage tea gargle can ease the mucous membranes of your larynx and boost your immune system. Pour 1 cup of warm water over 1 teaspoon of red sage and steep for 10 minutes. Strain, then gargle.

Maybe you were a little too enthusiastic yelling your lungs out on the soccer sidelines. Or maybe you had too much fun at the pub, shouting across the table and doing your always-popular rendition of "New York, New York." But when you woke up, you felt like you had tacks in the back of your throat, and instead of "Good morning," you said something like, "Grroo...murgh." Blame laryngitis, an inflammation of the vocal cords. It sometimes results from an infection, but usually it's simply a consequence of using your voice too much.

I Can't Hear You...

Check with your doctor if your laryngitis doesn't go away within a few days to a week. In the meantime, try these tips to start sounding like yourself again:

- **Give your voice a break.** The most effective treatment is silence. Don't use your voice at all—not even for whispering. Trying to express yourself in squeaks and croaks just aggravates your inflamed vocal cords, actually causing them to bang together, slowing your recovery.

- **Suck in some steam.** If you have an extreme case of laryngitis, try resting in a warm room with high humidity for a day or two. Use a humidifier if necessary, and let your worn-out throat soak up some moisture while you sleep.

- **Alleviate with elm.** Slippery elm is used by professional singers and speakers to recover their voices and keep their laryngeal tissues in tiptop shape. To make a tea, steep 1 heaping teaspoon of dried herb in 1 cup of hot water for 15 minutes. Strain, add honey and lemon if you like, and drink three or four cups per day.

Take Your Thyme

An herbal steam can help soothe respiratory passages and alleviate laryngitis pain. Put 3 or 4 drops of thyme oil in a bowl of steaming hot water. Bend over the bowl—but not close enough to burn your face—and tent your head and the bowl with a towel. Breathe in deeply.

It's a Wrap!

Place a warm, wet, cloth compress on your neck for 2 to 3 minutes, then replace it with a cold one. Wrap a wool scarf around your neck to keep the cold compress in place for 30 minutes.

The Carrot Cure

A carrot neck wrap may ease inflammation and help you recover your voice more quickly. Grate a carrot onto a length of cheesecloth, fold the cloth in half lengthwise, and moisten it with warm water. Wrap it around your neck, then wrap your neck with a warm towel. Leave it on for 20 to 30 minutes. For extra heat, sprinkle a pinch of red pepper on the grated carrot.

Sip It Warm

Drink lots of water or tea, but keep it tepid—not too hot or too cold, either of which could further inflame your vocal cords.

Keep It Bland

When your throat is under siege by laryngitis, be wary of what you put down it. Avoid very spicy foods, hot soups and beverages, and any other edible irritants.

Back Away from the Butts

The most serious cause of laryngitis is long-term smoking. If you haven't been convinced by now that smoking is a major health risk, let the damage to your delicate vocal cords motivate you. Look into all the aids to help you quit—from prescription medications and nicotine gum to group therapy. Ask your doctor to help you find the right method for you.

MODERN MARVEL

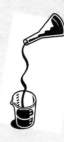

Calm a Cough

The more you cough, the more you irritate your sensitive larynx. If your cough is dry and unproductive, use an over-the-counter cough suppressant such as dextromethorphan to keep your larynx from further harm. Follow the package directions.

Menstrual Pain

Women used to refer to monthly periods as "the curse." It's easy to understand why a term usually used in relation to mummies and witchcraft came to summarize the clockwork fluctuations of a woman's hormones. More than half of menstruating women have menstruation-related cramps and low-back pain. The discomfort may begin before any bleeding, then peak in the next few hours, and usually stop in a day or two. The intensity of the pain, known as dysmenorrhea, varies among women and can even vary for the same woman from one period to the next.

Cramps are caused by uterine contractions, and many of the accompanying symptoms, such as fatigue, headaches, and bloating, are thought to be due to an imbalance of the hormones estrogen and progesterone. An excess of estrogen or a deficiency of progesterone can trigger discomfort.

Move Your Belly

If you've ever had an urge to explore the culture of the Middle East, here's your excuse: The movements taught in belly dancing are great for stretching your pelvis and keeping cramps at bay. In fact, any exercise that gets you moving and rocking your pelvis will bring relief.

Kill the Cramps

If you have severe menstrual cramps or changes in your normal flow, see a doctor. Most women, however, don't need medical technology to feel better. There are plenty of strategies for handling the pain that have been working for women for centuries. Here are the best:

- **Trust OTCs.** Aspirin and other nonsteroidal anti-inflammatory drugs are inexpensive and very effective for treating cramps. They block the production of prostaglandins, body chemicals that cause uterine contractions. Take the standard dose of two caplets every 4 to 6 hours, but no more than 8 in 24 hours. Avoid aspirin if you have heavy bleeding.

- **Put fish on the menu.** Anti-inflammatory compounds are also abundant in seafood. Have a daily serving of oil-rich fish, such as sardines, salmon, or cod, to help reduce your symptoms.

- **Avoid processed foods.** The more fresh fruits, vegetables, and whole grains you eat, the less room there will be in your diet for packaged and processed foods. That means you'll cut out a lot of sodium, which will reduce the discomfort of water retention and bloating. It also means that you'll eat fewer animal-based saturated fats, which have been linked to pain and inflammation. Plus, you'll get plenty of complex carbohydrates, which will keep your blood sugar levels steady and your mood on an even keel.

- **Crank up the calcium.** This mineral was voted by women as one of the top treatments for premenstrual syndrome because it can soothe cramps, low-back pain, bloating, food cravings, and mood swings all at once. Try taking 1,000 milligrams a day. Magnesium helps, too, but you might want to go easy on it (stick with 200 milligrams once or twice a day) because too much can give you diarrhea.

Bump up the Bs

Vitamin B_6 seems to have a positive effect on levels of serotonin, a feel-good chemical in the brain. Make sure it's in your daily multivitamin.

Alternate Heat and Cold

You can unkink menstrual cramps with compresses made by soaking washcloths in hot and cold water. First, place a hot compress on your abdomen for about 3 minutes. Replace it with a cold compress left in place for 30 seconds. Repeat the cycle two more times, always ending with cold. This simple technique is a very effective way to increase blood flow, which in turn reduces cramps.

Ease with Oil

A castor oil pack is a traditional way to ease the pain of menstrual cramps. First, spread castor oil on the skin of your abdomen and cover it with

dial the DOCTOR

Catch Bad Cramps

Certain types of cramps may signal a serious medical problem, such as endometriosis or fibroid tumors, that has nothing to do with menstruation. See your doctor if cramps don't disappear after your period ends; if the pain is on only one side rather than the entire abdomen; or if you don't get relief from aspirin, ibuprofen, or related drugs.

a layer of plastic wrap. Then heat the area with a warm, moist towel or a heating pad set on low. The gentle heat penetrates deeply into your abdomen and relaxes muscles as well as cramps. *Caution:* Don't use this remedy if you have heavy menstrual bleeding.

Experiment with Exercise

Studies show that exercise eases premenstrual and menstrual symptoms, but a high-impact workout may be uncomfortable if you're cramping. Take it easy for a few days and stick to low-impact forms of exercise, such as yoga, swimming, or tai chi. You may get relief from these moves:

■ **Stretch like a cat.** Yoga's great for menstrual problems because it's relaxing, and it increases circulation. One yoga pose in particular, called

Munch Pumpkin Seeds

They're loaded with essential fatty acids (EFAs) that lower levels of body chemicals responsible for muscle aches and menstrual cramps. You can get the same oils by eating ground flaxseed or cold-water fish, such as salmon and tuna. Plan on having at least one of these foods daily when your symptoms are flaring up. Or you can take EFA capsules or liquids, available in health food stores—but only if you're not taking aspirin or prescription blood thinners.

the Cat, is especially helpful because it targets the abdominal area. Get on your hands and knees on the floor. Moving slowly and gently, tilt your pelvis and tailbone toward the floor while arching your back toward the ceiling. Hold the stretch for a few moments, then go the opposite way: Tilt your pelvis upward and let your spine curve toward the floor.

- **Try the Child's Pose.** This is another yoga move that's good for menstrual discomfort. Kneel on the floor, then sit back on your heels. Lean forward, gently lowering your chest until it's resting on your thighs. Extend your arms in front of you until your palms touch the floor. Hold the pose for as long as you're comfortable, then slowly return to the kneeling position. It's very relaxing—and good for you, too!

Migraines

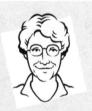

Ice is nice.
Grandma Putt reduced migraine pain by putting a cold pack against the part of her head that hurt. Keep it in place for about 10 minutes to shrink blood vessels and reduce the pounding.

It's true that migraines are a type of headache, but they really don't belong in the same category as garden-variety tension headaches. It's almost impossible to exaggerate how awful migraines can make you feel.

About 26 million Americans get migraines, and women are more prone than men to these miserable skull busters. They occur when blood vessels in your scalp dilate, or expand, and press against nearby nerves. Intense, throbbing pain is just one part of the picture. Many people are so nauseated during migraine attacks that they can't leave the bathroom. They may experience "auras"—sparkling flashes of light or zigzag lines in their field of vision. They may also have weakness or tingling in their face or other parts of their body. It's common for migraines to persist for hours—and sometimes even days—so putting a stop to the pain is a top priority.

Start Early

It's generally fine to take ibuprofen at the first sign of a migraine. Over-the-counter treatments are effective as long as you take them before the migraine really gets under way. Even if you have only "simple" migraines, you should talk to your doctor at some point. There are a number of prescription drugs that can stop migraines within minutes, and there are other treatments that can help keep them from recurring.

Beware the Rebound

A paradoxical thing about migraines is that the same treatments that make you feel better can also make things worse. If you take a lot of aspirin or other medication to control migraines, the pain may come back, or rebound, even more severely as soon as the medication wears off. The natural response is to take more medication, and the cycle continues. Obviously, you shouldn't stop taking a prescription drug without checking with your doctor first, but if you find yourself reaching for aspirin or ibuprofen over and over, you may end up aggravating your migraines, so speak to your doctor.

Allay the Agony

Most people with migraines don't have to spend a fortune on medical care. There are plenty of effective home-care approaches that can reduce

dial the DOCTOR

Pain Signals

If migraine pain doesn't retreat fairly quickly, you'll want to see your doctor. This is especially true if you've had a recent head injury, if the pain occurs on both sides of your head, or if it's accompanied by difficulty speaking or mental confusion. Migraines can be a symptom of serious underlying problems, such as a brain tumor or blood vessel damage, so don't delay in seeking medical help.

your need for high-powered medications. Here are two you may want to try:

- **Take a break.** Lie down immediately in a cool, dark place when you feel a migraine coming on. Moving around will only intensify the pain.

- **Try the caffeine-and-aspirin combo.** The combination of 130 milligrams of caffeine (that's about 1½ cups of coffee) and two aspirins relieves a headache 40 percent better than the pain reliever alone, according to the National Headache Foundation. In addition to starting your motor in the mornings, caffeine helps your body absorb medications. You'll feel the full effects within 30 minutes, and they'll last from three to five hours. Some headache remedies already contain caffeine, so be sure to check the ingredients.

Starve Your Migraine

Many people with migraines find that their attacks are connected to what they eat, and that they usually start 1 to 24 hours after a meal. Trigger foods include alcoholic beverages, particularly red wines and beer; aged cheeses; smoked fish; sour cream; yogurt; and, alas, chocolate, even though some people crave it just before an attack. Food additives and preservatives such as monosodium glutamate (MSG) and sodium nitrate (often found in lunch meats) are known triggers, as are sweeteners containing aspartame.

To figure out if food's fueling your headaches,

keep a simple diary. Write down what you eat and when, as well as when your headaches occur. You'll spot the connections. Another tip: Eating regularly, three times a day, may also help fend off migraines.

Eliminate the Triggers

Most migraines are triggered by external factors. Everyone's different, so you'll have to be a bit of a detective to identify the things that tend to bring yours on. Besides foods, common triggers include bright lights, changes in altitude, and even certain odors. Pay close attention to your environment when you feel a migraine beginning. Over time, you'll start to identify patterns, activities, or specific things that seem to invite these skull busters.

Strike Out Against Stress

A stressful situation can trigger a migraine immediately afterward—it's called a "letdown" migraine. If you are living a migraine lifestyle, you need to take stress reduction seriously. One way to do that is to take up regular aerobic exercise, such as walking, swimming, or bicycling. Besides taming stress, it helps maintain healthy circulation, which can also head off migraines. Whatever activity you choose, do it for 20 to 30 minutes every day, and you'll be healthier all over. Just be sure to check with your doctor before you start any exercise program.

Pamper Your Feet

Reflexology is a type of massage therapy in which pressure is applied to places on the feet that are believed to influence other parts of the body. Find a reflexology practitioner and give the treatment a try—it may just be the answer to your desperate migraine prayers. In a Danish study, regular reflexology treatments helped 81 percent of the participants find relief from their migraines. One-fifth were even able to go off their pain medication.

Live By the Clock

Being overtired can trigger migraines, so try to go to bed and get up at the same times every day. You may even want to eat at regular times, too, since low blood sugar from skipping a meal can bring on a migraine.

Nature's Aspirin

Willow bark contains salicin, which metabolizes in the body in the same way as aspirin, its synthetic cousin, does. To help calm a migraine, pick up some dried willow bark at a health food store, then follow the package directions to brew up a soothing tea. *Caution:* Don't use this herb if you're sensitive to aspirin, and don't combine it with aspirin or alcohol.

Muscle Cramps

One of nature's rules is that for every action, there's a reaction—and your muscles are no exception. Each time you step forward, bend your arm, or squeeze a loaf of bread to see if it's fresh, your muscles contract and then relax. Sometimes, though, they forget the second part of the equation. They contract tightly, then refuse to let go. The result: one heck of an agonizing cramp.

Muscles contract and relax in response to electrical signals generated by electrolytes, which are minerals such as magnesium, calcium, and potassium. Your muscles work normally when levels of these minerals are properly balanced. If there's an imbalance—because you're not getting enough of one or more electrolytes in your diet, your thyroid's out of whack, or the minerals have been depleted by hard exercise—the signals essentially get crossed. The result can be painful cramps.

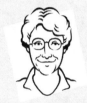

Grandma Says...

Stand for relief. Whenever I got one of those awful foot or toe cramps in the middle of the night, Grandma would have me stand up and put weight on my foot. This stretched the muscles and stopped the cramp, pronto.

Fix It Quick

Muscle cramps rarely last more than a few seconds, but they're not something you want to put up with. For one thing, they're excruciatingly painful. More important, cramps that happen at the wrong time—when you're at the deep end of the pool, for example—can be dangerous. The next time you're clamped by a cramp, try one of these to get out of its grip:

- **Help the muscle move.** A painful muscle cramp will eventually relax on its own, but the sooner you encourage it to do so, the sooner you'll get relief. Since the cramped muscle can't move itself, you'll need to use a free hand to straighten the affected leg, arm, or foot. Gently pull the muscle in the opposite direction from the cramp. Doing this a few times will usually relax the muscle and ease the pain.

- **Rub out the pain.** Some firm finger work will almost always ease a cramped muscle. During a

Eat Green

The greener your midnight snack, the less likely you are to be rudely awakened by middle-of-the-night cramps. Leafy green vegetables, such as spinach, okra, and turnip and beet greens, are chock-full of cramp-stopping electrolytes—especially magnesium, potassium, and calcium. A daily salad or stir-fry that includes these ingredients should keep cramps at bay.

cramp, muscle fibers stay contracted and forget how to relax. Massaging the cramped area will break up the contraction and loosen the muscle.

- **Put minerals in the bank.** Your muscles need healthful amounts of calcium, potassium, and magnesium to function properly. If your stores of these electrolytes have been depleted by exercise or a poor diet, your muscles will become much more prone to cramping. To prevent this, your best bet is to take a daily multivitamin/mineral supplement that contains these and other important minerals.

Soothe with Sour

Hot vinegar is great for relaxing stubborn muscle cramps that last longer than a few moments. Mix equal parts of water and vinegar in a saucepan, heat until comfortably hot, and soak a small towel in the solution. Wring it out and hold it against the painful area for 5 minutes, then replace it with a towel that's been soaked in cold water. Repeat the cycle three times, keeping the hot towel in place for 5 minutes and the cold towel in place for 1 minute, and always end with the cold treatment.

Gulp a Sports Drink

Drinks such as Gatorade contain the minerals that your muscles need in order to function properly. If your cramps are caused by a lack of

dial the
DOCTOR

The Cholesterol Connection

If you're taking cholesterol-lowering medication, report any muscle aches, pains, or cramps to your doctor immediately. They can indicate a rare, life-threatening condition in which muscle—including heart muscle—is being destroyed as a side effect of your medication.

nutrients, a swig of a sports beverage before and during exercise could prevent them from occurring (or recurring).

Stretch It Out

Stretching your muscles before you exercise is essential if you want to prevent cramping. It's especially important if you haven't been active for a while.

Water Your Muscles

Muscles that aren't properly hydrated are more prone to cramping. Drink at least six to eight glasses of water a day, and more if you're going to be sweating heavily. And don't wait until you're thirsty to drink—by the time you start to feel parched, you may already be dehydrated.

Change Position Often

Some cramps happen because a muscle group becomes fatigued after being in the same position for a long time. If you can schedule your day so that you can alternate long tasks with shorter ones, your muscles will appreciate the chance to switch gears. Get up from your desk a few times an hour. Rake leaves as a break from working on your knees in the garden. The more frequently you change position, the less likely you are to have cramps.

Nausea

Good food, good drink, good friends—who doesn't love to celebrate? But all that rich food and tasty libations can make you wish you'd spent the night at home alone, watching TV. While eating or drinking too much can often trigger nausea, all sorts of other things can also make your stomach go topsy-turvy. Among them are infections, stress, bad smells, long car trips, and—URP!—going sailing.

Quell the Queasies

Queasiness doesn't usually last very long, but it can make you mighty miserable in the meantime. Here are some ways to help your stomach settle down:

- **Snap up ginger.** Ginger is widely used as a remedy for upset stomach and nausea. You don't even have to chew the root; simply make a tea by boiling a quarter-size piece of ginger in a cup of water for 5 minutes, then strain.

Tea Time

A homemade infusion of dill seeds can help calm an upset stomach and ease nausea. Steep 1 teaspoon of seeds in 1 cup of hot water, covered, for about 15 minutes. Then strain and sip.

Whenever I was feeling queasy, my Grandma Putt would give me peppermint candies to suck on. The fact is, volatile oils in peppermint can help counteract nausea. A more direct approach is to simply uncap a vial of peppermint oil and inhale for a few seconds. If you're feeling up to a bath, add 4 to 6 drops to your tub and slide in. Just remember to breathe deeply while you're soaking.

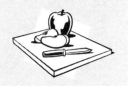

■ **Beat it with broth.** Mix together two 12-ounce cans of vegetable broth or bouillon (or 2 cups of water with three packets of instant vegetable bouillon), two quarter-size pieces of ginger, two cloves of minced garlic, and ¼ cup of soy or tamari sauce. Bring it all to a boil, turn down the heat, and let it simmer for 30 minutes. Sip it slowly by the spoonful.

■ **Soothe with the sweet.** For nausea caused by stress and anxiety, have a cup of meadowsweet tea. Steep 1 heaping teaspoon of the herb in 1 cup of hot water, covered, for 10 minutes, then strain. Sip it slowly to settle your stomach.

■ **Scratch and sniff.** If you're feeling queasy, head for the fridge. Grab an uncut lemon, and scratch into the peel. Then sniff the clean, fresh citrus scent. That's what they do in India to handle bouts of nausea!

Nip Nausea in the Bud

When you're feeling a bit green around the gills, these can help:

■ **Calm with the balm.** Bee balm leaves contain a compound called thymol, which helps ease nausea, vomiting, and even embarrassing flatulence. Simply combine 1 teaspoon of dried bee balm leaves with 1 teaspoon of black or green tea leaves. Put 1 teaspoon of the mixture into 1 cup of boiling water, steep for 5 to 10 minutes, and strain. Sweeten the tea with 1 teaspoon of honey, then sip.

Olives, Anyone?

Does sailing make you queasy and flying turn you green? The next time you launch yourself into major motion, take along some olives. At the first sign of motion sickness, eat a couple. Olives contain tannins that dry your mouth, which reduces the excess saliva that can trigger nausea.

■ **Focus on fluids.** For the first 12 hours after a bout of nausea, drink only clear liquids such as ginger ale, plain water, or soothing teas. Vomiting causes your body to lose a lot of liquid, and it's important to replace it.

■ **Bring on the bland.** When your appetite finally returns, scout around the kitchen for bland foods. Easy-to-digest applesauce, a little plain rice, dry toast, or even a mild cooked vegetable are all good choices.

Osteoporosis

Oil Away Pain

As osteoporosis progresses, the bones in your spine can begin pinching the nerves that run between them. St. John's wort oil works effectively on nerve pain. Massage a small amount into any painful areas two or three times daily. You can find the oil at health food stores.

For years, most of us have been trying to reduce the fat in our diets in order to lose weight and lower cholesterol. In our efforts to save our hearts, however, we may have done long-lasting damage to our bones.

The dairy industry used to have us all convinced that milk is the ideal food. In some ways it is, but in trying to reduce fat, a lot of us simply gave it up. The problem is, milk is among the best sources of calcium, the bone-building mineral that you need to keep your skeleton strong. So it's hardly surprising that osteoporosis—a serious condition in which bones get progressively weaker with age—has become so common in this country. Most women, who are at highest risk for osteoporosis, get only about 450 milligrams of calcium daily, which is nowhere near the 1,000 to 1,500 milligrams that most doctors recommend.

Good to the Bone

Although we can't see, hear, or feel it coming, osteoporosis can happen to anyone. While men generally have larger, stronger bones and don't experience a drop in bone mass the way women do after menopause, they're still at risk as their testosterone levels gradually decline. The good news? Osteoporosis is completely preventable. Here's how to help keep body and bone together:

- **Drink the moo juice.** As long as you buy low-fat or fat-free dairy products, you'll get all the calcium you need without putting weight where you don't want it. One glass of milk, for example, has about 300 milligrams of calcium, while a cup of yogurt has between 275 and 325 milligrams. As a bonus, milk is generally fortified with vitamin D, which you need to help your body absorb calcium.

- **Bite some bones.** No, not like a puppy, but like this: Eat a can of sardines or salmon with bones once or twice a week for a calcium boost. Just 3 ounces of canned salmon with bones has about 200 milligrams of calcium.

- **Pile on the tofu.** Add ½ cup of tofu made with calcium sulfate to salads and stir-fries to get 250 milligrams of calcium. As a bonus, tofu is rich in two major types of isoflavones, compounds that have weak estrogen–like effects and may protect your bones.

- **Go easy on the hooch.** Alcoholism is a major cause of osteoporosis in men. Alcohol poisons

dial the DOCTOR

The Test That's Best

Many women don't get bone density tests until something happens, such as a broken hip, and then it's too late to reverse the damage. You should have this easy test for the first time around age 60 and then each year thereafter to monitor for any changes in bone density. If you have risk factors, such as small stature, lack of exercise, or years of smoking, ask your doctor to give you this test soon.

the bone-forming cells called osteoblasts. If you do drink, do so in moderation. One drink a day for women and two for men is considered moderate.

Can the Soda

Many soft drinks are loaded with phosphorus, a mineral that interferes with calcium absorption. It's fine to have a cola now and then, but water is always a healthier choice.

The Lowdown on D

Your body needs vitamin D—which you can get from food, a supplement, or regular exposure to sunlight—to absorb calcium. Take 400 IU of vitamin D_3 each day if you are over age 50. If you are over age 70, you need 600 IU daily. The best food sources of D are salmon and tuna and some types of mushrooms.

If you spend sufficient time outdoors, you may not need a vitamin supplement. After age 50, however, our bodies have more difficulty manufacturing vitamin D from sunlight and absorbing it from food. So if you do want to soak it up from the sun, you should expose your face and arms for 15 minutes before you put on any sunscreen. But keep in mind that in northern climates, the sun's low angle from November to March prevents it from providing much benefit, so be sure to drink vitamin D–enriched milk during the winter months.

Get More Magnesium

This mineral helps promote bone health. The best sources are potatoes, seeds, nuts, legumes, whole grains, and dark green vegetables. Ask your doctor about supplements if you don't think you're getting enough in your diet.

Shake Dem Bones

When your bones are challenged, they rise to the occasion. Just 60 seconds of running during a brisk walk is enough to shift your bones into a strengthening mode. Since you need to perform at least 30 minutes of weight-bearing exercise three times a week, and the American Academy of Orthopedic Surgeons says running ranks the highest for bone building, hit the pavement to walk and run your way to better bones. If running isn't your cup of tea, don't despair. There are other surefire ways to get the weight-bearing exercise you need:

- **Get out in the garden.** According to a report in the *Journal of the American Geriatric Society*, moderate physical activity such as gardening reduces the risk of hip fracture by 20 to 60 percent. In fact, one study showed that women who did some form of leisure activity for more than three hours a week had about half as much chance of fracturing a hip as those who were sedentary. So grab a trowel and get gardening!

- **Stamp your feet.** No, don't have a tantrum— but do take up step dancing or get out the

Tea Time

Nettle, horsetail, oatstraw, alfalfa, dandelion, chicory, kelp, and bladderwrack can all be made into bone-boosting teas. Combine equal parts of two or more of these dried herbs, steep 1 heaping tablespoon in 1 quart of hot water for 10 minutes, and strain. *Caution:* Dandelion is rich in potassium and shouldn't be taken with potassium tablets.

When times were hard, Grandma Putt relied on penny-pinching recipes like bone soup. She didn't realize she was doing our bones a world of good with every bowl—just 1 pint of this soup can give you as much as 1,000 mg. of calcium. To make it, pick up beef bones at the meat counter. Put them in a soup pot with water, vegetables, potatoes, your favorite herbs and spices—and vinegar (it dissolves calcium from the bones).

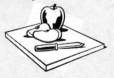

castanets and try some flamenco. With every step you take, the striking of your heel on a hard surface creates stress on your skeleton. In response, it strengthens and renews itself. Going down stairs is also ideal, as is ballroom dancing—especially if you do it for two hours several times a week.

■ **Build 'em with weights.** Regular strength training does more than just keep you fit: The pull of your muscles as you work out stimulates your bones to increase their density. In fact, in a landmark study, 20 sedentary postmenopausal women attended two weekly supervised weight-lifting sessions of about 45 minutes each. In just one year, they gained an average of 1 percent in bone density, while the control group, who didn't lift weights, lost about 2 percent in bone density. What's more, members of the weight-lifting group were soon in-line skating, playing tennis, gardening, shoveling snow, and walking—doing things they hadn't done in years! If you don't have dumbbells, you can hoist a couple of heavy cans of food. Just be sure both cans are the same weight.

■ **Hold up a wall.** Wall pushups are an easy way to strengthen the bones in your upper body. To perform this simple exercise, put your hands flat on a wall, level with and about as far apart as your shoulders, and take a step away from the wall. Lean into the wall, then push your body away from it. Repeat several times at least three times a week.

Pizza Mouth

We eat hot foods all the time without getting burned, so what is it about pizza that almost guarantees the occasional singed mouth? Eagerness obviously has something to do with it. Take one sniff of that delicious rising steam, and it's hard to resist diving right in before it cools. Then there's the molten cheese: It's not only hot right out of the oven, but it stays hot for a long time. Yow! Instant burn.

Stop the Singe

A burned mouth is no laughing matter. It takes only a second for hot foods to sear the delicate tissues in your mouth. The area will usually heal within a few days, but it can be hard to eat in the meantime. To reduce pain and help the burn heal more quickly, here are some tips to try:

- **Stick to cool cuisine.** The last thing your mouth needs after a close encounter with scorching pizza is even more heat. Remember, you've already burned off a protective layer of skin.

B for Burns

The next time you burn your mouth with hot pizza, make the second course a fresh green salad. Spinach, arugula, and other leafy greens are loaded with folate, a B vitamin that helps damaged cells grow and reproduce to repair damage. While you're recovering, take a supplement containing 400 micrograms of folic acid.

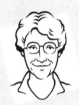

Grandma Says...

Chill out. Whenever I was a bit overeager to bite into hot pizza, Grandma Putt told me to suck on an ice cube to ease the pain of my burned mouth. Ice helps strip away the heat, numb the pain, and slow inflammation. You can also swish ice water around in your mouth for about 20 seconds.

Eating anything hot at that point will be doubly painful. So stick to cool foods for a day or two when you've got a bad burn. Cool soups are good choices, as are salads and sandwiches. And just say "no" to Mexican food. The chemical compounds that put the heat in salsa, chili, and other spicy foods will really irritate the burn.

- **Try a slippery swish.** Slippery elm is one of the best herbal remedies for pizza mouth. It's soothing, it reduces irritation and inflammation, and it shortens the healing time for burns. Buy the powdered form at a health food store, and mix it with water. Several times a day, swish the solution around in your mouth, then swallow it or spit it out.

- **Heal with St. John's.** To help a pizza burn heal more quickly, put a tiny amount of St. John's wort oil, available at health food stores, on your finger and dab it on the sore area once or twice a day.

Eliminate the Acids

Forget oranges, pineapple, tomatoes, and other acidic foods when you're recovering from pizza mouth. Apart from causing pain, they'll increase the time it takes the injury to heal.

Avoid the Crunchies

There's a good reason that people with pizza mouth often find themselves eating a lot of cot-

Heal with Bicarbonate

Rinsing with a baking soda solution will reduce acidity in your mouth. That's important because mouth acids cause additional pain, and their levels rise quickly after burns or other injuries. Add a level teaspoon of baking soda to an 8-ounce glass of water and swish the solution around in your mouth a couple of times a day until the discomfort is gone.

tage cheese and similar foods. Anything with hard edges, such as pretzels or carrot pieces, can jab against the roof of your mouth and make the pain worse.

Protect the Area

You can't stick a bandage on your tongue or the roof of your mouth, but you can cover the area with an over-the-counter adhesive gel such as Orabase. It will form a shield against irritation from acids and other pain-causing substances.

Nix the Salt Water

A traditional remedy for mouth burns is to gargle with salt water, but take this advice with a grain of salt. Salt water can actually increase discomfort and slow healing time.

Pneumonia

dial the DOCTOR

Listen to Your Lungs

Pneumonia kills more than 40,000 Americans each year. If you develop a fever, difficulty breathing, or chest pain, or if you begin coughing up blood, go to an emergency room right away.

As long as there have been scarves, parkas, and knitted hats, moms have been saying, "Dress warmly or you'll get pneumonia!" No offense to Mom, but cold weather actually has very little to do with it. Pneumonia is the general term for inflammation of the lungs. Like other infections, it can be caused by bacteria, a virus, or even a fungus or parasite. As you might guess, your lungs are protected by some pretty sophisticated defense mechanisms. When those defenses are weaker than they should be—because of smoking, for example, or the natural decline in immunity that occurs as we get older—germs are more likely to multiply.

Bad Luck for the Lungs

The symptoms of viral pneumonia are pretty much the same as those of the flu. You may have a fever, chest pain, coughing, chills, muscle pains, and fatigue. In addition, you'll find it increasingly difficult to breathe as the illness progresses. Your lungs simply can't function well when they're compromised by infection-related inflammation and fluid buildup. Even though many people with pneumonia naturally recover on their own, the fact remains that your lungs are pretty crucial pieces of equipment, and severe pneumonia is life-threatening. It doesn't pay to take chances: You must see a doctor if you even *suspect* that you have pneumonia.

Antibiotics and other medications can knock out bacterial pneumonia pretty quickly, but severe pneumonia requires ongoing care, either at home or in the hospital, to ensure that your lungs make a full recovery.

Save Your Breath

By now you're probably thinking that pneumonia sounds pretty scary. But it doesn't have to be. In most cases, you can get back on your feet without multiple visits to your doctor. Here are a few things you can do to help bounce back:

- **Stay close to water.** You should never be more than an arm's length away from a glass of water while you're recovering. So drink at least eight glasses a day. Drinking lots of water dilutes all the mucus your lungs produce when you have pneumonia. You'll breathe easier, and your lungs will recover more quickly.

- **Take plenty of downtime.** Your immune system needs every ounce of energy it can

From Grandma's Kitchen

Grandma Putt would often whip up something garlicky-good for me to eat when I had a chest cold. Now we know that garlic is one of the best herbs for strengthening our immunity and fighting infections. To get the most out of this powerful herb, take your garlic straight up by eating two raw cloves a day until the infection is gone. If that's too intense for you, lightly bake the garlic to sweeten it up a bit.

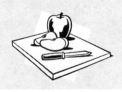

muster to defeat pneumonia, so it's important to get as much rest as you can.

- **Eat some eggs.** They come in single-serving packages (no leftovers!), and they're stuffed with easy-to-digest protein that your body needs to recover. They also build immunity and can help prevent flu as well as pneumonia.

Encourage Coughs

The chest-racking cough that accompanies pneumonia can be agonizing, but you don't necessarily want to block it with a cough suppressant. Coughing is your body's way of expelling the gunk that's clogging your lungs. The more mucus you cough up, the better you'll feel, and the more quickly you'll recover.

Of course, there are times when a cough is so severe that it interferes with your sleep or causes intense pain. In fact, people have even broken ribs during coughing attacks! So if your cough is really bad, go ahead and use an over-the-counter cough suppressant, following the label directions.

Heal with Humidity

A dry environment causes mucus to dry and thicken, impeding your recovery. Keep the air moist with a humidifier or bedside vaporizer, but be sure to get some fresh air at the same time. If you have a window where you're spending most of your time, keep it cracked open.

Dodge the Dairy

Milk, cheese, and other dairy foods are loaded with beneficial calcium and protein, but they also tend to thicken mucus—the last thing you need when you're recovering from pneumonia. So stay away from dairy products until the infection is gone.

Salt to the Rescue

Your nose and throat will probably feel intensely irritated when you're battling pneumonia. Sniffing salt water is a quick way to ease the discomfort because it draws fluid from the tissues and encourages the inflammation to clear up. You can buy ready-made saline solution at drugstores, or you can make your own by mixing a few teaspoons of salt in a few ounces of warm water. Cup some of the solution in your hand, sniff it into your nostrils, then blow it out.

Slurp That Soup

For one thing, soup increases the amount of lung-cleansing fluids in your body. In addition, it provides an abundance of healing nutrients, and it's easy to eat when you're sick and your appetite is low. Soup has even more benefits. The warmth helps loosen mucus in your chest, and the high protein content of chicken or other meat-based soup helps your body recover. There's also some evidence that chicken soup increases the activity of immune cells that help mop up infections.

Rashes

dial the DOCTOR

Don't Delay

Always check with your doctor when you discover a new, unexplained blemish on your skin. It's probably a rash (or maybe a mole), but it could be skin cancer. Be especially concerned if the "rash" displays any characteristics in "Know Your ABCDs" on page 288.

Are you one of those lucky people who have never had a rash? Nope, didn't think so. There are probably hundreds of potential causes of rashes, and no one's immune to all of them. Insect stings can obviously cause a rash. So can poison ivy. Eczema. Reactions to metal jewelry. Diet. Stress. The list goes on and on. Obviously, the best treatment will depend on what's causing the rash in the first place. Some rashes are just reddened skin. Others burn or sting. Still others are maddeningly itchy. It all depends on what's behind the rash, and how your skin reacts to it.

Take Action

If you keep getting rashes and you don't know why, you obviously need to see a doctor. Once you determine what's making you break out, then you can take steps to avoid it. If that's not possible, your doctor may advise you to take antihistamines or use topical steroids to control the symptoms. In the meantime, here are a few ways to defend yourself:

■ **Get your pencil ready.** A recurring rash has so many possible causes that it may take careful observation—and a lot of notes—to get to the root of it. Ask and answer as many questions about the rash as you can. Has it been there a long time, or did it just appear? Is it a reaction to something that touched your skin? Were there any recent changes in your diet, clothing, or environment that preceded it? The answers to these kinds of questions will help you determine the best way to respond.

■ **Say "ahh" with oats.** An almost instant way to ease a dry, itchy rash is to treat it to an oatmeal bath. You can buy a colloidal oatmeal kit at most drugstores. Add the finely ground oatmeal to warm (not hot) water, then settle in for a soothing soak. You can also fill an old sock with plain dry oatmeal, then fasten the open end to the faucet with a rubber band. Fill the tub with warm water, letting the water run through the sock. (You can fasten the oatmeal bundle and let it float in the bathtub when you're done filling it.) Oatmeal makes water soft and soothing—perfect for a painful rash.

■ **Mend with an herbal blend.** If your rash is wet and oozing, here's some help: Wash your skin, then help dry up the rash and prevent secondary infections by dusting it with an herbal powder. Mix equal parts of slippery elm powder and goldenseal powder, and gently dust the mixture on the rash for soothing relief and quick healing.

- **Fix it with flax.** People with skin conditions such as eczema are often lacking essential fatty acids. Ideally, you should get these kinds of fats (found in nuts, seeds, and cold-water fish) from your diet, but you can get quick relief by applying them directly to your skin as well. Rub a small amount of flaxseed oil into rashy areas before going to bed and after bathing, and sweet relief will soon be on its way.

- **Lose the heavy metal.** Earrings with nickel wires and posts commonly cause rashes in people with metal allergies. You'll know if you're one of them: A metal allergy will make you itch within 20 minutes, and a rash will usually appear within a day or two. To avoid both, make sure only stainless steel needles are used for ear piercing, and buy earrings with stainless steel posts. Although stainless steel does contain some nickel, it is bound so tightly to the steel that it is safe, says the American Academy of Dermatology. In addition to your jewelry, check buttons, fasteners, and zippers. If they touch your skin, they can cause a rash.

Stay Balanced

Very hot or very cold temperatures can aggravate a skin rash. Unfortunately, you won't find the perfect environment anywhere, except maybe in the next biosphere, but if you can, avoid exposing your skin to extreme heat and cold. Also avoid sudden changes in temperature or humidity, which can trigger a rash.

Check Your Cosmetics

Even if you've used the same brands of makeup for years without any problems, you can get a rash if the company changes the chemical ingredients. Choose products with no fillers, dyes, or added colors, and those labeled "hypoallergenic."

Keep a Diet Diary

A recurring or chronic rash could be triggered by something in your diet—dairy foods, wheat, corn, or citrus fruits, for example. Keeping a record of everything you eat over the course of several weeks and noting when the rash occurs and subsides may flush out the cause—or at least

MODERN MARVEL

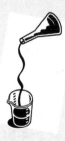

Calm It with Cream

Hydrocortisone cream is an anti-inflammatory steroid cream that is safe for self-care, says the American Academy of Dermatology. It blocks the allergic skin reactions that trigger some rashes, and it can speed healing of inflamed or cracked skin, regardless of the cause. You can find it at drugstores.

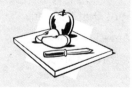
narrow the pool of suspects. Remember, a rash can appear 24 to 72 hours after you eat the problem food.

Heal with Hydrotherapy

This is just a fancy way of saying that you may want to use warm or cool compresses to get relief. If you have a rash that feels warm to the touch, for example, you may want to soak a small towel in cool water and drape it over the area to relieve the discomfort. If your rash feels dry and itchy, a warm compress may be more effective.

Get some R&R

Sometimes a rash appears because your body's overloaded with stress or irritating waste products. One of the best things you can do is take some time to relax and get the stress out of your life. Start by taking an hour a day to just play. Go to the zoo, head for the pool, or dig in the dirt. That may be enough to make the rash disappear.

Make Time for Marigolds

Marigold (a.k.a. calendula) blossoms are skin-friendly botanicals that are great for stopping a rash in its tracks. The next time a rash appears, dab on marigold oil with a cotton swab or clean cloth. Keep applying the oil, available at health food stores, until the rash is gone.

Shingles

Consider yourself lucky if you never had chickenpox when you were a kid. Apart from the fact that you were spared those ugly, itchy, red bumps that could have kept you housebound for a few weeks, you'll never have to worry that a sneaky virus is lurking somewhere in your body. You see, the virus that causes chickenpox never goes away altogether. It just goes into hiding. Sooner or later, it may reappear to cause a painful, blistering disease known as shingles.

Painfully Ugly

If you've had chickenpox, there's about a 40 percent chance that you'll eventually have an attack of shingles. The virus that causes the original infection isn't completely destroyed by your immune system. Instead, it slips deep into the nerves and remains there in a dormant state. In some people, it stays dormant; in others, it wakes up, travels up the nerves to the skin, and causes

Tea Time

Hot tea made with rose hips is good for you when you have shingles. It's high in vitamin C, and taking the time to enjoy a cup of tea will help you relax and maintain immunity. Drop a teaspoon of dried rose hips into a cup of boiled water. Steep for 15 minutes, strain out the herb, and enjoy your tea.

A Rash Approach

If you're over age 50, there's a good chance that nerve damage caused by the shingles virus will cause lingering pain known as postherpetic neuralgia.

It's worth seeing your doctor right away. You may need pain-killers or other medications to tide you over. In addition, there are drugs that can shorten the duration of attacks if they're given within 24 hours of the start of blisters.

a painful, blistery outbreak. The sores usually appear in a band across the torso or buttocks, and sometimes on the face.

The good news is that shingles isn't dangerous in most cases, and it does clear up on its own. To reduce your discomfort in the meantime, take the following tips to heart:

- **Be serious about cleaning.** Wash the blisters twice a day with regular soap and water to prevent infection. Resist the urge to cover them up with a bandage. And hang in there—the rash usually runs its course in three weeks or so.

- **Rub away the itch.** If the touch of clothing against your skin drives you crazy, here's a way to defuse the sensitivity: Rub the area with a clean towel for several minutes—after you've gotten the okay from your doctor.

- **Nix nerve pain.** St. John's wort oil may reduce any nerve pain that lingers once the shingles have cleared up. Apply the oil directly to your skin two or three times daily.

- **Pop a few aspirin.** Over-the-counter remedies such as aspirin and ibuprofen can help control shingles pain.

- **Add some vitamin C.** When you're battling the shingles virus, extra vitamin C, which is an immune booster, is helpful as long as you don't have kidney or stomach problems. Check with your doctor about the amount that's right for you.

Try an Alphabet Combo

A potent nutrient combo that will strengthen your immune system and help shingles blisters heal more quickly includes vitamins A, C, and E, plus the mineral zinc. Look for a supplement that contains each of these important nutrients and follow the label directions.

Fight Back with Herbs

Enlist these herbal helpers in your battle with shingles. Some help fend off the virus while others soothe its symptoms:

- **Echinacea.** It's one of the most powerful herbs for strengthening the immune system, and it will gear up your defenses to fend off the shingles virus. Echinacea is more effective in the early stages, so start taking it as soon as you notice symptoms. It's available in capsule form at health food stores and drugstores; follow the label directions. *Caution:* Don't take it if you have an autoimmune disease such as rheumatoid arthritis, lupus, or multiple sclerosis, or if you're pregnant or nursing.

- **Chickweed.** Don't let the name fool you: The herb chickweed is no mere weed. It's a wonderful anti-itch herb. You can buy creams or salves made with chickweed at health food stores.

- **Valerian.** This herb sedates the nervous system and helps put a damper on the pain of shingles. It's especially useful when you are having difficulty sleeping because of the pain. To make a soothing tea, steep 1 heaping teaspoon of the herb in 1 cup of freshly boiled water for 10 minutes, then strain. Drink one cup after dinner and one before bed. *Caution:* Do not use valerian with pain relievers or anti-anxiety or antidepressant medications.

Ease it with Ice

A fast way to reduce the itching and pain of shingles is to wrap a few ice cubes in a washcloth or small towel, and hold them against the tender spots. Ice acts as a local anesthetic by temporarily numbing the skin. If you have trouble keeping the ice pack in place, make a cold "slush pack" that conforms to the shape of your body. Mix 1 part rubbing alcohol with 4 parts water, fill a few plastic zipper-lock bags with the mixture, and put them in the freezer. After they're chilled, take one out and use it on your shingles for up to 20 minutes at a time.

Pepper Away Pain

Rubbing hot-pepper ointment on your painful skin may not sound as though it would put out the fire, but apparently it does. The American Academy of Dermatology says that ointments made with capsaicin, the element that provides the heat in hot peppers, can help some people with shingles. Apply it three or four times a day, and within one to two weeks, the pain should gradually ease. Check with your doctor about what strength to buy, and when you apply it, be careful not to get it near your eyes or any area of broken skin.

Soak in Oats

A warm bath spiked with a cup of colloidal oatmeal can help keep itchy shingles from driving you crazy. You can buy it at most drugstores and supermarkets. Or you can fill a sock with regular dry oatmeal, fasten the sock to the faucet with a rubber band, and let the water run through it as you fill the tub. If you don't have oatmeal, add a cup of baking soda to the water.

Baby Those Blisters

Shingles blisters are a lot more painful than the kind you get from too much hiking or working in the yard. They can be so sensitive, in fact, that even the pressure from heavy clothes can be agonizing. Until they're gone, get in the habit of wearing loose, light clothing.

Don't Be a Typhoid Mary

Shingles blisters are packed with live viruses that can potentially cause chickenpox in people who haven't had it. Don't let anyone touch the blisters, and take the time to clean them every day with soap and water.

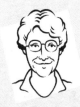

Grandma Says

Think pink. It's been on drugstore shelves almost forever, and was Grandma Putt's favorite cure for itchy skin. I'm talking about calamine lotion, best known for its vivid pink hue. It can ease the itch of shingles and reduce pain, as well. Apply the lotion after a shower or bath, and several more times during the day.

Shin Splints

If you've always been a casual athlete—you enjoy staying in shape but aren't exactly fanatical about it—you'll probably never get shin splints. Serious athletes, on the other hand, get them all the time. Some even consider them a badge of honor. As if there's anything honorable about agonizing pain!

The term shin splints, incidentally, isn't a medical term. Truth be told, doctors don't even know how this particular pain in the front of the lower leg—pain that's aggravated by exercise—got its name. They do know what causes it, though. What probably happens is that you strain or slightly tear one of the tendons in your lower leg. This usually happens at either end of the athletic spectrum: Elite athletes who push themselves really hard often get shin splints, and so do beginners who aren't quite as fit as they think they are. The good news is that shin splints don't need medical attention.

Your Wakeup Call

Shin splints hurt, but usually not as much as a serious sprain or strain—and the pain almost always goes away once you get a little rest. Consider the pain of shin splints to be a warning that it's time to take things a bit easier. In the meantime, try these tips to recover more quickly and prevent future problems:

- **Lie low for a while.** You're likely to get shin splints only when you're dishing out more stress than your body is able to handle. For instance, if you're a weekend warrior who tends to push yourself hard, you're a candidate. The solution, obviously, is to rest. For most recreational runners (shin splints are a problem mainly for runners), taking a week off is usually enough to eliminate the pain.

- **Do the cube cure.** Ice cubes are your best friends when you're coping with shin splints, since putting cold on your lower leg will help

MODERN MARVEL

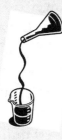

Protect Your Arches

If you have flat or fallen arches, you may be at risk for shin splints. One of the easiest solutions is to drop by a drugstore and pick up some orthotic shoe inserts, which will support your feet and help keep your lower legs pain-free. You can also visit an orthopedic doctor to be fitted for custom inserts.

reduce swelling as well as pain. Apply a cold pack or ice cubes wrapped in a washcloth or small towel to the area that hurts. Keep it in place for 20 minutes and repeat the treatment every hour or two until you're feeling better.

- **Get new shoes.** Running shoes that are badly worn are a common cause of shin splints, so plan on replacing your shoes about every 300 miles. In addition, don't settle for shoes that don't fit perfectly, because they give poor support and put excessive strain on the muscles and tendons in your lower legs.

- **Stay level.** One of the quickest solutions for shin splints is simply to run on level ground—a running trail, for example, or the track at a local high school or college. Runners who stay off rocky or uneven terrain often improve right away and stay pain-free in the future.

The Sour Solution

Moist heat is a great treatment for shin pain, and adding vinegar to the mix increases the anti-inflammatory power. Heat a mixture of equal parts vinegar and water, soak a small towel, wring it out, and apply it where you hurt. Leave it on for about 20 minutes. If you don't have any vinegar in the house, you can get similar results with castor oil. Rub the oil onto your sore shin, cover the oil with plastic wrap, then top that with a hot, moist towel. Leave it on for 20 minutes, then wash off the oil with soap and water.

Go Half-and-Half

You're more likely to get shin splints if you run every day. A better approach, especially if you're just beginning a workout program, is to run one day, take a day or two off, then run again. Giving your muscles a little recovery time means that you'll be less likely to limp home with shin splints. A great way to loosen up your legs and prepare them for an injury-free run is simply to walk for a few minutes. It gets your muscles nice and warmed up before strenuous exertion.

Walk into a Wall

Well, stretch into one, anyway. If ice and pain pills don't make you feel better, you may want to try some gentle stretching. It helps the muscles relax and flushes away waste products that contribute to the pain. Here's a stretch that will help: Stand in front of a wall with your legs shoulder-width apart and one foot a step or two in front of the other. Bend the knee of your front leg while keeping your rear leg straight, then lean into the wall, keeping both heels flat on the floor. Hold the stretch for 5 to 10 seconds, then switch leg positions and repeat.

Sinusitis

Tea Time

Nothing clears your sinuses faster than a bite of horseradish root. If that's too intense, make a tea by grating 1 teaspoon of fresh root into 1 cup of hot water. Steep for 5 minutes, then strain. Drink three cups a day.

Has anyone ever told you that you have holes in your head? We usually use this humorous expression when someone's a little absent-minded, but there's also some literal truth to it. We do have holes in our heads. They're called sinuses, and they're simply empty spaces found above and below the eyes and on either side of the nose.

Actually, life would be better sometimes if the sinuses really were empty, but that's not always the case. All too often, the mucous membranes that line the sinuses provide a safe haven for harmful bacteria. The resulting infection can cause fever, facial pain, and unbelievably painful headaches.

The sinuses normally produce a steady flow of mucus that traps dust particles and other airborne irritants, and keeps them out of the lungs. When you have a cold or allergies, however, the resulting congestion can prevent mucus from getting out. Bacteria love all that stagnant fluid, and they multiply like crazy. That's when you start holding your head and looking for a quiet place to lie down.

Save Your Sinuses

In most cases, sinusitis clears up on its own, usually within a week. If you're sick for longer than that, check with your doctor. You may need antibiotics to clear up the remaining infection. In the meantime, though, the trick to beating sinusitis is to restore the normal flow of mucus. Here's how:

■ **Whack it with wasabi.** This powerful Japanese horseradish, which could blow the lid off a manhole, will empty your sinuses. It's available at Asian restaurants and grocery stores, as well as some health food stores. Use it as a dip for sushi—or take it straight, if you dare!

MODERN MARVEL

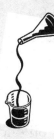

Clear the Air

Keep your environment as dust-free as possible by using an air-filtering system. If you can, keep your home and car air-conditioned to help filter out the pollens and allergens in the outside air. Your sinuses will thank you for it.

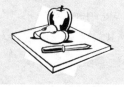

■**Snort some salt.** Use a saline nasal spray several times a day to remove mucus that could harbor bacteria. If you can find one that contains eucalyptus, so much the better, since eucalyptus kills bacteria.

■**Apply deep heat.** When your sinuses are acting up, place a hot, damp towel over the top half of your face and let the heat penetrate into your nasal cavities. Leave it there for 15 minutes, then repeat three or four times a day to promote drainage and increase blood flow.

■**Breathe tropical air.** Inhaling steam is one of the best ways to clear clogged sinuses. Boil a pot of water and remove it from the stove. Drape a towel over your head to trap the steam, lean over the pot (being careful not to scald yourself), and breathe in the steam. Add eucalyptus leaves to boost the penetrating power.

A Peachy Cure

If you've come down with sinusitis, pick up a peach. One small study found that people with sinusitis may not be getting enough glutathione, an antioxidant compound found in peaches and other fruits, such as watermelon and oranges.

Add Some Oils

To open your nasal passages, use a sinus oil once or twice daily. First, soak a washcloth in hot water and apply it to your face to increase circulation to the area. Keep the cloth in place for 5 minutes, resoaking it to keep it as hot as you can tolerate. Then apply a thin layer of olive oil to your frontal bone, above your eyes and cheekbones, below your eyes, and on the bony part of your nose. Next, place a couple of drops of eucalyptus oil on your fingers, and rub it into the same areas. Finally, place the hot cloth over your face again and rest for 15 minutes.

Fry up Some Salt

It sounds strange, but it's a traditional Russian remedy for sinusitis. Heat some salt in a frying pan, then spread it on a towel or clean cloth. Fold the cloth and put it over the bridge of your nose. The heat will open your sinuses.

Watch What You Drink

While you need to keep hydrated when you've got sinus trouble, don't drink milk. Along with the rest of the dairy family, milk thickens mucus. Since you already have enough of that clogging up your sinuses, avoid milk and dairy products until you're better. Instead, put water to work. Drink at least eight glasses a day to thin out your nasal mucus and improve its ability to drain.

Sore Throats

It's amazing what your throat puts up with on an average day. Dust and pollen, to start with, along with the occasional swarm of bacteria or viruses. Then there's hollering at the top of your lungs at concerts, or singing "O Solo Mio" in the shower. It's no wonder that your throat gets a little sore sometimes.

See a doctor if your sore throat lasts longer than about a week. You could have a bacterial infection that needs antibiotics.

Tame the Pain

Fortunately, most sore throats get better on their own, but they can make you mighty miserable in the meantime. Here are some time-tested remedies that really work wonders:

- **Load up on lozenges.** Use throat lozenges or hard candies to keep your throat moist. Look for cherry lozenges with benzocaine to numb your throat temporarily and help with swallowing. Slippery elm lozenges work well, too.

dial the DOCTOR

The Strep Trap

If your sore throat is accompanied by white spots in your mouth and throat or by difficulty swallowing, see your doctor immediately. You may have a strep infection, which can lead to serious complications if not treated appropriately.

- **Shhh.** The less work your throat muscles and membranes have to do, the better you will feel. Save the speeches until your throat has healed. Better skip the choir rehearsals, too.

- **Quell it with calendula.** For a speedy end to soreness, paint your throat with fresh calendula juice or tincture. Simply dip a cotton swab in the calendula juice and apply it thoroughly to the back of your throat, paying particular attention to the sides. Too unpleasant for you? Make a strong infusion of calendula and gargle with it. Steep a heaping teaspoon in ½ cup of hot water for 10 minutes, strain and let cool, and use as needed.

- **Pucker up.** No cough drops or candy handy? Soak half a lemon in salt water, then suck on it for a while. This treatment moistens your throat and relieves soreness.

- **Ease it with violet.** Violets are not only beautiful, but they're medicinal, too, helping to ease the pain of a sore throat caused by a cough. Simply steep 1 heaping teaspoon of violet flowers in 1 cup of hot water for 10 minutes, then strain. Drink two or three cups a day, sipping slowly to bathe your throat.

Swig Some Juice

If you own a juicer, now's the time to rev it up. Juices are a great source of the extra fluids and natural healing substances your body needs to

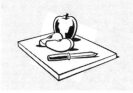

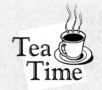
help cure a sore throat. All fruit juices are beneficial, but papaya, orange, and pineapple are good choices because they're loaded with vitamin C. Other throat-comforting produce includes carrots, spinach, blueberries, and dark cherries. The juice will be especially soothing if you warm it slightly before drinking it. If the flavor is too intense, just add a bit of water.

Ace It with A and C

Both of these nutrients strengthen immunity and increase the activity of specialized cells that fight infection. Take a multivitamin that contains both—plus (if you don't have stomach or kidney problems) 500 milligrams of vitamin C twice a day.

Gobble Garlic

This herb is one of the best remedies for sore throats, as well as for colds and flu, because it has anti-inflammatory, antiviral, and antibacterial properties. The problem with garlic, of course, is that you'd have to eat a fair amount to take advantage of its healing properties—and that can give you a powerful aroma. To get the benefits without the stink, take odor-free garlic capsules. Look for a supplement that provides about 10 milligrams of allicin, the active ingredient.

If you're a true garlic fan, though, go ahead and enjoy the real McCoy. Plan on eating one or two cloves a day. Raw or lightly steamed garlic provides more allicin than garlic that has been thoroughly cooked. Just don't decide to visit with the neighbors until you've showered and brushed your teeth!

An E-Z Answer

Enlist echinacea and zinc in your battle against a sore throat. The herb echinacea is like a general who rallies the troops: It stimulates the immune cells that fight off throat-burning infections. You can brew echinacea tea, but it's easier to take capsules. The recommended dose is 350 milligrams three times a day. *Caution:* Don't take echinacea if you have an autoimmune disease such as rheumatoid arthritis, lupus, or multiple sclerosis, or if you are pregnant or nursing.

It may be at the end of the mineralogical alphabet, but zinc comes first when you need to

Lick It with Licorice

Licorice root is loaded with natural chemical compounds that soothe inflammation anywhere in your digestive tract, including your throat. Don't bother with licorice candy, though; it has only licorice flavor, not real licorice. What you want is licorice capsules, so visit your local health food store, then take 100 milligrams three times a day. Since a substance in licorice called glycyrrhizic acid can cause high blood pressure in some people, look for deglycyrrhizinated licorice (DGL) products.

soothe a sore throat. It makes your throat feel better, and boosts your immune system. So suck on zinc gluconate lozenges, available at most drugstores.

Axe Those Allergies

If you tend to get sore throats during ragweed season (ragweed is one of the most common allergy triggers), you may want to take herbal supplements that contain nettle. The herb blocks the action of histamines, natural chemicals that fire up allergic reactions. Take 200 milligrams three times daily until your allergies—and your sore throat—are better.

Simmer Some Soup

Your throat will heal faster if you don't overuse it by swallowing solid food. And if you happen to have a cold, you'll bounce back faster if your body doesn't expend a lot of energy in digestion. So stay away from heavy, fatty meals and instead keep them light and liquid. In other words, this is the best time to eat a bland diet that includes plenty of liquids and easy-to-digest foods. Broths are a great choice. An important bonus: Liquids help make your mucus thinner and more watery, so it will drain more easily and cause less throat irritation.

Splinters

You don't have to be a carpenter to have a close encounter of the splintery kind. The danged things are everywhere—on worn windowsills, old garden tools, and Grandma's old table, to name just a few possibilities. And it's amazing how much a teeny-weeny, hardly-nothin', sliver-of-somethin' can hurt. Yow. Ouch. And maybe even *$#@!!

There's a good reason splinters hurt so much. It's because your fingertips, the usual places you get splinters, are filled with sensitive nerve endings. That's what makes your fingers so deft at knitting or putting puzzles together, but it's also what makes them sting like the dickens when a sliver of wood gets under your skin.

First-Aid Basics

Splinters aren't exactly a medical emergency. Unless the area is badly infected or the splinter is lodged under a nail or somewhere else

From Grandma's Kitchen

Grandma Putt would tape a slice of raw potato onto a splinter and leave it on overnight. If the splinter was in her finger or toe, she'd hollow out the potato and slip the spud on. In the morning, she'd easily pluck out the splinter.

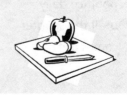

where you can't get at it, there's no reason to call a doctor. You can remove most splinters in the time it takes to read this chapter. But read it anyway, just to be sure that you get the nasty thing out—or not, in some cases—with a minimum of discomfort:

- **Ignore it.** If the splinter is lodged close to the surface of the skin, and the area isn't bleeding or painful, it's okay to just leave it alone. Your body will probably work it out of there on its own. But it's best to keep an eye on it to be sure it isn't digging deeper into the skin or becoming infected.

- **Tweeze to please.** Don't use a needle to root out a splinter. Tweezers work better. Wash the area around the splinter with soap and water, sterilize the tweezers with rubbing alcohol, then grip and pull. And here's a helpful piece of advice: Pull the splinter out of the hole at the same angle that it went in at. This will reduce the chances that it will break off in the skin.

- **Move it out with marshmallow.** Marshmallow ointment can coax a stubborn splinter to the surface of your skin. Dab some ointment (available at health food stores) on the site, bandage it, and leave it alone for a few hours. When you remove the bandage, the splinter will have inched close enough to the surface for you to easily pluck it out.

- **Rub away the pain.** If a splinter hurts like the dickens, but you can't find a way to remove it right away, simply press or rub the skin close to the sliver. The pressure signals travel faster than pain signals, so they get to the brain first. They get all the attention, and you feel less pain.

Clean Like Crazy

Once the splinter's been removed, be sure to keep the skin around the injury clean. Wash the area gently with soap and water once or twice a day, and cover the area with a bandage if it's likely to get dirty. Check the site of the injury for signs of infection—redness, pus, swelling, and so on. You can treat a minor infection with some triple antibiotic ointment, but see a doctor if it doesn't clear up in a day or two.

Soothe with a Soak

The skin where a splinter was embedded will hurt the most right after the sliver has been

MODERN MARVEL

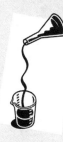

Treat Them Like Warts

The powerful salicylic acids in wart removers can also help you get rid of a splinter. The superficial layers of skin break down and become soft from contact with the acid. Use wart remover disks; they have a higher salicylic acid content than liquid wart removers do.

removed. For quick relief, soak the area in warm water for 10 to 15 minutes. You can also use warm soaks to help propel difficult-to-remove splinters to the skin surface.

To promote healing and ease the sting of splinters, try this triple herbal wash. Combine equal parts of dried calendula, echinacea, and comfrey, which you can find at health food stores. Add a heaping tablespoon of the mixture to a pint of freshly boiled water, and steep for 20 minutes. Strain the liquid, let it cool, and use it to wash the area thoroughly.

Tetanus Alert

Had a tetanus shot lately? Probably not. Do you need one? Probably. Why? Because any sort of break in the skin could be an entrance for tetanus. The tetanus germ can cause painful and potentially fatal muscle spasms, and it tends to live on wood or rusted metal. If you haven't had a tetanus shot in the past 10 years, you're probably due.

Sprains and Strains

Okay, here's a test. What's the difference between a sprain and a strain? Answer: Who cares? They're pretty much alike. Pain is pain, and the treatments for sprains and strains are, for the most part, the same. Just in case you still want to know the answer, a sprain is an injury to the ligaments that support your joints, and a strain is a pulled or overworked muscle. They're usually a result of overextending or twisting your arm or leg beyond its normal range of motion. You end up with pain when you move the limb, as well as swelling and pain in the involved joint. It feels tender to the touch, and you'll probably get black and blue.

Halt the Hurt

Sprains and strains almost always get better on their own, usually within a week or two. Here's what you need to do in the meantime:

Get Comfort with Comfrey

Comfrey wraps work wonders for speeding recovery from a sprain or strain. Blanch two to four leaves and place them on the injured area. Apply an elastic bandage over the leaves, and keep the wrap on all day.

■ **Start with RICE.** It stands for rest, ice, compression, and elevation. In other words, stop the activity and rest the injured body part. Apply a cold compress or ice wrapped in a towel to decrease swelling. Wrap your injured limb in an elastic bandage, or use a splint or sling. And keep the injured part elevated above the level of your heart. Don't use heat until at least 48 hours after the injury. And by all means, seek medical attention if the pain or swelling is severe.

■ **Add herbs to ice.** For a cooling, warming, and healing experience all wrapped in one, add herbal oils to your cold pack. First, fill a bowl with ice-cold water. Sprinkle several drops of oil into the water—try camphor, eucalyptus, chamomile, or rosemary. Next, soak a clean washcloth in the bowl and wring it out well. Lay it over the sprained area and cover with an ice pack. Limit the ice treatment to 10 to 20 minutes to avoid frostbite.

■ **Heat it up.** Once the swelling is gone, you can apply a heating pad set on low or a warm compress. The warmth will penetrate into the tissues and help improve the flow of nutrients to the area, while promoting the outflow of pain-causing substances. Always end warming treatments with an ice pack for 5–10 minutes.

■ **Keep up the pressure.** If you have leg swelling that persists for more than a few days, you may want to get a compression stocking from your doctor or a medical supply store (the ones sold in drugstores aren't measured as precisely). It won't come loose and require rewrapping the way bandages do. Compression stockings provide different amounts of pressure. Get one labeled "25–35," which provides about the same amount of pressure as an elastic bandage.

Down the Drain

A lot of the pain of sprains can come from the buildup of fluids in the area. A quick way to reduce swelling is to gently move the area through its full range of motion now and then. Keep going for a minute or two, but don't push yourself to the point of severe pain. Try it a few times a day while you're recovering.

Fish for Relief

The essential fatty acids (EFAs) found in the oils of cold-water fish such as salmon and tuna help suppress inflammation and speed recovery. These oils also stabilize cell membranes that may have been damaged by the injury. It's a good idea to eat fish three or four times a week until you're feeling better. If you aren't a fish fan, you can get healing amounts of EFAs by eating a tablespoon of ground flaxseed daily. Try sprinkling it on cereal or mixing it with yogurt.

Tea Time

Witch hazel can help shrink the swelling from a sprain or strain. Brew a tea by tossing 1 teaspoon of dried leaves or 2 inches of root into 1 cup of boiling water. Steep for 10 to 15 minutes, then strain. Soak a clean washcloth in the cooled tea and apply it to the affected area several times a day.

Stomachaches

Most stomachaches don't actually occur in your stomach at all, even though that's where the trouble usually begins. For various reasons, your stomach doesn't always do a great job of digesting its contents. When undigested food travels into the intestine, you're likely to experience cramps or painful gas. Thus, a stomachache is really an intestine ache—one that occurs when your bowel has to deal with your stomach's unfinished business.

Temper Tummy Troubles

A stomachache isn't always a routine problem. In fact, there's a long list of medical conditions that cause pain somewhere in the belly, and some of them are serious. You'll want to see your doctor if your stomachache lasts more than a day or two. In most cases, though, you can get relief without fancy tests or high-priced consultations. Here are a few things that are sure to help:

- **Mix a "lawn salad."** Dandelion greens are a traditional remedy for stomach problems of all kinds. Eaten before a meal, the pleasantly bitter leaves stimulate digestive secretions and curb cramps. Be sure to pick your greens from an area that hasn't been treated with chemicals. The leaves are most tender when they're picked just before the flowers bloom.

- **Sniff and settle.** Sometimes all it takes to settle an upset stomach is the right scent. The next time your gut's in a knot, scratch the peel of an uncut lemon and take a few whiffs, or open a bottle of peppermint oil and take a deep sniff. The odors travel to your brain and seem to help keep your stomach from going all topsy-turvy.

- **Add some heat to your diet.** Many pungent spices can help relieve stomach problems. Ginger, turmeric, cumin, coriander, clove, cinnamon, and garlic all promote good digestion. And you don't have to eat tons of these spices to get the benefits.

Get Extra Enzymes

If your stomach's not doing an effective job of digesting your meals, you'll know it because you're sure to get heartburn or a stomachache. Supplemental digestive enzymes can help. Many different digestive enzymes are available at health food stores, including bromelain and papain. Take them before you eat, following the directions on the label. They're particularly

**dial the
DOCTOR**

More Than Belly-Achin'

Stomachaches are rarely serious, but there are plenty of exceptions. The basic rule is this: A stomachache that clears up within a day probably isn't a problem. If the pain lingers, is accompanied by fever or vomiting, or keeps coming back, see your doctor. You'll probably need some tests to find out exactly what's going on.

good for reducing that after-meal bloated feeling. *Caution:* Don't use bromelain if you take blood thinners.

Pre-Empt the Ache

Sometimes stomachaches are predictable, often occurring after you eat, or while you're taking certain medications. If that sounds like your usual pattern, these might help:

- **Hold off on the liquids.** If you tend to get stomachaches after eating, give up drinking water or other liquids with your meals, because they dilute the stomach's acid secretions. And it's the acid that helps you digest food.

- **Boost beneficial bugs.** Your gut is loaded with beneficial bacteria that break down and digest food. Sometimes these bacteria get depleted—if you've been taking antibiotics, for example— resulting in painful abdominal cramps. An easy way to boost their numbers back to healthful levels is to take supplements that contain acidophilus. One or two acidophilus capsules is often all you need to calm the upset feeling. A serving of yogurt is another great way to load your gut with more beneficial bacteria. Look for brands that contain live cultures.

- **Drop the dairy.** If you tend to get stomachaches after drinking milk or eating other dairy products, it's probably because you don't produce enough of the enzyme needed to digest lactose,

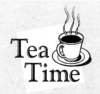

Tea Time

Chamomile is one of the world's most popular teas, and for good reason: It's been used as a stomach soother for centuries. Just be sure to wait 15 minutes after meals before drinking it. Otherwise, the liquid will dilute the acids needed for proper digestion. As long as you're not allergic to ragweed, you can make tea by adding a tea bag or a teaspoon of dried herb to a cup of freshly boiled water. Steep for 10 minutes, remove the tea bag or strain out the herbs, and drink.

a sugar found in dairy products. One solution is to give up dairy altogether. Another is to buy reduced-lactose dairy foods. In addition, having small servings—say, half a glass of milk instead of a full pint—may allow your stomach to handle dairy without discomfort.

Listen to Kitty

Everyone knows what catnip does to our feline friends. In humans, however, the herb is actually quite soothing. It has a mild sedating quality, calms the gastrointestinal tract, and decreases cramping. Take catnip in capsule form when you have a stomachache, following the directions on the label. Or make a tea by adding a teaspoon of dried herb to a cup of freshly boiled water. Steep for 10 minutes, strain, and drink.

Lemon Aid

To prevent stomachaches from getting started, squeeze a little lemon juice into a glass of water and sip it before meals. It will stimulate digestive secretions and get your stomach ready for action.

Give Up Antacids

While they're great for occasional bouts of heartburn, antacids won't do you any good when you have a stomachache. In fact, they can cause side effects, including constipation or diarrhea, that will make you feel even worse.

Stress

Prices rise, roofs leak, cars break down, kids get sick. Bosses yell, bills mount, deadlines pass, keys get lost. Sound familiar? Probably. And what do all of these events have in common? They all produce stress! Of course, stress is unavoidable in modern life. A survey by the Gallup and Harris organizations reported that 25 percent of participants said that the stress in their lives was bad enough to put them on the verge of losing their temper—if not worse!

While a little stress can improve productivity, the hormones generated by extreme or chronic stress can do some serious damage to your physical and emotional health. In fact, studies show that your risk of a heart attack is tripled within two hours of an extremely stressful incident or major meltdown. What's more, the flood of stress hormones can actually warp your brain!

Avoid a Meltdown

Since we can't eliminate all stress from our lives, the smart approach is to change the ways we respond to it. Here's how:

- **Put it in perspective.** Suppose that the IRS just informed you that it wants to audit your taxes for the past five years. Now *that's* stressful! One way to calm yourself down is to ask yourself these questions whenever you find yourself in a tough spot:

    - Is this really important to me?

    - Would a reasonable person be this upset?

    - Is there anything I can do to fix the situation?

    - Would fixing it be worth the cost?

  If you answer yes to all the questions, then take action. But if you answer no one or more times, just take a deep breath and ride out the stressful situation.

Switch mental gears. If you are strumming your fingers on your desk as you pore over a report that is already late and not as good as you'd like it to be, get up and walk away from it. Just take a break and shift to something mindless—even if you're on a deadline. You'll come back less stressed and better able to concentrate.

- **Rub it out.** Get a professional massage whenever you can, even once a month, if you can afford it. According to researchers at the University of Miami, massage can cut cortisol

Tea Time

Choose one of the following herbs to make your own tension-tamer tea: lemon balm, chamomile, passionflower, vervain, wood betony, or skull-cap. Try them each for a week at a time until you find your favorite. Then, every time you feel stressed, steep 1 teaspoon of your preferred herb in 1 cup of hot water, covered, for 10 minutes, then strain. Drink one to three cups a day. *Caution:* Avoid chamomile if you're allergic to ragweed.

levels, lower blood pressure, and boost immunity. To find a licensed therapist near you, contact the American Massage Therapy Association at www.amtamassage.org.

- **Get moving.** Studies have consistently found that even a single exercise session can make you feel less stressed. A simple morning walk at a brisk pace enhances the flow of brain chemicals that block the effects of stress. In a pinch, even a dash up and down some stairs will help.

Unclench

Lots of people clench their teeth when they're uptight. Here's an easy exercise to relax your jaw, face, and neck. Take a deep breath and drop your jaw right now. Next, open your mouth and exhale with a long "haaaaaaa" sound. Finally, gently close your lips. Repeat this exercise throughout the day. You'll soon become aware of how often your jaw clenches—and how that tightness moves tension down into your neck and shoulders.

Visualize Relief

When you feel your stress level rising, close your eyes, breathe deeply, and visualize a peaceful scene from nature. Keep the scene in your mind for 15 to 20 minutes. You'll find that you feel a lot more relaxed afterward.

Sunburn

The source of sunburn is no big mystery, but here's something you might not know. The brilliant rays of the sun that you see on a bright, sunny day aren't really the ones to worry about. Most of the damage comes from the invisible ultraviolet rays. They pack so much energy that even brief exposure causes your skin to darken—or, if you stay out too long, turn a painful, blistering red.

Burn Busters

It almost goes without saying that severe burns—whether you get them in the kitchen or on the beach in Acapulco—always need to be treated by a doctor. Most sunburns aren't this serious, of course. Here's what you need to do to ease the pain and, more importantly, to avoid getting fried in the future:

- **This enzyme is fine.** An enzyme called photolyase, which is made from ocean algae and added to some sunburn products, is said to be

Take the Capsule Cure

For a mild sunburn, mix your own soothing oil by adding the contents of six capsules each of vitamin A and vitamin E to 1/4 cup of flaxseed oil. Apply frequently to the burned areas. You may also add this combination to 1/4 cup of aloe juice, and smooth it over your skin.

Burns That Go Too Far

Most sunburns are only minor annoyances, but sometimes they're serious enough to require emergency care. If your skin blisters or develops open sores, or you feel dizzy or nauseated, go to a doctor immediately. Severe sunburn can also cause chills or fever, which are early signs that you may be going into shock.

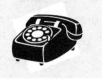

the magic elixir for a painful sunburn, reversing some of the critical DNA damage caused by soaking up too much ultraviolet light. In fact, studies have shown that photolyase reduced skin redness and DNA damage by as much as 45 percent.

■ **Pop an analgesic.** Aspirin, ibuprofen, or other pain relievers won't help heal your sunburned skin, but they're very effective at reducing pain while nature takes its course.

■ **Soak and cool.** Cool water is a refreshing treat for sunburned skin. As soon as you can, soak a washcloth, wring it out, and apply it to the burned area, or simply lounge in a cool bath or shower. Apart from providing nearly instant relief, cool water helps hydrate your skin and prevents it from drying out.

Get Extra C

If you're a sun worshiper, vitamin C is the nutrient you need most. For one thing, your body uses it to build healthy skin that's somewhat resistant to the sun's burning rays. Vitamin C is also an antioxidant that blocks the damaging effects of free radicals, which are harmful oxygen molecules that are produced in profusion when the sun toasts your skin. Finally, C helps repair sunburn damage. As long as you don't have stomach or kidney problems, you should already be taking supplemental vitamin C every day. The Daily Value is 60 milligrams, which is enough under normal circumstances, but not if you've gotten burned. Then you'll need a lot more; your doctor can tell you exactly how much and the best way to take it.

Add Some E

Another sun lover's nutrient is vitamin E. Like vitamin C, it's a protective antioxidant that helps prevent, or at least minimize, skin damage. Take 800 IU daily when you're nursing sunburn. You can also apply vitamin E cream or oil directly to the burned areas of your skin. They'll heal more quickly, and you'll be less likely to have permanent scars.

MODERN MARVEL

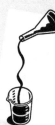

Buy the Right Screen

Did you get burned even though you slathered on sunscreen? It's possible that you used the wrong product. Most sunscreens protect against UVA and UVB, the sun's two types of burning rays, but they don't necessarily give all the protection you need. When you buy sunscreen, buy only products that contain zinc oxide or Parsol 1789 (also called avobenzone). They provide optimal protection against both types of rays. Choose a sunscreen with a sun protection factor (SPF) of 30 or higher. Use a waterproof brand if you'll be swimming or you perspire heavily. And be sure to reapply sunscreen every two hours, no matter what it says on the label.

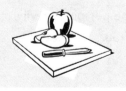
Bottom's Up!

Sunburns remove part of your body's natural moisture barrier, so you'll need to drink plenty of water to compensate. Drinking water also helps your body repair the burn and keeps your immune system in good shape to repel any bacteria that invade through the damaged skin. Drink as much as you can hold—anywhere from four to eight glasses a day.

Skin Savers

Despite your best efforts, your day at the beach resulted in a painful burn. Don't lose hope—try these skin soothers to help you heal:

- **Let the soap slide.** For the first day or two after getting burned, don't use soap on the painful areas. It dries the skin and can actually make the pain worse.

- **Wallow in aloe.** The aloe plant may have been put on Earth just to help heal sunburned skin. Aloe thrives in any container, in any room, in any part of the country. If you get burned, break off a leaf, squeeze out the gel, and apply a generous amount.

- **Slather on a moisturizer.** Moisturizers pump healing fluids back into the skin and create a temporary cooling sensation. Just make sure the moisturizer you choose is fragrance-free, to avoid skin irritation.

Temporomandibular Disorder (TMD)

If it sounds like someone's cracking walnuts every time you open your mouth, or if your jaw occasionally freezes in either the open or closed position, you almost certainly have temporomandibular disorder. This condition, also known as TMD, isn't always painful, but no one likes going through life hearing clicking and popping sounds every time they yawn.

The temporomandibular joint is the hinge that allows your jaw to move up and down. Like any other joint in the body, it's vulnerable to things such as arthritis and sprains. The joint can also be looser than it should be, which can make it jump out of place on occasion.

Lube That Hinge

If TMD is causing you a lot of pain, or your jaw is locking up with some regularity, you may need surgery to repair the joint. In the vast majority of cases, however, you don't have to

dial the DOCTOR

Have it Checked

Check with your doctor if your jaw is sometimes painful or seems to be grinding instead of moving smoothly. Even if you don't have jaw-related problems, you should suspect TMD if you have frequent headaches, neck pain, or earaches.

pay out big bucks to treat TMD. You can usually ease or even eliminate it with creative home care. Here's how:

■**Pack in the vitamin C.** This helpful vitamin is an antioxidant nutrient that helps prevent harmful molecules called free radicals from damaging your joints. It also promotes the growth of collagen, a tissue that helps keep joints healthy. Take 3,000 milligrams of vitamin C daily. Be aware that doses this large may cause diarrhea or other side effects, and they may be harmful for people with stomach or kidney problems, so check with your doctor before you start. You can minimize digestive problems by taking the total amount in divided doses at different times during the day. Taking vitamin C with food also helps.

■**Have a cuppa ice.** Flare-ups of TMD are usually accompanied by inflammation, which is what causes the pain and swelling. Probably the quickest way to reduce inflammation is to immediately apply cold to your jaw to make blood vessels constrict, or narrow, which reduces swelling. Fill some paper cups with water and keep them in the freezer. When TMD strikes, tear off part of the cup or push out an inch or two of ice, then apply it right where it hurts. You can apply the ice for about 20 minutes every few hours throughout the day.

■**Warm your jaw.** You don't want to apply heat to your jaw joint right away because it can

Modern Marvel

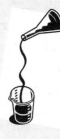

Supplement the Joint

Two over-the-counter dietary supplements, glucosamine and chondroitin, encourage the growth and repair of cartilage and other protective tissues in the joints. They may also help prevent age-related joint damage that can lead to TMD. The recommended dose is 500 milligrams of either (or both) three times daily. Most drugstores carry combination supplements, but avoid them if you're allergic to shellfish.

increase swelling. After a day or two of cold treatments, though, heat will increase circulation and help remove any buildup of fluids and painful toxins. Soak a washcloth in hot water, wring it out, and hold it to your jaw until it cools. Then dip the cloth again and repeat the treatment as often as necessary for relief.

Sleep with a Splint

Don't worry, it sounds worse than it really is. One of the most successful strategies for easing TMD is to use an oral splint that guides the jaw back into its proper position. The splints are custom made by doctors and dentists, and they're usually worn only at night—although if your TMD is serious, you may have to wear a splint night and day for a while. It takes time to get used to a splint, but it works very quickly.

Nibble, Don't Chomp

When TMD is acting up, it's important to give your jaw a rest, just as you'd stay off your feet after spraining your ankle. Stick to foods that are easy on your chops and avoid those that require a lot of jaw action, such as apples and corn on the cob. And by all means, let the silverware do the work. Cut food into small pieces so you don't have to chew as much.

Straighten Up

No slumping while you work! Postures that create the least stress on your upper body will also produce the least stress on your jaw. This means standing and sitting up straight and always making an effort to keep your head and neck in line with the rest of your body. It really does help!

Tame Tension

Any kind of emotional stress makes TMD worse because it makes muscles tense. It also increases levels of body chemicals that aggravate pain. Whatever it is that you do when you relax, do it even more often when TMD is acting up. Things like meditation, yoga, or just getting away for a while can make a big difference.

Rub It Right

You can't always rub out TMD, but you can almost always rub it the right way. When you first notice pain, put your fingers on the side of your jaw, then open and close your mouth. The thick muscle that you feel is the one that controls your jaw. Put one finger on either side of the muscle and knead it gently, working all the way from your ear to your jaw. This is one of the best ways to prevent—or ease—painful spasms.

Tennis Elbow

The elbow seems to be one of those joints that's always looking for trouble. Apart from the fact that your elbows jut out from the rest of your body, making them vulnerable to painful knocks, they also do an awful lot of bending. Raise a glass, pull a weed, or scratch your head—then give thanks to your elbows for doing all the hard work.

All that constant movement comes with a price, however. Even if you've never picked up a racket in your life, you've probably experienced tennis elbow. Here's what happens: The strain of repetitive movements causes the muscles or tendons to become inflamed, causing pain that can range from a dull throb at your elbow to an ache that radiates down your arm. Often, the pain starts off as a minor twinge, and it may or may not flare into major agony. It all depends on what you do next.

Cream It with Calendula

Want fast, natural relief from an ouchy elbow? Grab a jar of calendula cream, available at health food stores, and rub 1/2 teaspoon into the muscles surrounding your elbow. It can reduce the ache and help you heal more quickly.

Dark berries, such as blueberries, blackberries, and boysenberries, contain natural chemicals called bioflavonoids that relieve pain and inflammation. It's also a good idea to eat plenty of other fruits and vegetables while you're healing to pump even more bioflavonoids into your system.

Ax the Ache

In extreme cases, tennis elbow will go away only if you take powerful drugs to reduce the inflammation. Occasionally, it's necessary to have steroid injections or physical therapy to get things working properly again. But unless your symptoms persist for a few weeks or more or steadily get worse, you can almost always treat tennis elbow at home simply by putting down the tennis racket (or whatever it was that caused the pain). Here are a few quick ways to reduce the discomfort and help the muscles and tendons heal more quickly:

- **Stop the bends.** Since moving your elbow too much is what causes tennis elbow, it makes sense that keeping it still will help it get better. You may want to pick up an arm brace at a drugstore or medical supply store to protect the injured joint and keep it from moving in an inappropriate (and painful) direction.

- **Wait it out.** You shouldn't rush back into action as soon as your pain is gone. Wait a few days or a week to be sure you're really better. The tissue's still healing, and you don't want to aggravate it.

- **Rebuild with protein.** When you're recovering from tennis elbow, you're going to need a lot of protein—the nutrient that your body uses to repair muscle damage. The usual rule is to get 0.8 gram of protein for each kilogram of body weight. Here's an easy way to figure out how much you need: Divide your body weight by 2.2 (there are 2.2 pounds per kilogram), then multiply that number by 0.8 to get your daily target for protein. Thus, if you weigh 150 pounds, you'll need 54 grams of protein. That's roughly the amount you'd get in a cup of tuna salad, a cup of long-grain white rice, and a cup of milk.

Heed the Signals

You probably remember this old joke: A patient says to his doctor, "It hurts when I do this," and the doctor says, "Well, don't do that." Okay, it's a groaner, but there's a lot of truth behind it. The best thing you can do is find the movements that cause or aggravate the injury, and then quit doing them. Pain from tennis elbow tends to be very specific: It hurts when you move your arm one way, and it doesn't hurt when you move it a different way. Limit your movements to the nonpainful ones, (try some of the movement tips here), and let the healing begin:

▪ **Stretch it out.** Some slow, gentle stretching will help your elbow heal and strengthen. First, extend your arm straight in front of you, palm down, and slowly bend your wrist so the back of your hand moves toward you. Then lower your hand and flex your wrist so that your fingers point down. Next, hold your arm out, palm up, and slowly bend your elbow so your palm moves toward you. Repeat both of these stretches a few times a day, but quit if

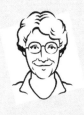

Grandma Says...

Freeze it fast. As soon as the pain starts, reach for an ice pack (with the other arm). Grandma Putt knew that you can't beat ice for reducing inflammation and numbing pain. For the first few days after the injury, apply ice for 20 minutes at a time every few hours.

they cause real pain. It's okay for stretches to be slightly uncomfortable, but they shouldn't hurt. If they do, you're overdoing it.

- **Turn to weeds.** Two common garden plants, chickweed and comfrey, are traditionally used to relieve swelling and pain. Pick a handful of chickweed and one or two large comfrey leaves. Blanch them in hot water and apply to your elbow, using chickweed as the first layer and holding it in place with the comfrey leaves.

- **Try indirect massage.** When you have tennis elbow, direct pressure may make the sore area hurt even more, but massaging the surrounding area is fine.

Get a Drop on Pain

St. John's wort oil is an excellent pain reliever that can be applied directly to the aching area.

MODERN MARVEL

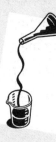

Heat is Neat

Smooth some hot-pepper cream over your sore joint, and you'll begin to feel relief. The heat from capsaicin, the stuff that gives peppers their bite, brings more blood circulation to the area. You can buy a cream containing 0.025 to 0.075 percent capsaicin at drugstores. Use it up to three times a day, but be careful not to get it in your eyes or on areas of broken skin.

For an extra boost, add 4 to 6 drops of arnica oil and 2 or 3 drops of wintergreen oil. *Caution:* Do not use arnica on broken skin.

Reach for Omega-3s

Essential fatty acids, especially the omega-3 fatty acids in cold-water fish such as salmon and tuna, help suppress the inflammation that causes the pain. You can also get plenty of omega-3s by eating a few tablespoons of ground flaxseed or—unless you're taking aspirin or prescription blood thinners—taking 1 to 3 grams of fish oil or flaxseed oil.

Pop a Pineapple Pill

Pineapple does more than add delicious sweetness to fresh fruit platters. It's also rich in bromelain, a substance that acts as a natural painkiller. In fact, bromelain has been shown to reduce the swelling around muscles and tendons that causes the pain of tennis elbow. Since you can't get healing amounts of bromelain by eating fresh pineapple, a better approach (as long as you're not taking blood thinners) is to take supplements; the usual dose is 375 milligrams three times a day. Don't take them with meals, though, because their enzymatic activity will be used to digest your food rather than reduce inflammation.

Toothaches

It's a wonder we all don't get toothaches more often, since the tiny nerves inside our teeth are just a fraction of an inch from the outside world. They don't cause any pain as long as they're well shielded, but when they lose some of their protective armor, watch out!

Think about what happens when there's a breach in the protective tooth enamel, or if your gum line recedes even a tiny bit. The incredibly sensitive nerves are then exposed to air—or, in some cases, assaulted by inflammation or infection. They let you know what's happening immediately by causing excruciating pain.

Stop the Pain

There's a curious thing about toothaches, though. It seems that they never happen when it's easy to see your dentist. They have an unfortunate way of cropping up late at night or at the beginning of three-day weekends. When that happens, you have to find ways to ease the agony until you can get some help. Here are a few terrific tips to try:

- **Fight it with floss.** As simple as it sounds, sometimes a toothache is caused by a particle of food lodged between your teeth or between your teeth and gums. So it's worth it to take a few minutes to gently floss the area to see if anything pops out.

- **Don't quit brushing.** Even if it hurts a little when you brush, it's essential to keep your teeth clean until you can see a dentist. That's because food and debris can collect on your tooth and make the pain worse. Just brush slowly and don't use a lot of pressure.

- **Spread on some spice.** Relief from a raging toothache may be as close as your spice rack. Folk healers often advise people to spread a little ground ginger or red pepper around the tooth. Add a little water to the spice to make a paste, then spread it liberally all around the point of pain. You may notice relief in as few as 5 minutes.

- **Hit it with ice.** You wouldn't think that placing a cold pack—or a washcloth wrapped around some ice cubes—on the outside of your mouth would have much effect on a toothache, but it does seem to help. Hold it against the tender area for 15 to 20 minutes every few hours until you can see your dentist.

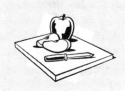

Take a Painkiller

The analgesics in your medicine cabinet are more effective for tooth pain than you might think. Acetaminophen can sometimes ease a toothache as effectively as mild prescription drugs, and as long as you're not sensitive to them, aspirin and ibuprofen may be even better. They reduce inflammation and stop the body's production of pain-causing prostaglandins.

Wet Your Mouth

Toothaches can get worse when your mouth is dry. Until the pain is gone, it's important to drink a lot of water to keep your mouth lubricated. Have a glass of water handy at all times and keep taking small sips. If your mouth is always a little dry, it's probably time to make a list of all the medications you're taking and review them with your dentist. Anywhere from 200 to 400 common drugs, such as heart drugs, antihistamines, and anti-anxiety medications, cause mouth dryness.

Ease It with Cloves

Clove oil has been used for generations for easing toothaches, and there's good evidence that it works. Buy the oil at a health food store or drugstore, then dip in a cotton swab and rub the oil on the sore tooth. In many cases, the pain will disappear almost instantly.

dial the DOCTOR

Ache No More

It's not unusual for toothaches to disappear on their own, but you can bet that the pain's going to come back—probably sooner rather than later. You may as well bite the bullet and make an appointment to see your dentist. Toothaches are often caused by decay, so there's a good chance you'll need a filling or even a root canal. Once the damage is repaired, the toothache will be gone for good.

Ulcers

Here's a little factoid that boggles the mind: The digestive acids in your stomach are nearly as strong as battery acid. How is it that these acids are strong enough to dissolve the heaviest meal into a digestible soup of nutrients, but somehow they don't digest the stomach at the same time? Nature, it turns out, designed the stomach to withstand constant acid onslaughts by giving it a thin, protective lining that prevents damage to the tender tissue underneath. Of course, this system works only if the protective barrier is intact.

That's where germs come in. Helicobacter pylori, a type of bacterium that commonly inhabits the stomach and intestine, digs into this protective lining. If you're infected with H. pylori, your stomach lining may be pitted with tiny holes that permit stomach acid to leak through. The result: small, painful little sores known as ulcers.

Tea Time

The next time an ulcer flares, soothe it with cinnamon. This aromatic spice appears to help knock out ulcer-causing germs, so brew yourself a cup of cinnamon tea. The German Commission E, which studies herbal medicines in Europe, says it really works.

Cool the Burn

Along with treatment you'll get from your doctor, there are a few lifestyle approaches that do make a difference when you're suffering from ulcer pain:

- **Don't depend on antacids.** When the burning pain of ulcers flares, your natural instinct is probably to pop a few antacids. There's nothing wrong with this approach in some cases, but some doctors suspect that quenching stomach acid with antacids may make ulcers worse in the long run, because you need stomach acids to kill ulcer-causing bacteria.

- **Say hello to aloe.** Aloe vera is one of nature's great healers, and it's especially good for ulcers because it coats irritated tissues and may promote faster healing. You can buy aloe juice at health food stores, or if you grow aloe at home to treat minor injuries, just break open a leaf and squeeze some juice into your mouth. You can take aloe up to a couple of times a day.

- **Get extra nutrients.** If you don't eat a lot of fruits and vegetables, you may not be getting enough of a few key nutrients—mainly vitamins A, C, and E—that are needed to repair damaged tissues throughout your body, including the stomach lining. If you have a history of ulcers, it's a good idea to take a daily supplement that provides the recommended daily amounts (RDA) of each of these important nutrients.

Take a Fish Pill

Doctors and nutritionists almost beg Americans to eat more fish, in part because it's a rich source of essential fatty acids that help quell inflammation. If you have ulcers, however, eating too much fish may cause an increase in stomach acid—and pain. Instead of eating fish, people with ulcers should take fish-oil supplements. Unless you take aspirin or prescription blood thinners, pick up some capsules at a drugstore or health food store, then follow the label directions.

Peel Some Relief

Having an ulcer is no reason to hold the onions. In fact, it's all the more reason to add them to salads, sandwiches, soups, and so forth. Onions contain sulfur compounds that seem to help eliminate ulcer-causing bacteria, so try to include them in at least one meal a day.

Load Up on Licorice

This sweet-tasting herb (not the candy) is powerful medicine. It reduces inflammation and appears to help ulcers heal more quickly. You can buy licorice-root tea bags or powder at health food stores. As long as you don't have high blood pressure, you can drink two or three cups of tea a day to ease the pain of ulcers and help keep them from coming back.

Also look for chewable DGL tablets, which

Protect with Slippery Elm

The herb slippery elm soothes the lining of the digestive tract. This may protect small ulcers from further acid damage and may help them heal more quickly. Slippery elm is available in powdered form at health food stores. Add a teaspoon of powder to a glass of water or juice and drink one or two glasses daily when ulcers flare up.

are made from licorice that's had the blood pressure–raising compound removed. Chewing these tablets between meals will speed pain relief and aid in healing an ulcer. Be sure to follow the package directions.

Hide the Hooch

And while you're at it, give up cigarettes if you're a smoker. Alcohol and tobacco tend to make ulcer pain worse, they weaken the stomach's protective lining, and they inhibit your body's ability to heal the damage. People who smoke and drink are more likely to get ulcers than those who don't indulge.

Chill

Even though emotional stress doesn't cause ulcers, it does increase levels of stomach acid while reducing the stomach's secretion of protective mucus, which can make the pain worse. Stress reduction should be part of every anti-ulcer strategy. When you feel your stress level rising, close your eyes, breathe deeply, and visualize a peaceful scene from nature. Keep the scene in your mind for 15 to 20 minutes. You'll find that you feel a lot more relaxed afterward—and you'll have less discomfort.

Urinary Tract Infections (UTIs)

There are plenty of things men will never understand about women—why their dress pants never have pockets, for example, or why they need three or four shampoos and conditioners when the average guy gets by with the same brand year after year. They also have a hard time relating to urinary tract infections (UTIs). Men rarely get them, but they're among the most common, and annoying, health issues women deal with. About a third of American women will get a urinary tract infection at some point in their lives, and some women get them over and over again.

Easy Access

Most UTIs occur when bacteria that normally live in the area surrounding the anus make their way inside the urethra. Once they get into that warm, moist environment, they quickly multiply, and sometimes they even work their way

> ### *Heat Away the Pain*
>
> To quickly ease the localized discomfort of UTIs, apply a warm compress to the urethral opening and the surrounding area. Moist warmth can reduce muscle spasms that result in pain. A long soak in a warm bath has similar soothing effects.

Stop the Spread

Most urinary tract infections are merely uncomfortable. Call your doctor immediately, however, if your infection is accompanied by fever, blood in the urine, or back pain. These are signs that you may be developing a kidney infection, which can be life-threatening without prompt treatment.

up to the bladder. Men sometimes get UTIs, but their extra inches of anatomy make it harder for bacteria to get inside. Women don't have that protection, so they're a lot more vulnerable.

The infections can occur anywhere in the urinary tract, but usually affect the urethra—the tube through which urine leaves the body—or the bladder. The main symptom is a burning sensation, along with urinary urgency—the sudden, overwhelming need to urinate.

No More Infection

If you think you have a UTI, or even if you're sure you do (women who get them know the symptoms all too well), see your doctor right away. You're going to need antibiotics to knock out the germs and relieve the symptoms. In the meantime, now's the time to think about ways to prevent future infections, and take steps to keep your current discomfort to a minimum. Here's what to do:

- **Spoon up some blueberries.** They're bursting with tannins, which are compounds that boot out the bacteria responsible for UTIs. Researchers have found that tannins prevent the germs from attaching to the bladder wall, where they thrive.

- **Fight back with cranberries.** Harvard scientists have found that women who drink a little more than a cup of cranberry juice daily for a month may be only 42 percent as likely to have a UTI as women who don't. Look for a drink that's 27 percent cranberry juice, preferably one without too much added sugar.

- **Cut the sweets.** Sugar can be a real problem if you get frequent UTIs. It encourages the growth of bacteria, and it reduces the ability of your immune system to battle infection. And it's not only sweets such as candy that cause problems, but all sources of sugar, including juices, fruits, and the sugar in packaged foods. Read labels so you know what you're getting.

Break the UTI Cycle

If you have a urinary tract infection, you want fast relief. Here are steps you can take to ease the discomfort and make another UTI far less likely to happen:

- **Imbibe less.** The bacterial colonies that cause UTIs love alcohol because it's converted into sugar in your body. Give up the drinks until the infection is gone.

- **Load up on protein.** You need plenty of protein to keep your immune system healthy. To make sure you're getting enough, divide your weight by 2.2 to get your weight in kilograms, then eat 0.8 gram of protein daily for each kilogram of body weight. As long as you eat a healthy diet that includes plenty of whole grains, legumes, and lean meat and fish, you're almost guaranteed to get enough protein to boost your defenses against UTIs.

Grandma Says...

Don't hold it. When your body tells you it's time to find a restroom, do it. Grandma knew that holding urine in the bladder for too long gives bacteria the chance to multiply.

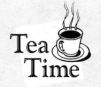

Tea Time

To help your body fend off UTIs, whip up a homemade immune system strengthener. Mix equal parts of dried echinacea, goldenseal, and licorice root. Put about a tablespoon of the mixture in a tea ball and steep in hot water for 10 to 15 minutes. Drink two or three cups daily until the infection is gone. *Caution:* Omit the licorice root if you have high blood pressure, and avoid echinacea if you have an autoimmune disease or are pregnant or nursing.

- **Take the C cruise.** Vitamin C is helpful because it supports the immune system. When you have a UTI, plan on taking 500 milligrams of vitamin C every two hours. Vitamin C in large amounts may cause diarrhea. If you're having problems, cut back on the dose until you find a level that works for you. If you have kidney disease or stomach problems, discuss using vitamin C with your doctor before giving it a try.

- **Try an herbal combo.** Treat a UTI with a combination of uva-ursi (sometimes called bearberry), buchu, echinacea, and goldenseal, which are available at health food stores. Take 200 milligrams of each three times daily for a week. *Caution:* Skip the echinacea if you have an autoimmune disease such as rheumatoid arthritis, lupus, or multiple sclerosis, or if you are pregnant or nursing.

Drink Like a Fish

The more water you drink, the more bacteria will be flushed from your bladder. So drink at least 2 quarts of water a day. That may seem like a lot, but if you carry water and sip it throughout the day, you won't even realize how much you're drinking.

Clean from Front to Back

It's an unfortunate fact of anatomy—the proximity of the anus and urethra—that makes women vulnerable to bacterial invasions. If you always wipe from front to back after using the toilet, you'll be less likely to push bacteria somewhere where they can cause problems.

Take a Bathroom Break

Some women find that they get UTIs after sex because intercourse can push bacteria where they shouldn't go. Urinating after intercourse can flush out any germs that may have worked their way into the urinary tract.

Stock Up on 'Shrooms

Most supermarkets offer several tasty varieties of gourmet mushrooms. You should definitely stock up on them when you have a UTI, because they boost the ability of your immune system to combat infections. Different mushrooms stimulate different aspects of the immune system, so it's good to combine them. Look for shiitake, reishi, and maitake mushrooms.

Protect with Citrate

If you take supplemental magnesium or calcium, be sure to get the citrate form. Citrates are easier for your body to absorb, and they make the urine more alkaline, which can help prevent UTIs.

Varicose Veins

Do your legs start hurting as the day goes by? Do you find yourself wearing long pants even on 95° days? Maybe you're one of the millions of Americans with varicose veins—and no matter what you hear, they're not just a cosmetic problem.

Even though nearly everyone has some varicose veins, there's a lot of confusion about what they really are. As doctors sometimes explain, they're nature's proof that gravity only pulls one way. Confused? Let's take a look.

A varicose vein is a blood vessel that doesn't have quite enough strength to push its cargo of blood uphill and back into circulation. When blood leaves your heart, it's traveling at tremendous velocity. The initial speed, combined with gravity, means that blood doesn't have any trouble reaching the blood vessels in your legs. Now consider the return trip. This time, the blood has to go uphill, without the heart's pumping action to help it along. As it moves upward from veins in your legs—assisted by the pumping action of your leg muscles—the blood passes through tiny one-way valves, which snap shut behind it at intervals. Basically, it moves uphill in stages. Sometimes, the valves aren't strong enough to support the weight of the blood, so it slips backward, forming pools inside one or more veins. After a while, the accumulated blood causes the vein to swell, and the result is a varicose vein.

Get That Blood Moving

You can see that you have to do something when you have varicose veins. If you really hate the way they look, or they're causing a lot of physical discomfort, surgery and other techniques can remove them. In most cases, however, you can bolster your veins with some simple home strategies that cost little or nothing to do. Start by checking out the Legs for Life Program online at www.legsforlife.org for information about free screening for leg circulation problems. Then give some of these a try:

- **Firm up with stockings.** Snug-fitting hose, called compression stockings, are available from drugstores and medical supply stores. They provide extra support to the walls of blood vessels in the legs, which helps keep blood moving

dial the
DOCTOR

Better Safe Than Sorry

Varicose veins can make your legs feel tired and achy. That's the most common problem, but there's also a risk that the poor circulation that accompanies varicose veins can cause ulcers on your lower legs. Less often, the swollen veins can promote the formation of blood clots that are potentially serious. If varicose veins are bothering you, talk to your doctor about your options.

upward. Your doctor should write a prescription for the right kind of hose for you. Over-the-counter compression stockings work well, but they may not provide the exact amount of pressure that you need.

■ **Raise your legs.** The blood in your legs has to fight gravity to climb all the way back to your heart. Why not reverse the situation and let gravity work for you? To do it, raise your feet above the level of your heart for a couple of hours each day, or sit with your legs propped up on pillows. About 10 minutes after you elevate your legs, the ache will go away.

■ **Point your feet.** Sleeping with your feet raised a few inches will give your veins a boost all night. You can prop your feet on a flat pillow or put some boards under the foot of your bed. Check with your doctor before you try this, though, since this sleeping position may aggravate some health problems.

■ **Sit and put your feet up.** If you spend most of your day on your feet, your varicose veins may feel as if they're going to pop out of your legs by the time the day's over. Don't wait until you get home from work to give your legs a breather. Think about ways to baby your legs, such as taking breaks as often as possible. If you stand a lot, take some time to relax in a comfortable chair. Put your feet up on a desk if you can.

Stop Vein Pain

Here are more steps you can take to relieve the discomfort of varicose veins:

- **Dress loosely.** Compression stockings are designed to give your veins the kind of pressure they need, but other garments that put pressure on your legs can interfere with circulation. Avoid tight panty hose, girdles, and other kinds of restrictive clothing.

- **Exercise often.** Having varicose veins isn't an excuse for not exercising. In fact, it's all the more reason to be active. The more fit you are, the better your circulatory system will be able to cope with the diminished capacity of your leg veins. Try yoga, swimming, or walking, which doesn't put excessive pressure on the lower extremities.

- **Beat the heat.** You don't want your legs to get too hot when you have varicose veins, because it could result in tissue-damaging inflammation. You should avoid long, hot baths and other activities that make your legs hotter than usual.

Strength Training

You can improve the pumping action of leg veins with a technique called contrast hydrotherapy, in which you alternate between hot and cold treatments. First, soak a cloth in hot water, wring it out, and place it over the area where

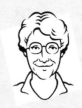

Grandma Says...

Cool the ache.
My Grandma Putt used cold witch hazel to soothe her aching veins. It's simple: Chill a cup of witch hazel in the refrigerator for an hour, then soak a washcloth in it, and apply to the parts of your legs that hurt. Keep the compress in place for 15 minutes while elevating your legs.

you have varicose veins. Leave it in place for 3 minutes, then replace it with a cold cloth for 1 minute. Repeat the cycle two or three times, always ending with the cold cloth. It's helpful for relieving congestion and promoting healthy circulation—and it makes your legs feel good!

Rub 'Em Right

There's nothing like a massage for soothing tired legs (or tired anything, for that matter). Besides making you feel good, massage can improve your circulation, which is a big plus if you have varicose veins. To help ease the ache even more, add a few drops of your favorite essential oil to a few tablespoons of olive oil, then give yourself a soothing oil massage. The essential oil will boost circulation and help your leg discomfort fade a lot faster.

Warts

In *The Adventures of Huckleberry Finn*, Tom and Huck debated about several ways to get rid of warts—most involving prowling around town at midnight. But the most effective, they agreed, was to take a dead cat to the grave of a recently deceased, "wicked" person. At midnight, they said, a devil would come to take the wicked person's body away. "You heave your cat after 'em and say, 'Devil follow corpse, cat follow devil, warts follow cat, I'm done with ye!' "

Folklore is full of wart remedies, simply because the unsightly little bumps are tough to get rid of. There are more than 50 types of warts that can appear anywhere on your body, but hands and feet are the most common sites. And, as if one weren't bad enough, they sometimes appear in groups. They're caused by the human papillomavirus, which stimulates rapid cell growth on the outer layer of your skin.

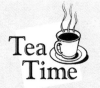

Tea Time

The development of warts can signal a weakened immune system. You can give yourself an antiviral boost with astragalus tea. To make it, simmer 1 heaping teaspoon of dried root in 1 cup of water for 20 minutes, then strain. Drink two cups daily.

Say Goodbye to Bumps

Fortunately, warts appear less frequently as we age—possibly because we develop immunity to the virus that sprouts them. If you do happen to get them, and dragging dead felines through a cemetery seems just a bit much, consider the following ways to get rid of them:

- **Keep your feet covered.** The wart virus is everywhere, and you can pick it up easily by (literally) following in someone's footsteps in a shower, locker room, or public pool. These little growths are also acquired through direct contact with an infected person. So don't shower in the same stall with someone who has warts, and wear flip-flops or sandals when you're walking around in locker rooms or at public pools.

- **Leave them alone.** Picking at a wart just spreads the virus that causes it. It will grow back anyway, so let nature take its course.

- **Clobber them with cedar.** Yellow cedar, also known as thuja, contains potent oil in its leaves that makes an excellent wart remedy. Fill a small jar with thuja leaves and cover them with olive oil. Add the contents of a capsule of vitamin E oil. Let the jar sit in a sunny window for 10 days, shaking it well each day. Strain the oil, then store it in a cool, dark place. (If you keep it in the refrigerator, it will last for four to six months.) Apply the oil to the surface of the wart two or three times daily.

MODERN MARVEL

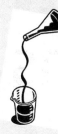

Ax 'Em with Acid

Warts will usually disappear on their own, but if you're impatient, head for the drugstore. An over-the-counter acid solution can help, say doctors at the Mayo Clinic. You'll have to apply the remedy twice a day for a few weeks, or it won't be effective. Look for a product that contains salicylic acid, which will peel off the infected skin, but be aware that the acid can be irritating. Try a 17 percent acid solution on your hands (or the end of your nose) and a 40 percent solution on your feet. If you're pregnant, ask your doctor if a wart remedy is safe to use.

Bark Up the Right Tree

Folklore from Michigan suggests that you find yourself a nice birch tree and cut off a strip of bark. (You can also get birch bark in some health food stores.) Soak the bark in water until it softens, then tape it directly to your wart. Nobody knows why it works, but folks point out that birch bark contains salicylates, the basis of some FDA-approved wart treatments.

Yeast Infections

dial the DOCTOR

Make Sure

Most women are all too familiar with the symptoms—usually pain, itching, or a bad odor—that accompany yeast infections. If you've never had one before and you experience any of these symptoms, check with your doctor.

In some ways, germs aren't a whole lot different than people. They like warm places where there's an abundance of moisture, plenty of protection, and lots of tasty treats. Once these basic needs are met, they tend to stay right where they are and multiply like crazy until the body's mechanisms step in to keep them in check.

The yeast fungus normally lives in your body, but under normal circumstances, there's not enough of it for you to notice. When something upsets your body's internal ecosystem, though, the fungus, called candida, may grow out of control. Thus, you can think of vaginal yeast infections as a sign that something's not quite the way it should be. Changing levels of hormones can allow it to thrive. So can changes in acidity. Women who take antibiotics often get yeast infections because the drugs kill beneficial organisms that normally keep the fungus in check.

Stop the Yeast Feast

For the most part, your body is pretty good at getting this all-too-common problem under control, and most infections will clear up even if you do nothing. But why suffer? There are many over-the-counter treatments, and they're very effective. Since drugs don't work instantly, though, and they won't prevent future problems, take a look at the following remedies. Unlike drugs, these strategies can help you get to the root of the problem and keep yeast infections from recurring:

■ **Switch methods.** Birth control pills are at the top of the list for causing vaginal yeast infections. You're more likely to have trouble with pills that contain a high percentage of estrogen. If you have recurrent yeast infections, ask your doctor if you should try a different type of pill or perhaps even switch to a different form of birth control.

■ **Spoon up some yogurt.** Whether you want to prevent a yeast infection or relieve an existing one, the solution may be in your fridge. Eating a cup or two of live-culture yogurt daily will replenish your body's healthful bacteria, helping keep the bad bugs under control.

■ **Change your diet.** Recurring, recalcitrant, or unresponsive yeast infections may require even more drastic dietary changes. Eliminate all refined starches, such as bread and pasta, from your diet. Avoid foods that contain yeast or

Tea Time

Studies in
Germany show
that echinacea
tea can prevent
yeast infections.
Make a cup of the
tea by putting
1/2 teaspoon of
dried echinacea
in 1 cup of boiling
water. Steep for
about 10 minutes,
then strain out
the herb. The tea
loses its effect
after eight weeks,
so stop for a
month, then start
drinking it again.
Caution: Don't use
echinacea if you
have an autoim-
mune disease such
as rheumatoid
arthritis, lupus, or
multiple sclerosis,
or if you are preg-
nant or nursing.

fungus, such as beer, leavened pastry products, aged cheeses, and mushrooms. You'll also want to give up fermented foods, such as vinegar, pickles, and sauerkraut, and eliminate all forms of sugar, including fruit and juice.

Soak the Itch

A quick way to ease the discomfort of a yeast infection is to soak in warm water. Fill your bathtub, add a handful of colloidal oatmeal, and relax for a while. If you don't have colloidal oatmeal, it's fine to sprinkle in some baking soda, or you can use plain oatmeal. Just fill an old sock with a cup or two of oatmeal, fasten the open end to the faucet with a rubber band, and let the water run through it as the tub fills up. Oatmeal "softens" the water and helps soothe irritation.

Get Tested

Women who get frequent yeast infections sometimes have underlying blood sugar problems. Elevated blood sugar levels caused by diabetes can greatly increase the risk of infections, so if you keep getting them, ask your doctor to test you for diabetes just to be sure.

The Garlic Fix

Garlic has powerful antifungal properties. Raw or lightly cooked garlic delivers the biggest kick. Chop up a few cloves and throw it into just-cooked foods if you can't stand to eat it raw.

Keep Cool

Heat and hot water will aggravate a yeast infection. You may want to shower in lukewarm water until the infection is gone. Another thing to keep in mind: Summer's heat always makes yeast infections more uncomfortable, but even in winter, panty hose or tight clothing can trap heat and increase itching and other symptoms. It's a good idea to wear loose clothing made from cotton or other natural fibers, at least until the infection is gone.

Flush After Sex

Some women tend to get yeast infections after intercourse. It's not really the man's fault, it's just that semen is a bit alkaline and can alter the acidity of the vagina. Less acid means more yeast. To help restore a normal chemical balance after sex, either urinate soon afterward or take a quick shower and flush out the area.

Tame It with Tea Tree

Tea tree and peppermint oils are powerful fungus fighters. You can buy capsules at a health food store, then follow the label directions. Be sure to buy oil that is meant for internal use, and don't put it anywhere but in your mouth.

If You're Pregnant...

Pregnancy is another condition that predisposes women to yeast infections, so if you are pregnant, consult your doctor or health care provider before trying to treat a yeast infection on your own.

Index

turmeric, 20–21
Antiviral medications, 175–176
Apples, applesauce, as remedy
for asthma, 27
for bad breath, 41
for constipation, 127
for diarrhea, 156, 157
for nausea, 273
Apricots, 357
Arginine, 118
Arnica
contraindications, 335
as remedy
for arthritis, 19
for back pain, 38
for bruises, 77
for tennis elbow, 335
Aromatherapy, 317
Arthritis, 15–21
Artichokes, 55, 224–225
Artificial tears, 121–22, 162
Asparagus, 55
Aspirin. *See* Pain relievers, over-the-counter
Aspirin allergy, 227–228
Asthma, 22–27, 73
Astragalus, 111, 353
Athlete's foot, 28–32, 54

B

Baby wipes, 210–211
Back pain, 33–39
Bad breath, 40–43
Baking soda, as remedy
for body odor, 61
for calluses and corns, 99
for insect bites and stings, 44

for oral hygiene, 40, 42–43, 190
for pizza mouth, 281
Bananas, as remedy
for diarrhea, 156
for high blood pressure, 216
for kidney stones, 246
Bandages
for burns, 90–91
for bursitis, 93
for cuts and scrapes, 135–136
for splinters, 311
Barley, 158, 221
Basil, 188
Bath oils, 165
Baths. *See also* Epsom salt baths; Footbaths; Oatmeal baths
contraindications, 351
as remedy
for anal pain, 13
for bronchitis, 76
for constipation, 127
for hemorrhoids, 209
for sunburn, 324
for UTIs, 343
Beach walking, 86, 99
Beano, 185
Beans, 187, 223
Bearberry, 346
Beds and bedding, effects on
asthma, 25
hay fever, 196
headaches, 201–202
insomnia, 240, 241
Bedtime routines, 239–240
Bee balm, 272
Beer, for dandruff, 143
Belly dancing, 257

Benadryl, 122, 227
Benecol, 220
Benzoperoxide, 230
Bergamot, 42
Berries. *See also specific berries*
as anti-inflammatory, 95, 332
hives from, 228
Beta-carotene, 165, 357
Bilberry, 160
Bioflavonoids, as remedy
for bruises, 81
for bursitis, 95
for tennis elbow, 332
for varicose veins, 350
Biotin, 141
Birch bark, 355
Birth control pills, 357
Bites and stings, 44–46
Blackberries, 195, 332
Blackberry root, 155
Black cohosh, 39
Black current oil, 68
Black eyes, 47–49
Black tea
breast pain and, 67
as remedy
for acne, 1
for asthma, 22
for black eyes, 47
for blisters, 52–53
Bladderwrack, 277
Blisters, 50–54
Bloating, 55–60
Blood clots, in hemorrhoids, 211
Blood in stool, 209
Blood sugar levels, 358
Blood thinners, prescription, 24
Blueberries, as remedy

H

CITY

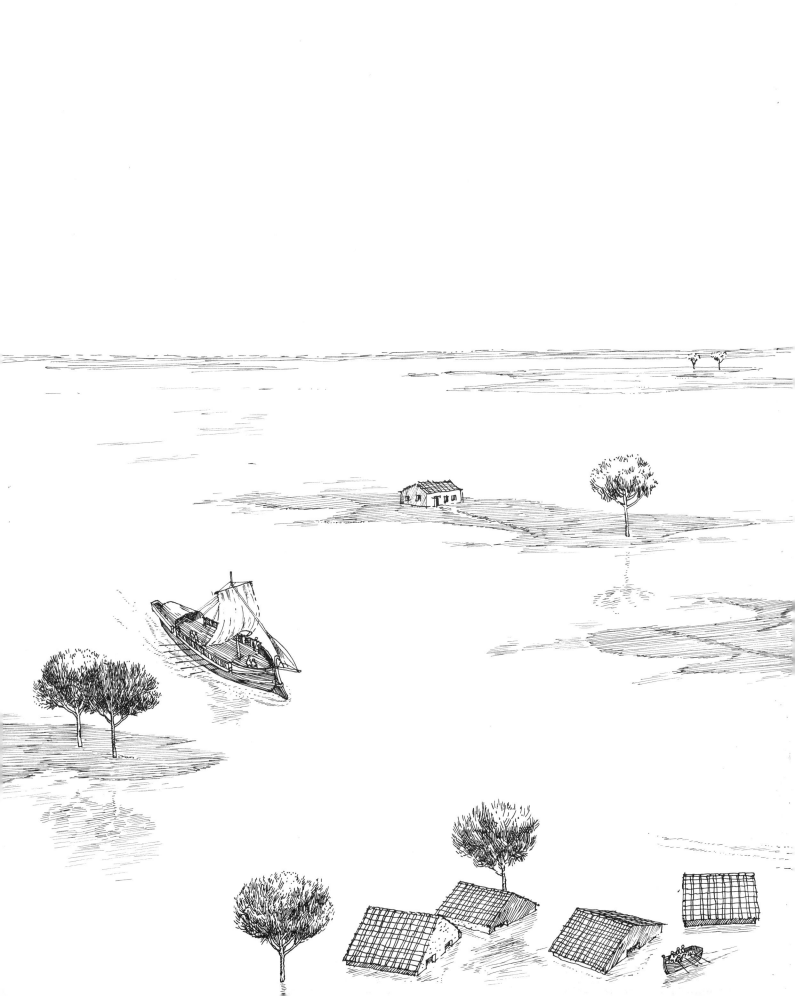

CITY

A Story of Roman Planning and Construction

DAVID MACAULAY

HOUGHTON MIFFLIN COMPANY BOSTON

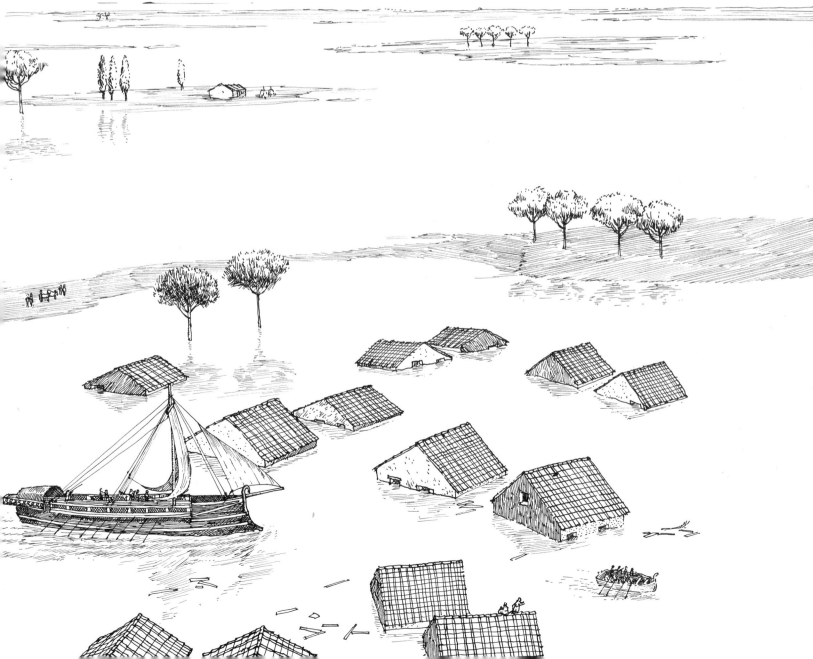

For Janice
and things to come

special thanks to Hardu, Mary,
Sidney, Bill, my parents,
Melanie, Walter and Vitruvius.

Library of Congress Cataloging in Publication Data

Macaulay, David.
   City; a story of Roman planning and construction.

   SUMMARY: Text and black and white illustrations
show how the Romans planned and constructed their cities
for the people who lived within them.
   1. Civil engineering — Rome (City) — Juvenile literature.   2. Rome (City) — Antiquities — Juvenile literature.
3. Building — Rome (City) — Juvenile literature.
4. Cities and towns — Planning — Rome (City) — Juvenile
literature.   [1. Civil engineering — Rome (City)
2. Rome (City) — Antiquities.   3. Building — Rome (City)]
I. Title.
TA80.R6M3   711'.4'0937   74-4280

ISBN: 0-395-19492-X (Cl)
ISBN: 0-395-34922-2 (Pa)

Printed in the United States of America

Cl H Pa. M 10 9

By 200 B.C. soldiers of the Roman Republic had conquered all of Italy except the Alps. In the following three hundred years they created an empire extending from Spain to the Persian Gulf. To insure their hold over these lands the Roman soldiers built permanent military camps. As the need for military force lessened, many camps became important cities of the Roman Empire. The Romans knew that well planned cities did more to maintain peace and security than twice the number of military camps. They also knew that a city was more than just a business, government, or religious center. It was all three, but most important, it had to be a place where people wanted to live.

Because cities were built either where no city previously existed or where a small village stood, the maximum population and size were determined before construction began. The planners then allotted adequate space for houses, shops, squares, and temples. They decided how much water would be needed and the number and size of streets, sidewalks, and sewers. By planning this way they tried to satisfy the needs of every individual — rich and poor alike.

The planners agreed that when a city reached its maximum population a new city should be built elsewhere. They recognized the danger of overpopulation. A city forced to grow beyond its walls not only burdened the existing water, sewage, and traffic systems but eventually destroyed the farmland on whose crops the people depended.

Although Verbonia is imaginary, its planning and construction are based on those of the hundreds of Roman cities founded between 300 B.C. and A.D. 150. No matter what brought about their creation, they were designed and built to serve the needs of all the people who lived within them. This kind of planning is the basis of any truly successful city. The need for it today is greater than ever.

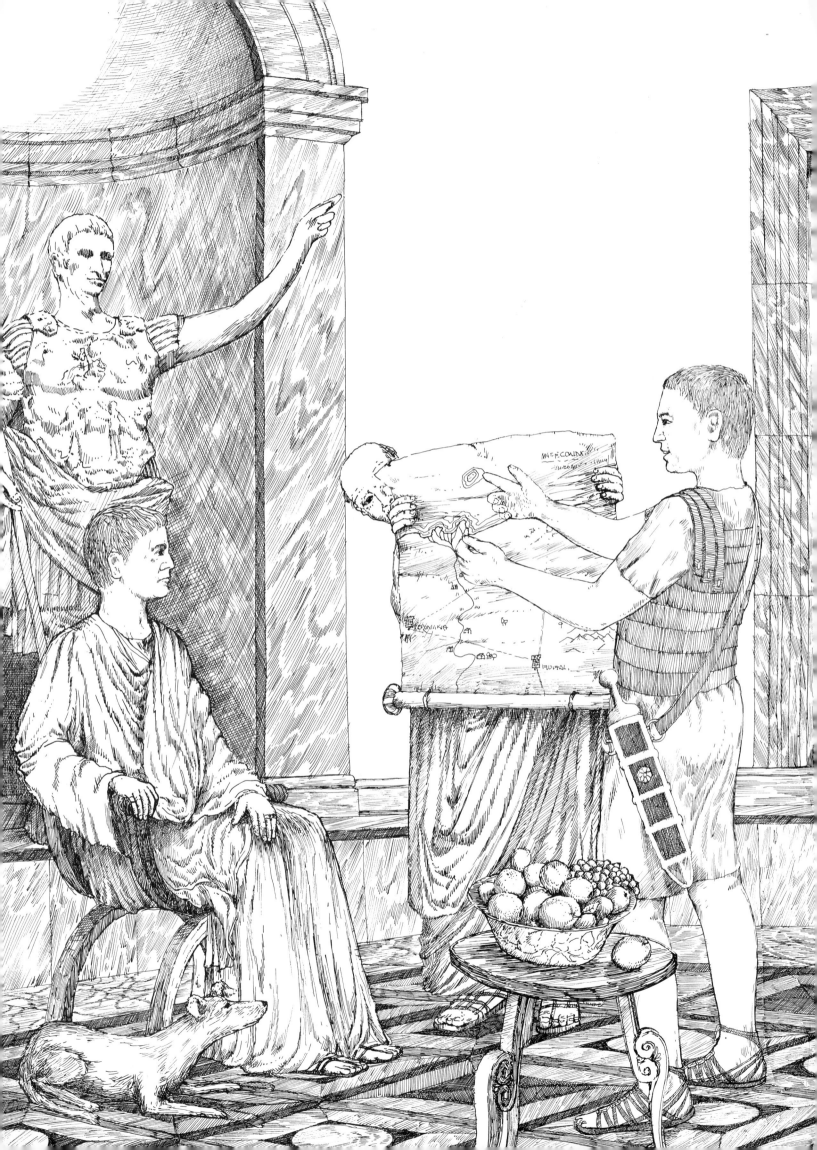

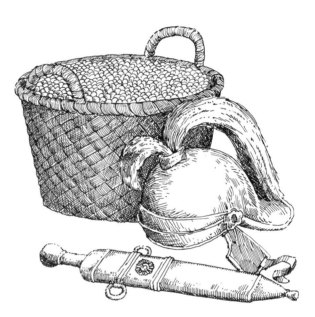

For almost two hundred years the wheat and grapes of northern Italy's fertile Po Valley had been collected in small trading villages and shipped to Rome. In 26 B.C. a disastrous spring flood destroyed the villages along the Po riverbanks as well as an important bridge. When news reached the Emperor Augustus he immediately dispatched to the stricken area forty-five military engineers, including planners, architects, surveyors, and construction specialists. They were to supervise the building of a new bridge and new roads and to lay plans for a new city. The city was named Verbonia, and — in honor of the Emperor — Augusta Verbonia.

Augustus hoped to combine all the remaining trading villages into one secure and efficient trading center and so increase the amount of produce coming into Rome. To speed up development of the new city, he retired to the area two thousand soldiers, who would not only help build Verbonia but also become its first citizens.

First the surveyors selected the place where the city would be built. They chose a flat but sloping site (to insure good drainage) that was high enough to avoid future floods. A Roman priest examined the livers of a rabbit and a pheasant from the area to find out if it would be a healthy place in which to live. When the animals were found to be without fault and an investigation of the land turned up no stagnant pools, the gods were thanked and the choice of the site was officially confirmed.

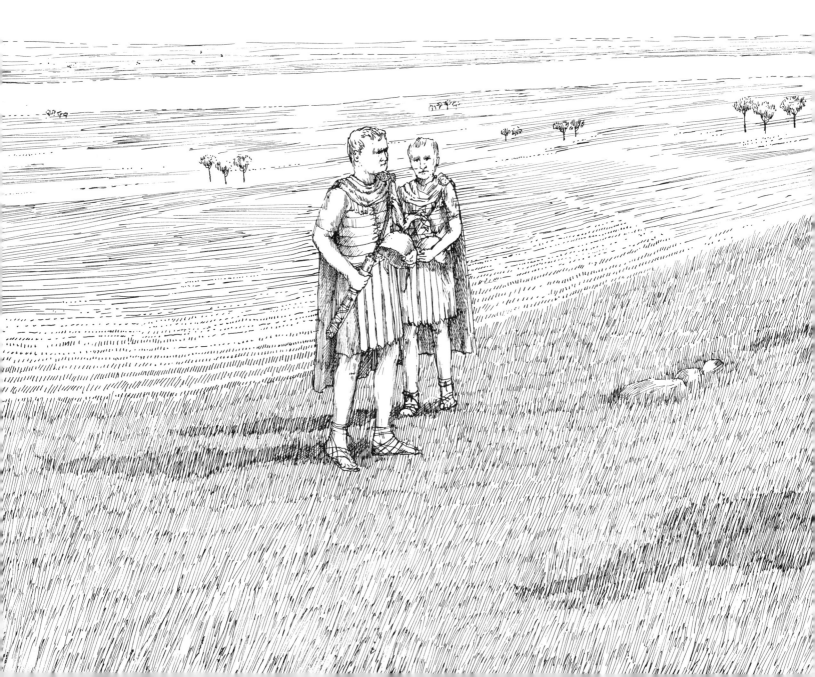

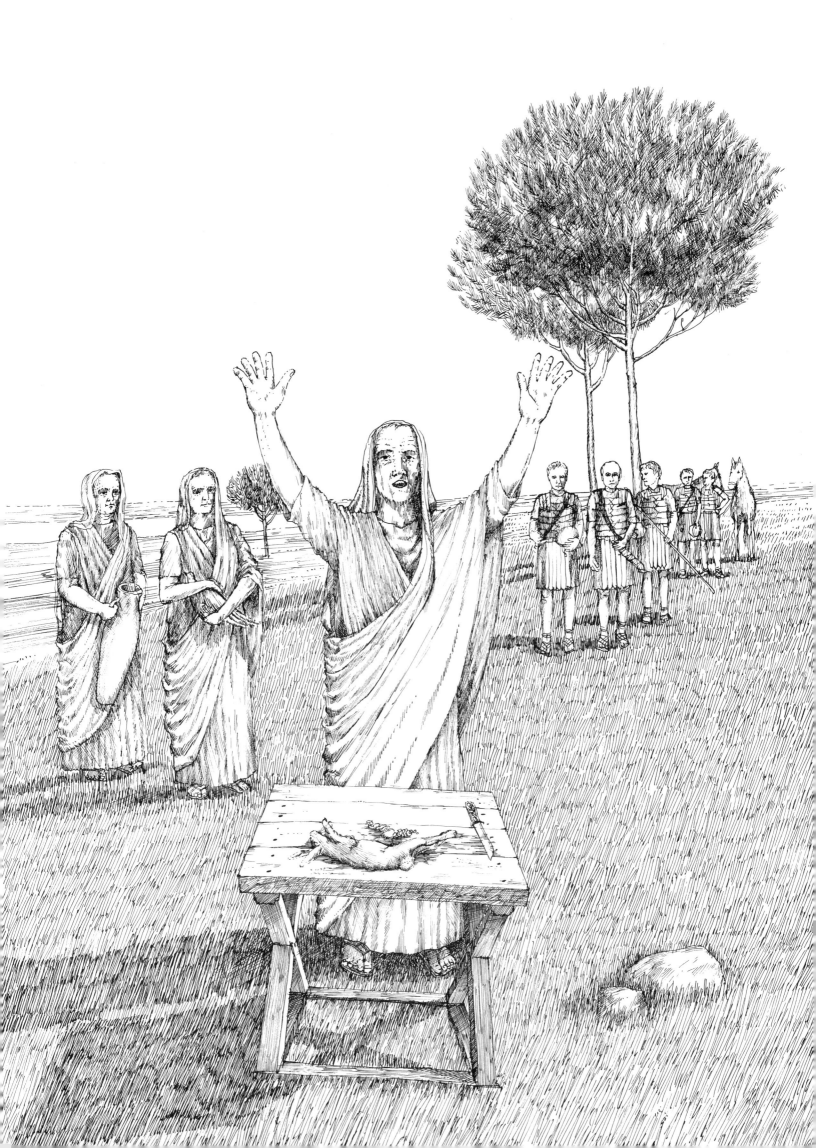

The soldiers and the slaves who traveled with them then set up a military camp called a castrum. First they dug a protective ditch and erected a stockade fence around a rectangular area. Next the two main streets were marked off — one running from north to south, the other from east to west. They crossed at right angles above a long open space called the forum where the soldiers would gather daily to receive their orders. At one end of the forum the

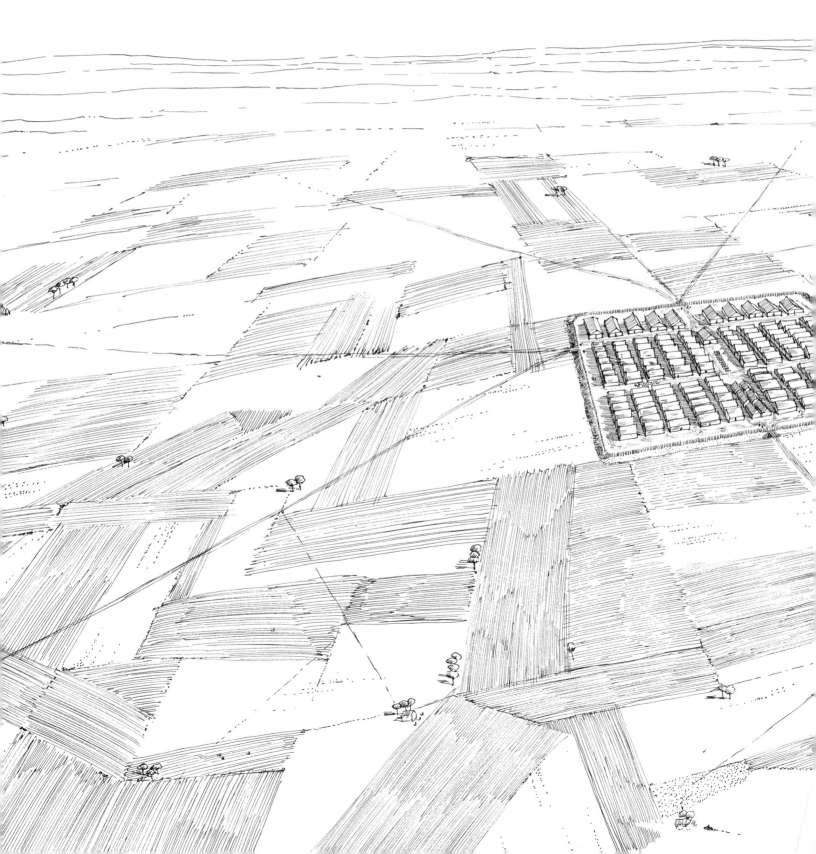

commander's tent was pitched. The tents for soldiers, slaves, and supplies filled the remainder of the castrum and were grouped in rows. In the following months all the tents were replaced by more permanent wooden shelters and a temporary bridge was constructed over boats anchored side by side across the river.

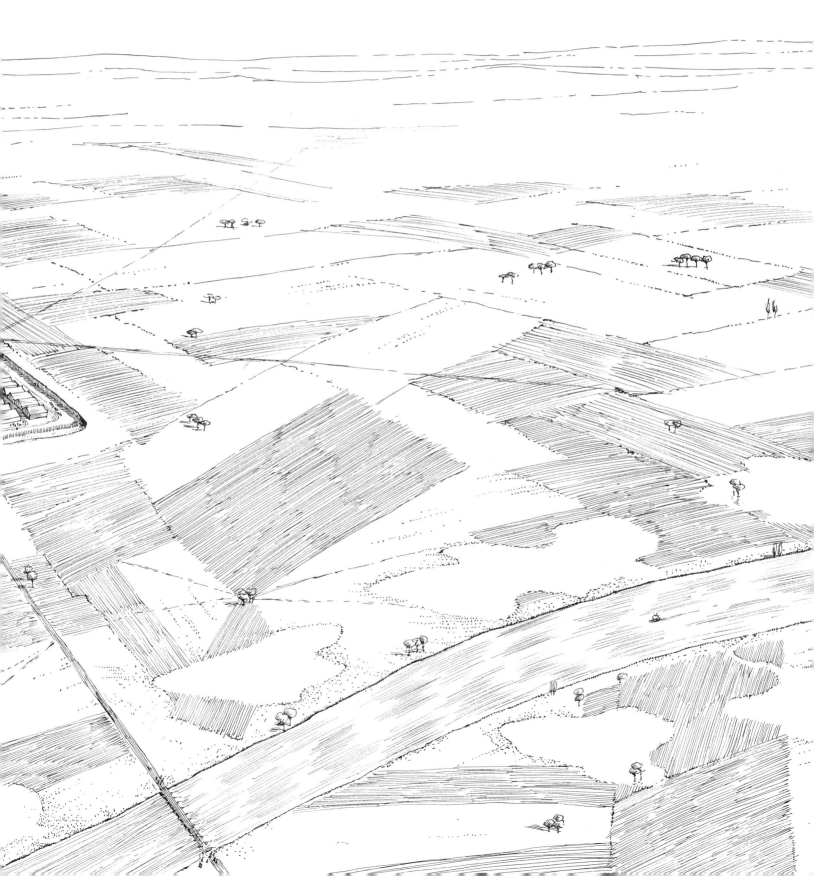

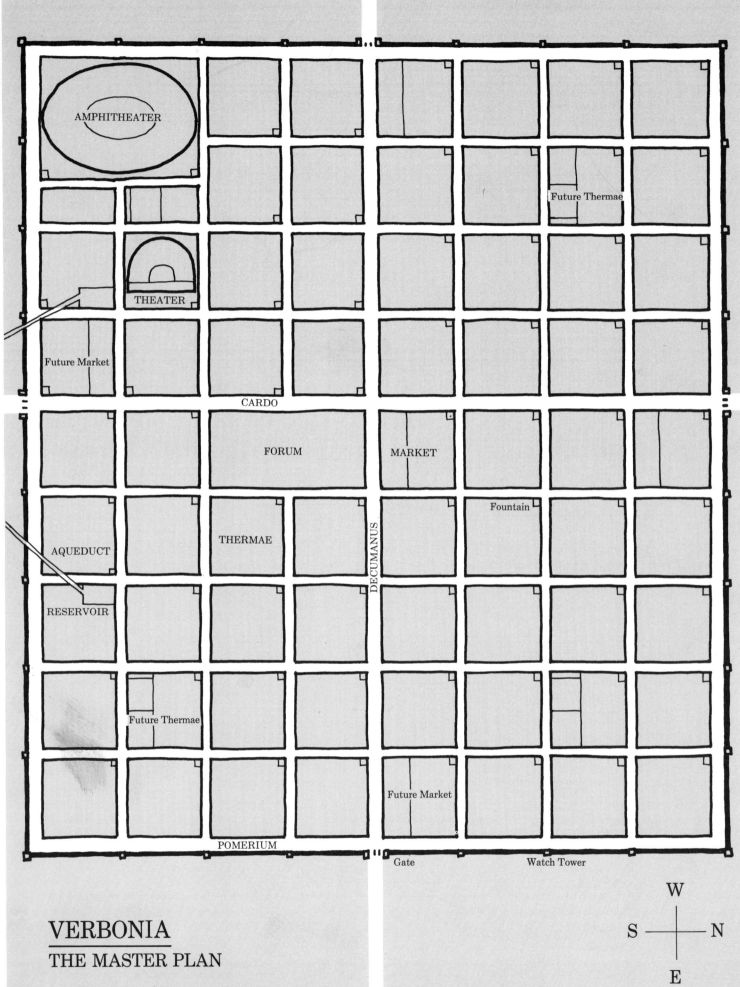

AMPHITHEATER

Future Thermae

THEATER

Future Market

CARDO

FORUM

MARKET

AQUEDUCT

THERMAE

DECUMANUS

Fountain

RESERVOIR

Future Thermae

Future Market

POMERIUM

Gate   Watch Tower

VERBONIA
THE MASTER PLAN

W

S —|— N

E

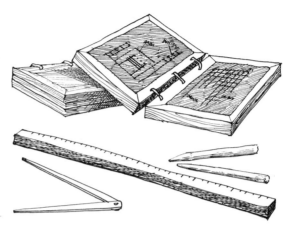

The engineers worked throughout the winter measuring, designing, and drawing. By the spring of 25 B.C. (the Roman year 728) the master plan for Verbonia was ready. The center of the castrum became the center of the city. The main street running from north to south was now called the cardo, the one from east to west, the decumanus. Both were widened and lengthened and the rectangular area of the camp was increased to seven hundred and twenty yards long by six hundred and twenty yards wide. This space allowed a maximum population of approximately 50,000. A greater number, the planners believed, would make the city too large and unable to meet the needs of the people.

The entire area was divided by roads into a chessboard pattern. Almost all of the blocks, called insulae, were eighty yards square. A high wall was designed around the city in which fortified gates were located where the main streets cut through. Around the city but inside the wall a thirty-foot-wide strip of land called the pomerium was marked off. It represented the sacred boundary of the city within which the land was protected by the gods.

The city planners indicated those facilities which served all the residents. They designed a new and larger forum which was to become the government and religious center of the city. They located public water fountains, the aqueduct that would bring the water, a central food market, public baths and toilets, and an entertainment center made up of a theater and amphitheater. They also set aside spaces for future buildings.

No privately owned building, they decreed, could be higher than twice the width of the street on which it stood. This insured that sunlight always reached the streets. They also required all persons whose buildings faced one of the main streets to build, at their own expense, shelter over the sidewalk for the comfort and protection of all pedestrians.

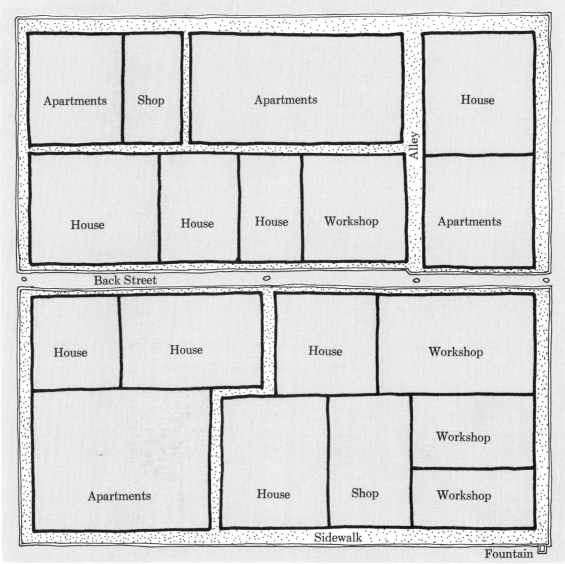

TYPICAL INSULA

The master plan allowed much freedom for the residents to determine the appearance and character of the city through the buildings they would construct for themselves. Each insula, left deliberately empty on the plan, would eventually be filled with buildings of all sizes and be crossed by narrow back roads and alleys.

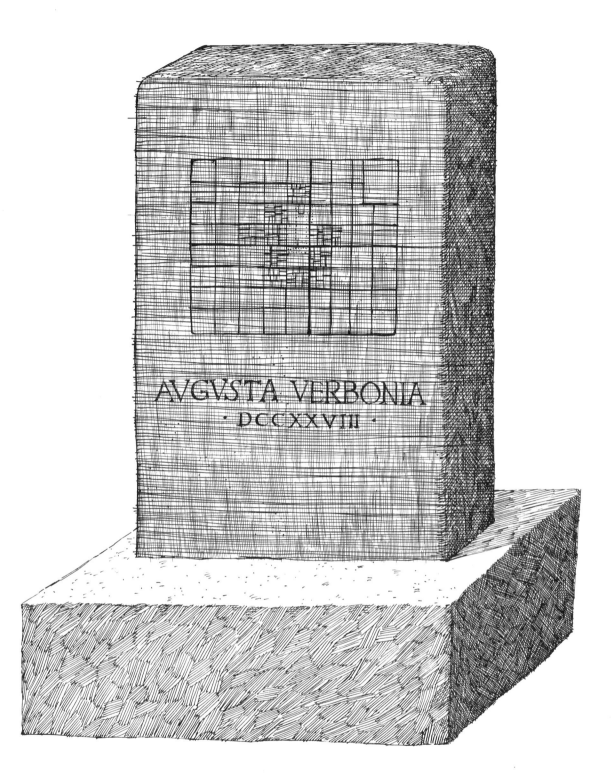

Some of the insulae designated for private ownership were divided up among the soldiers, traders, and farmers. The names of the owners and the sizes of their holdings were inscribed on the plan and sent to the land office in Rome. A copy of the plan was carved on marble and stood in the forum for everyone to see. Even though land was given to Verbonia's first settlers, each person had to pay for the construction of his own house.

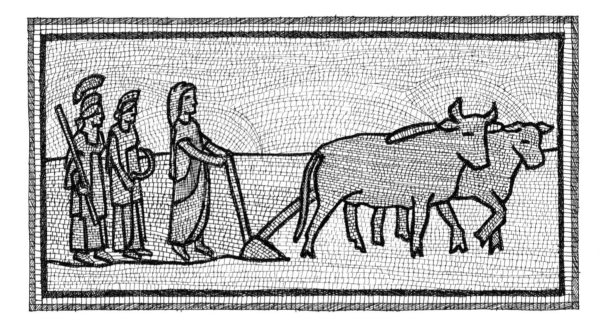

In the early summer of 25 B.C. a plow drawn by a white cow and a white bull guided by a Roman priest cut a furrow around the site. This solemn religious ceremony marked the location of the city wall and insured further protection by the gods. The plow was lifted only where gates were to be built.

Following the ceremony the surveyors marked off the roads using an instrument called a groma to make certain that all roads intersected at right angles. The groma was a pole about four feet high on top of which a cross was laid flat. When weighted strings hanging from each end of the cross hung parallel to the center pole the groma was known to be perpendicular to the ground. The streets could be accurately marked off by sighting down the intersecting arms of the cross.

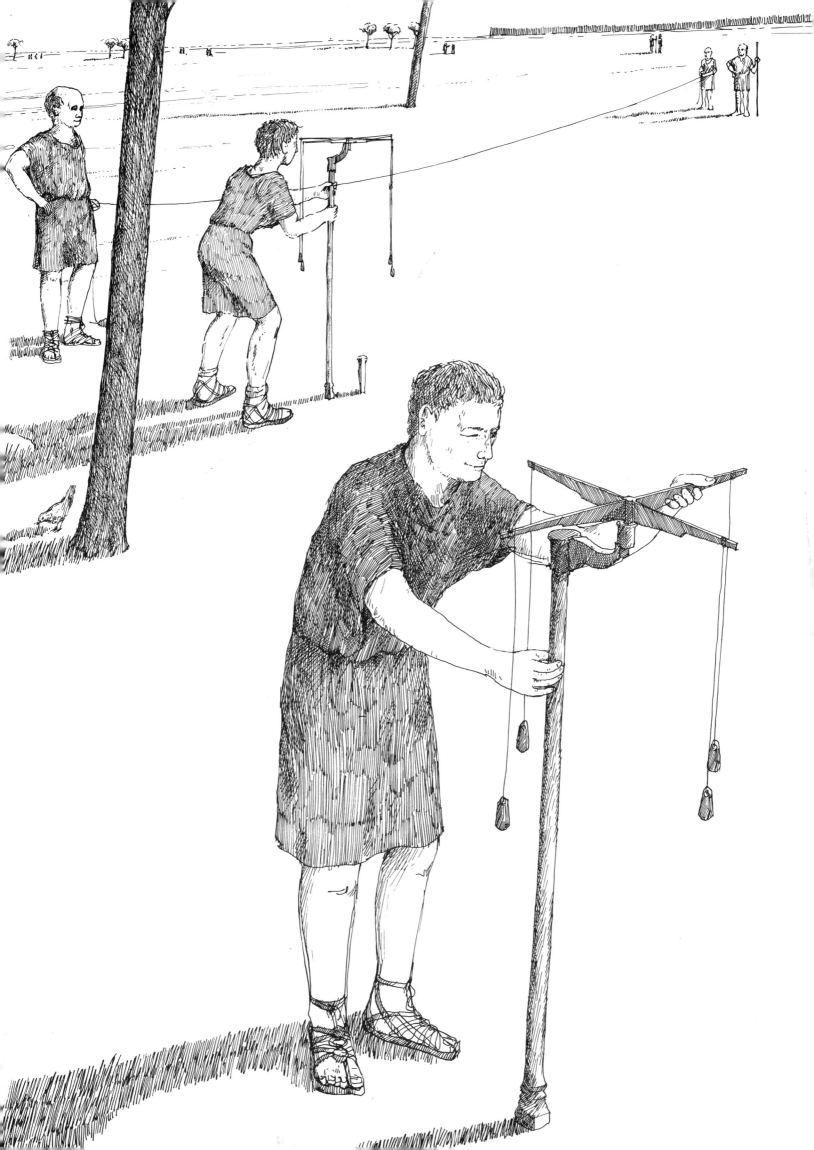

The same method was used to mark off roads and farmland outside the city.

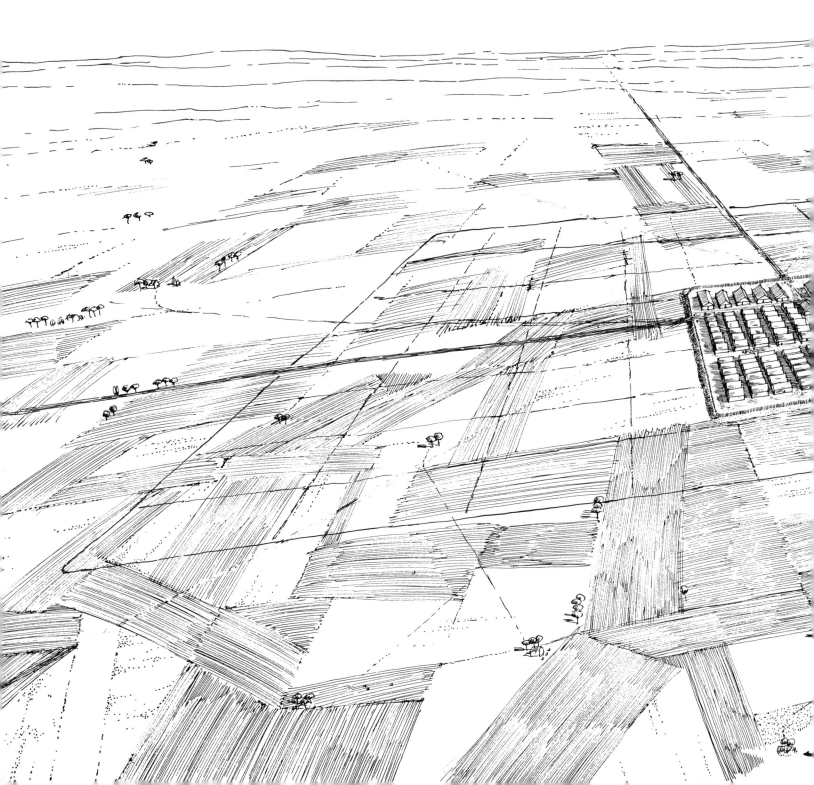

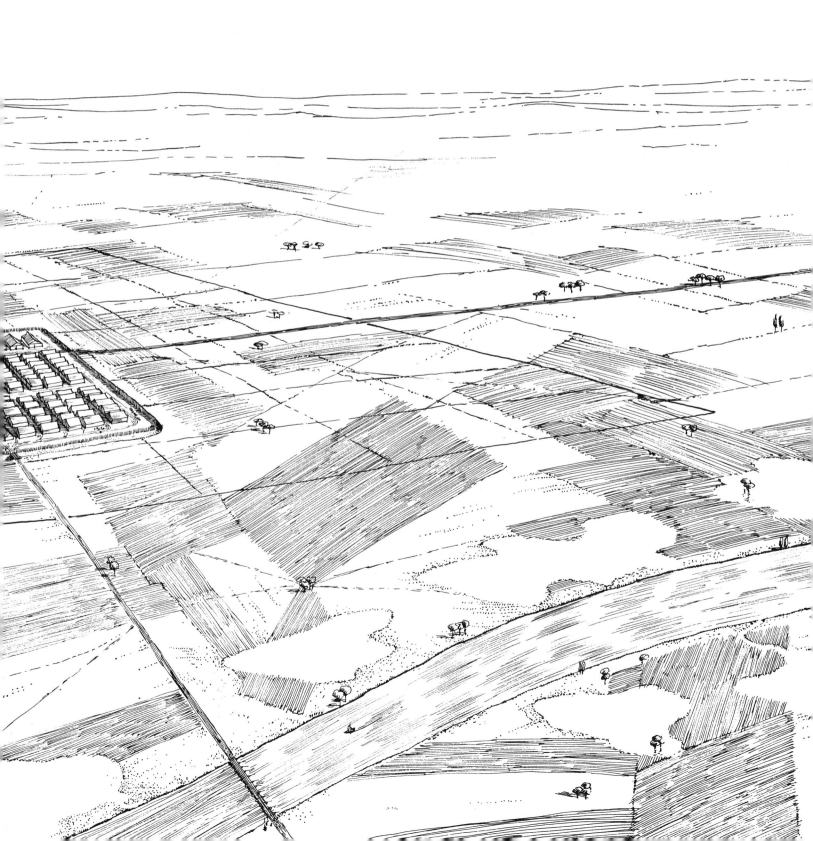

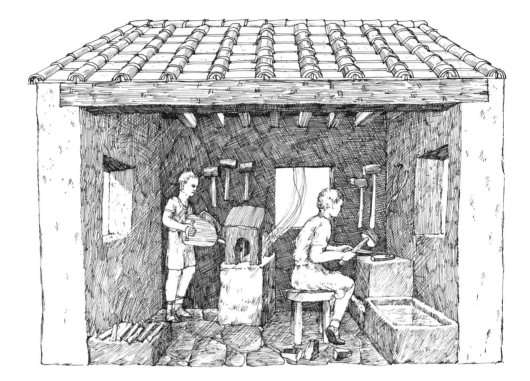

The materials used most in the construction of Verbonia were stone, clay, mortar, and wood. The stone came from a limestone quarry owned by the government. Besides many work sheds, the quarry contained a forge for making and repairing tools and a carpenter's shop in which cranes and pulleys were built.

The skilled laborers cut, polished, or carved inscriptions in the stone. The unskilled workers separated and lifted the huge blocks from the earth. The stone was usually cut with a saw. When the stone was very hard, the blade used in the saw had no teeth; sand and steel filings were placed under the blade and the back-and-forth motion of the saw ground away the stone.

When the stone could not be sawed, a row of holes was drilled where it was to be divided. Wooden stakes were then jammed into the holes. When water was poured over the stakes, they swelled, splitting the stone along the line of holes.

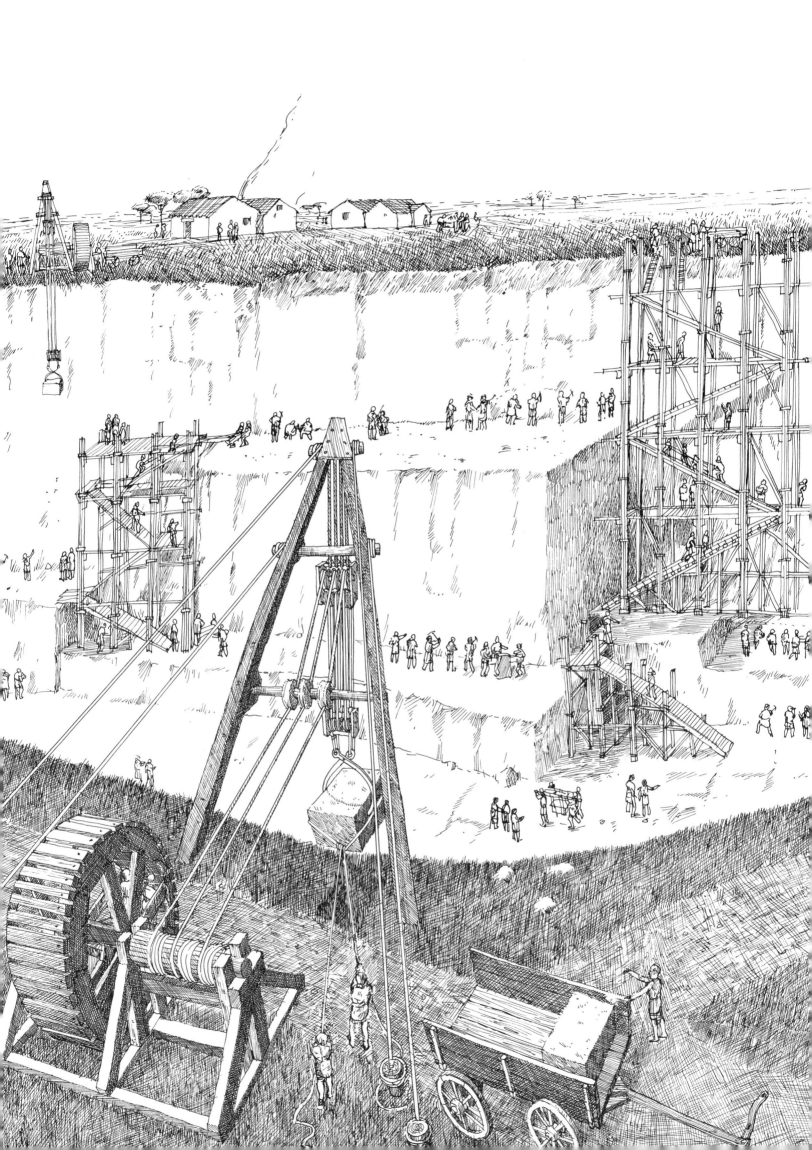

The clay was made into bricks and tiles in factories near Arretium. The clay, dug out of large pits in the ground, was formed into standard shapes and sizes using wooden molds. The mold was then removed and the wet clay placed in an oven to dry and harden. All bricks and tiles were stamped with the name of the factory owner and the name of the Emperor.

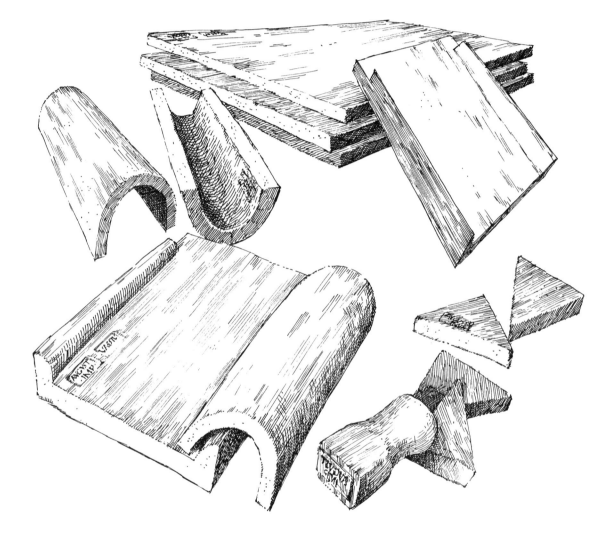

The mortar used between bricks and stones and in concrete was a mixture of sand, lime (a powder obtained by burning limestone), and water. When mortar was used in construction underwater, a gravelly substance called pozzolana was added which made the mortar become extremely hard when it set.

The wood used for scaffolding and roof framework came from a forest at the foot of the Apennine mountains to the south.

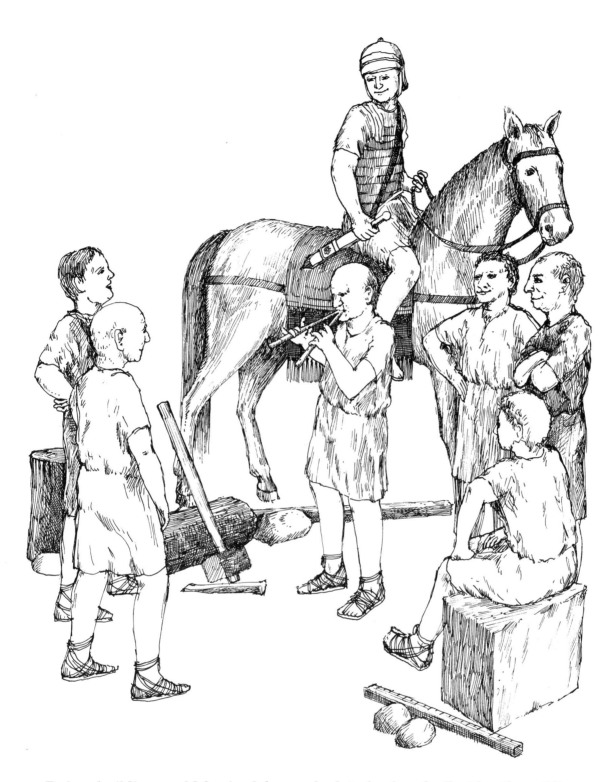

Before building could begin, laborers had to be found. Besides the soldiers many poor farmers from the countryside came to work and settle in the city. The majority of workers however were slaves, either owned by the state or by wealthy businessmen, or they were prisoners of war from Gaul, Greece, or Egypt. Unless they were skilled, the laborers were formed into work gangs to do jobs requiring no particular skill. To maintain as high a level of work as possible the laborers were treated almost as well as the soldiers.

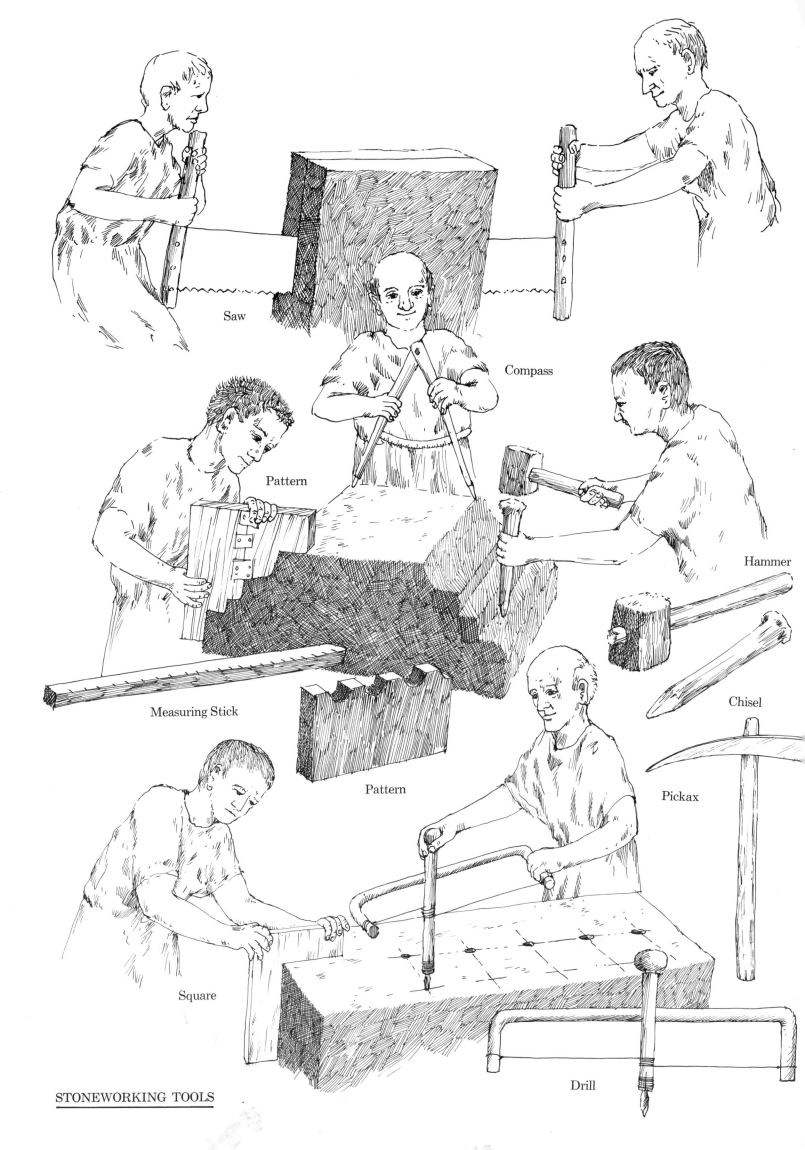

Saw

Compass

Pattern

Hammer

Measuring Stick

Pattern

Chisel

Pickax

Square

Drill

STONEWORKING TOOLS

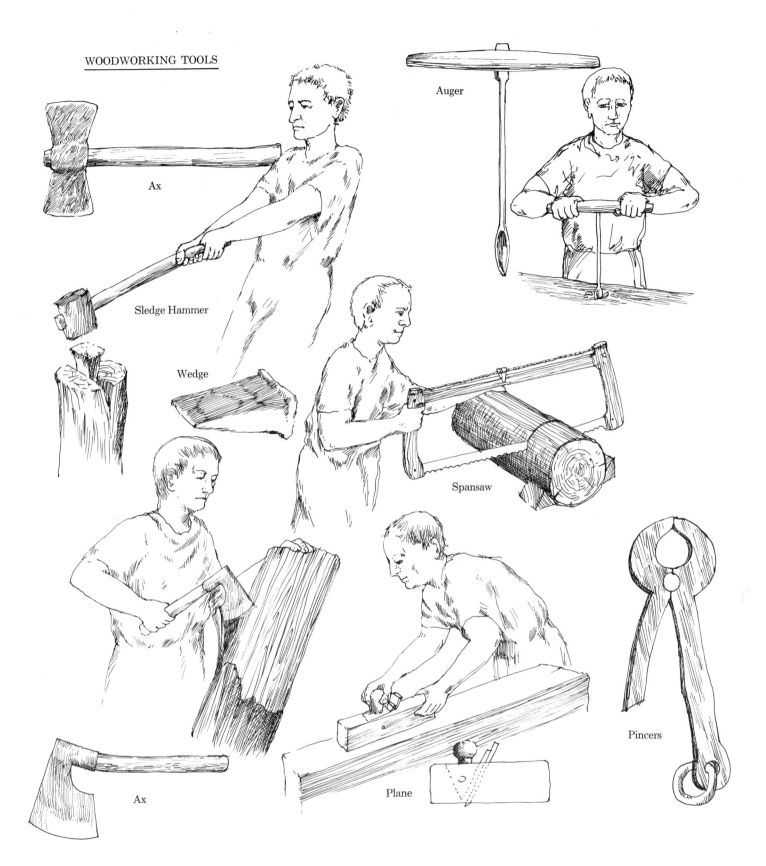

WOODWORKING TOOLS

Ax

Auger

Sledge Hammer

Wedge

Spansaw

Ax

Plane

Pincers

A great variety of tools was needed throughout the construction of the city. Most were made in forges and workshops on the site. The more precise measuring instruments and squares were brought from Rome.

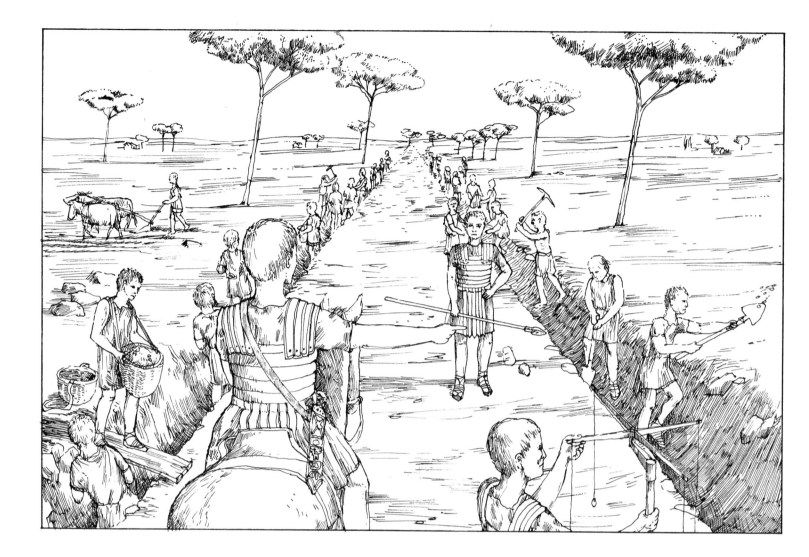
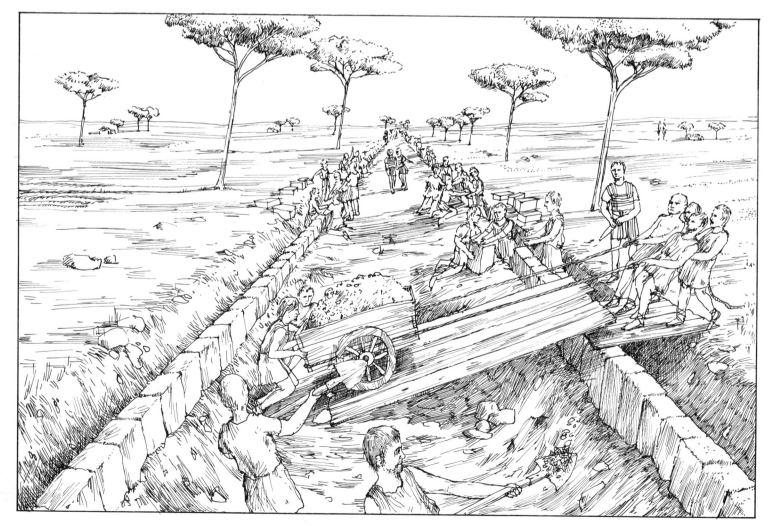

The new roads and bridge were completed before work began on the city itself. Once the surveyors had marked out a road with stakes, a ditch was dug on each side into which a row of curbstones was set. A deeper ditch was then dug between the two rows of curbstones which was filled with layers of stones of varying size. The top layer formed the pavement of the road and rose slightly in the center to force the rainwater into the side ditches. The pavement was constructed of flat stones that were carefully fitted together. Any spaces left between them were filled with smaller stones or pieces of scrap iron.

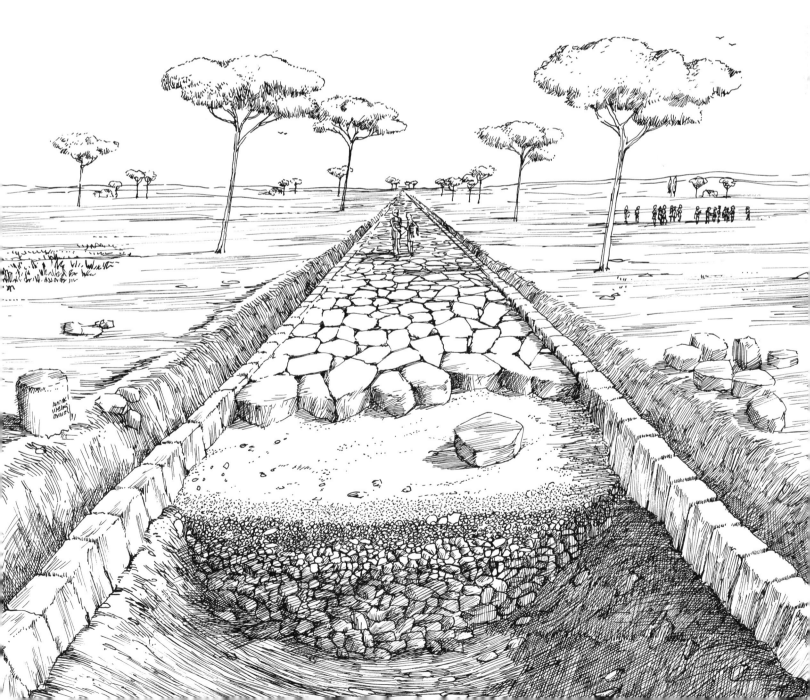

From the boat bridge work began on the permanent bridge. It was to be made of wood and supported on five stone towers called piers which were to stand in the river. Cofferdams were built so the laborers could erect the piers without having to work underwater. First, piles were driven into the riverbed. These were oak tree trunks, with all the bark scraped off, chiseled to a point at the bottom. They were chained together vertically in a shape around which the river could easily flow. When the gaps between the piles had been filled with clay, the water was pumped out of the enclosed area.

Each pier stood on a foundation of tar-covered piles and was constructed of carefully cut stones on the outside and smaller uncut stones on the inside. The mortar used between the stones contained pozzolana. When the piers reached a height of thirty feet above the river, wooden arches were hoisted into place between them.

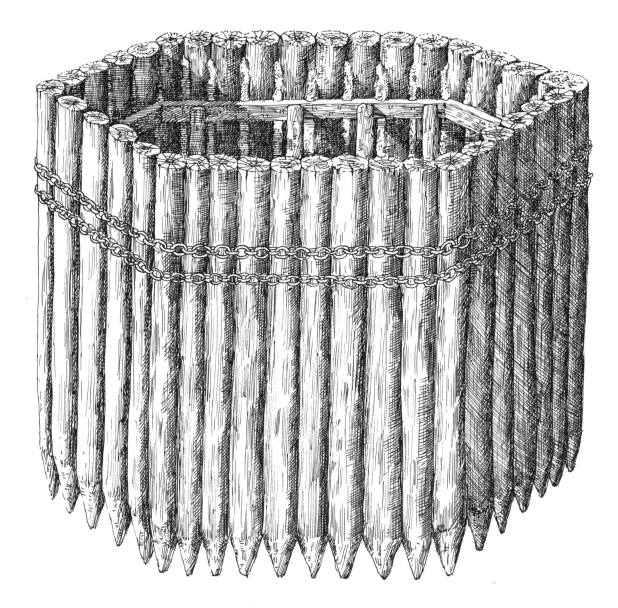

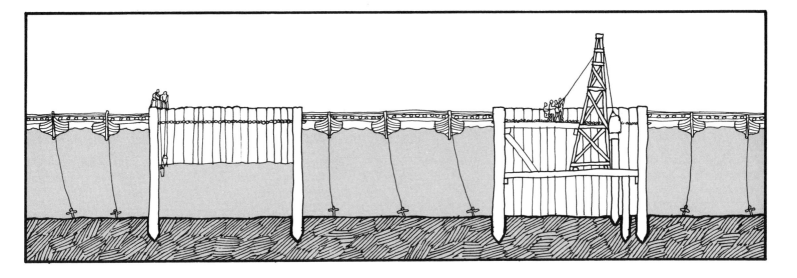

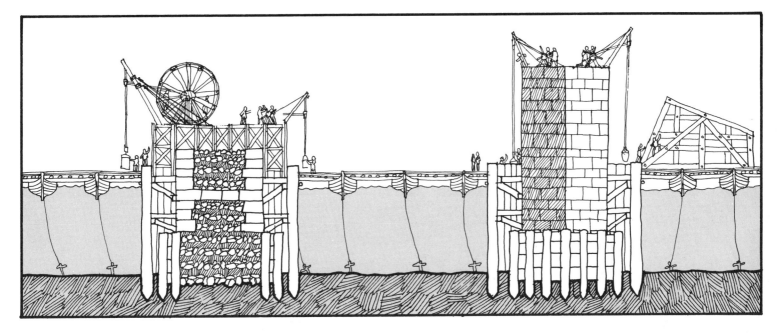

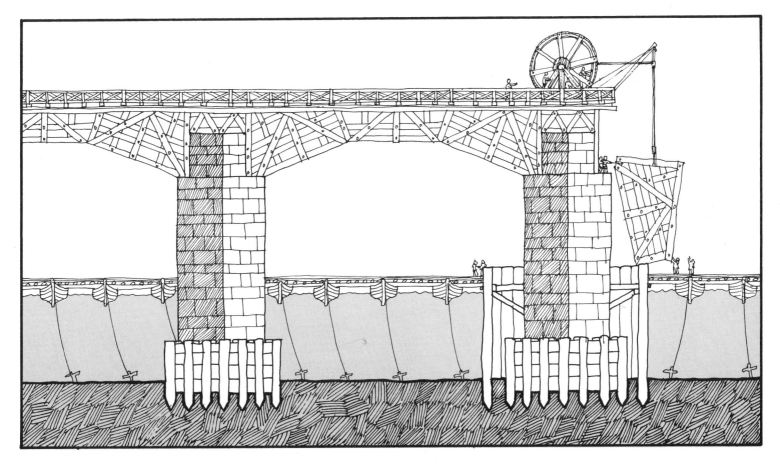

A wooden road was nailed to the arches and covered with a layer of earth. The finished road stood almost sixty feet above the river.

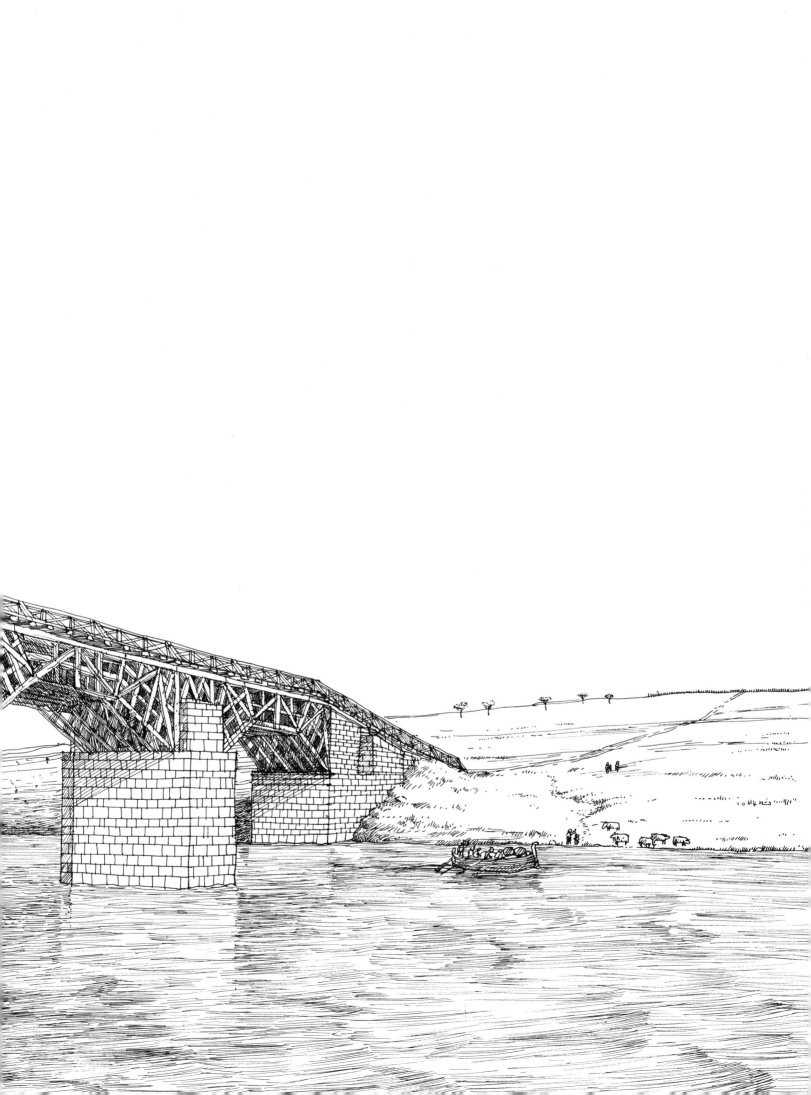

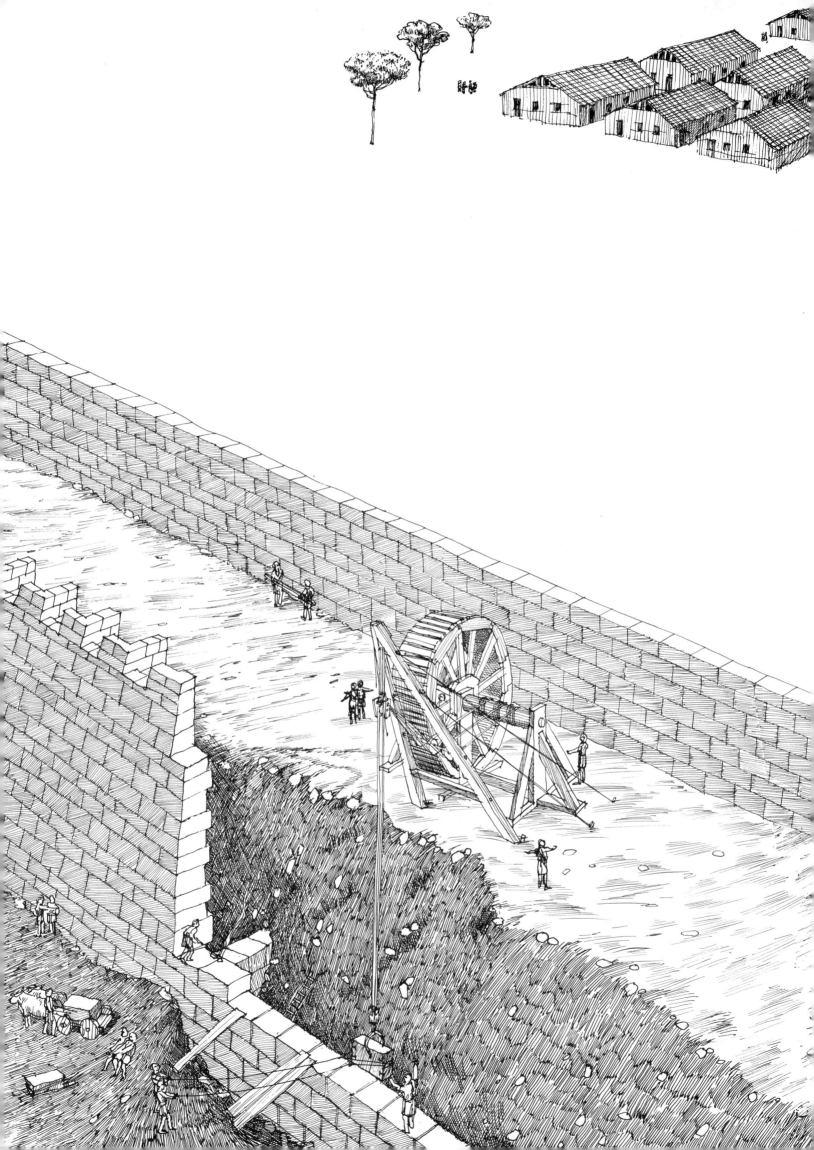

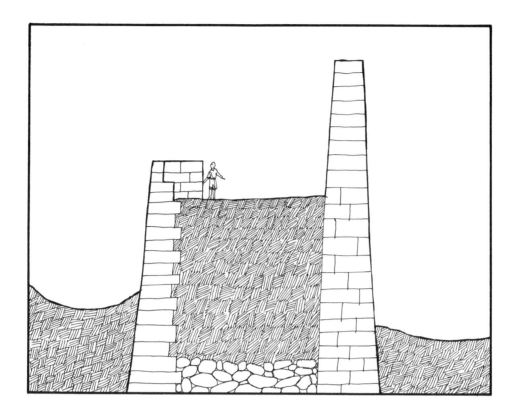

The city wall was built next. Two large ditches were dug along the furrow and the dirt was heaped into a high mound between them. A stone wall was built against each side for additional strength. The base of the outer wall went down thirty feet below ground level, making it almost impossible for anyone to tunnel under. On top of the outer wall alternating high and low sections called crenelations were built. The soldiers were protected behind the high sections while firing their weapons over the low sections. The inner wall was several feet higher than the outer wall to block the path of rocks and arrows that might be fired into the city.

Cranes on top of the mound lowered the stones into place. Four men standing inside a wooden wheel at the base of the crane provided the power. As they walked forward the wheel turned, rotating an axle which wound the rope. The engineers constantly checked to make sure each course of stones was level.

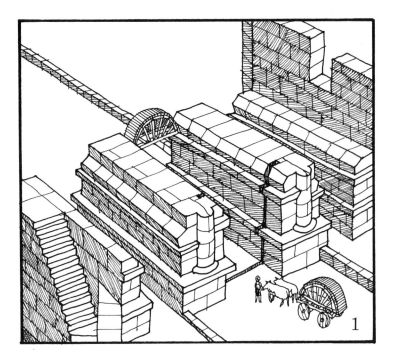

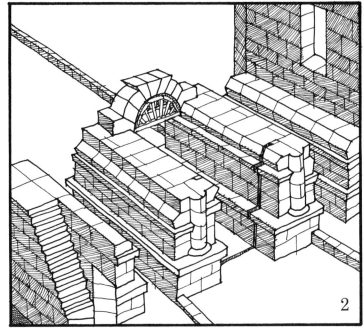

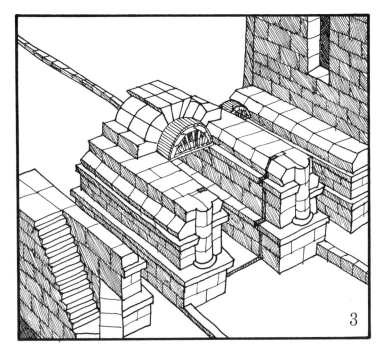

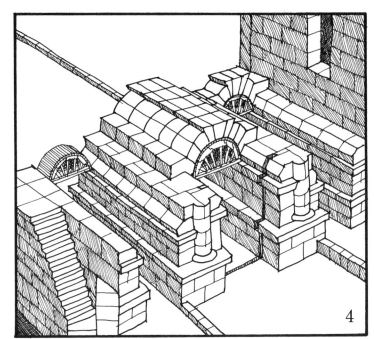

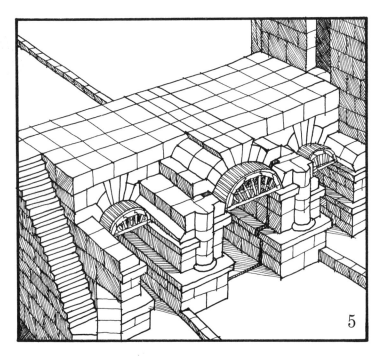

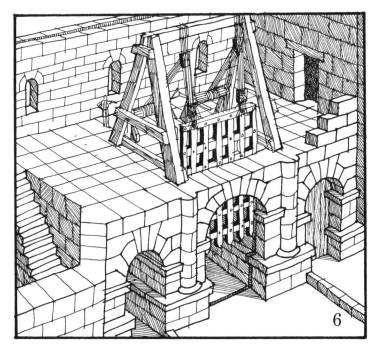

Each gate contained three vaulted openings, one for the road and another for each sidewalk. When the walls on both sides of the road were finished, a wooden arch called a centering was supported between them on projecting stones. The masons, working from both sides, then placed wedge-shaped stones on top of the centering. When the keystone was inserted in the center, the arch was complete. The centering was then moved sideways and another arch was constructed next to the first. This process was repeated until the entire passageway was covered by a semicircular roof called a tunnel vault. The sidewalks were covered in the same way.

The openings in the gate were sealed by heavy wooden doors. The central opening was also protected by a wooden grate called a portcullis, lowered from a room above the street. Both the doors and the portcullis were covered with bronze plates.

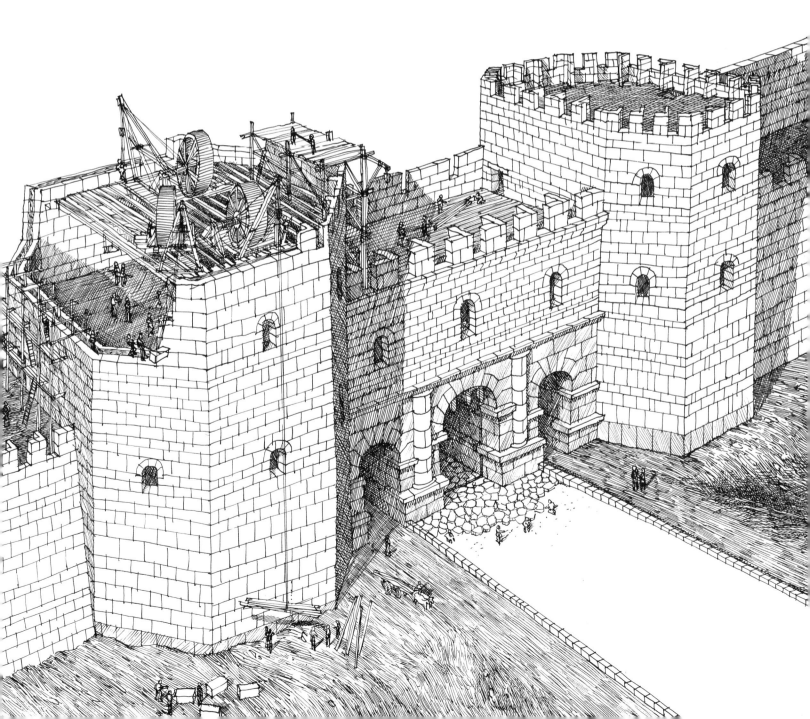

Along the wall and on each side of the main gates high watchtowers were built for additional protection.

At first, Verbonia's drinking water came from several deep wells within the city walls. But the planners knew that as the population increased the wells would no longer be sufficient. A pipeline called an aqueduct was proposed to bring water from the mountain lakes thirty-eight miles to the south.

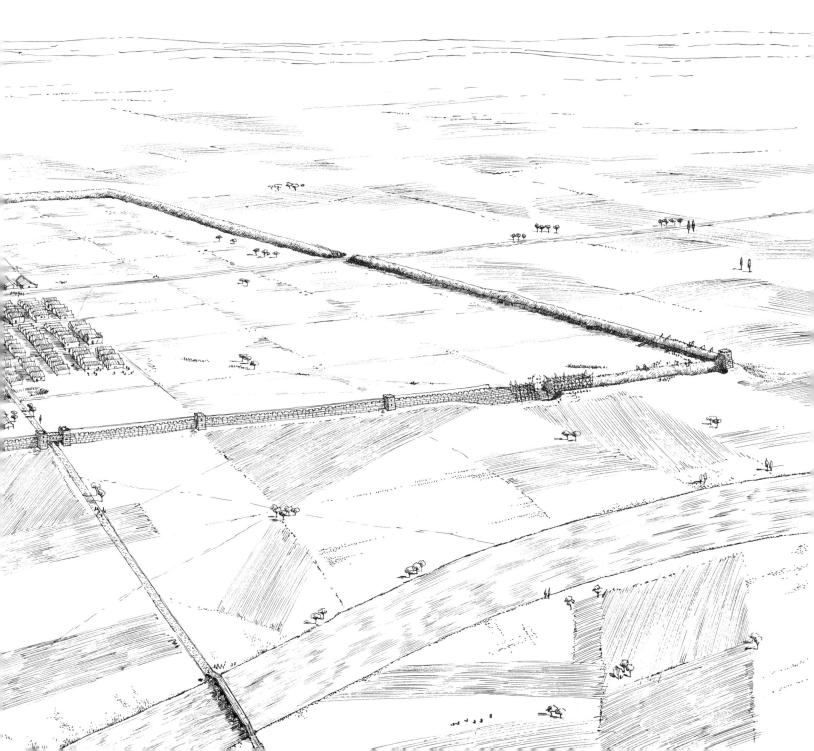

When the best route for the aqueduct had been chosen, a profile map of the land was drawn showing the hills and valleys. To determine the profile, surveyors used leveling instruments called chorobates. The chorobate was known to be level when weighted strings fastened to the horizontal bar hung parallel to the legs. This was double-checked by pouring water into a groove on top of the horizontal bar. When the distance between the top of the water and the top of the bar was the same all around the groove, the instrument was level.

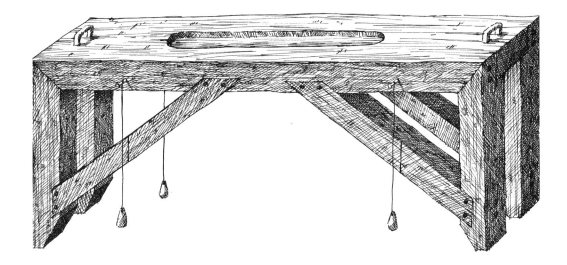

By sighting along the chorobate the surveyors were able to create an imaginary horizontal line over the entire route of the aqueduct. Every forty feet along this line the vertical distance between it and the ground was recorded. When the line was drawn on parchment the vertical distances were marked below it. By connecting all the marks with a single line the mapmakers obtained an accurate profile of the land. By then drawing the line of the aqueduct on the plan the engineers could easily see whether it would sit on the ground, cut through the ground, or rise above the ground.

The aqueduct had to be built with a constant slope from beginning to end to keep the water moving.

To prevent people from stealing or poisoning the water, most of the aqueduct was raised about fifty feet off the ground. It was supported by a continuous row of arches built on tall square piers which rested on deep foundations.

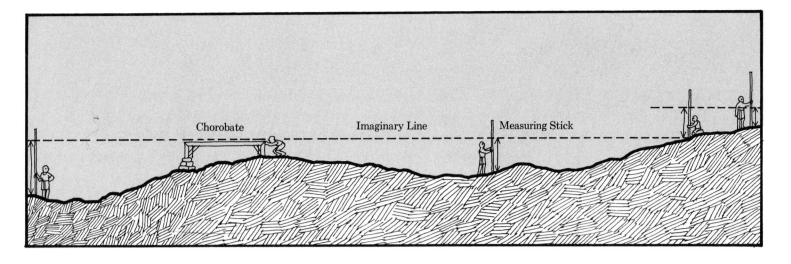

Chorobate   Imaginary Line   Measuring Stick

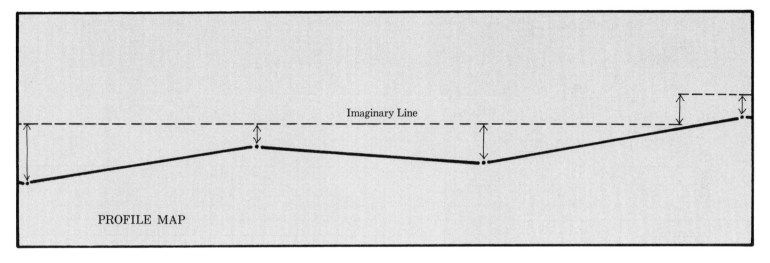

Imaginary Line

PROFILE MAP

Proposed Aqueduct

Arch

Pier

Foundations

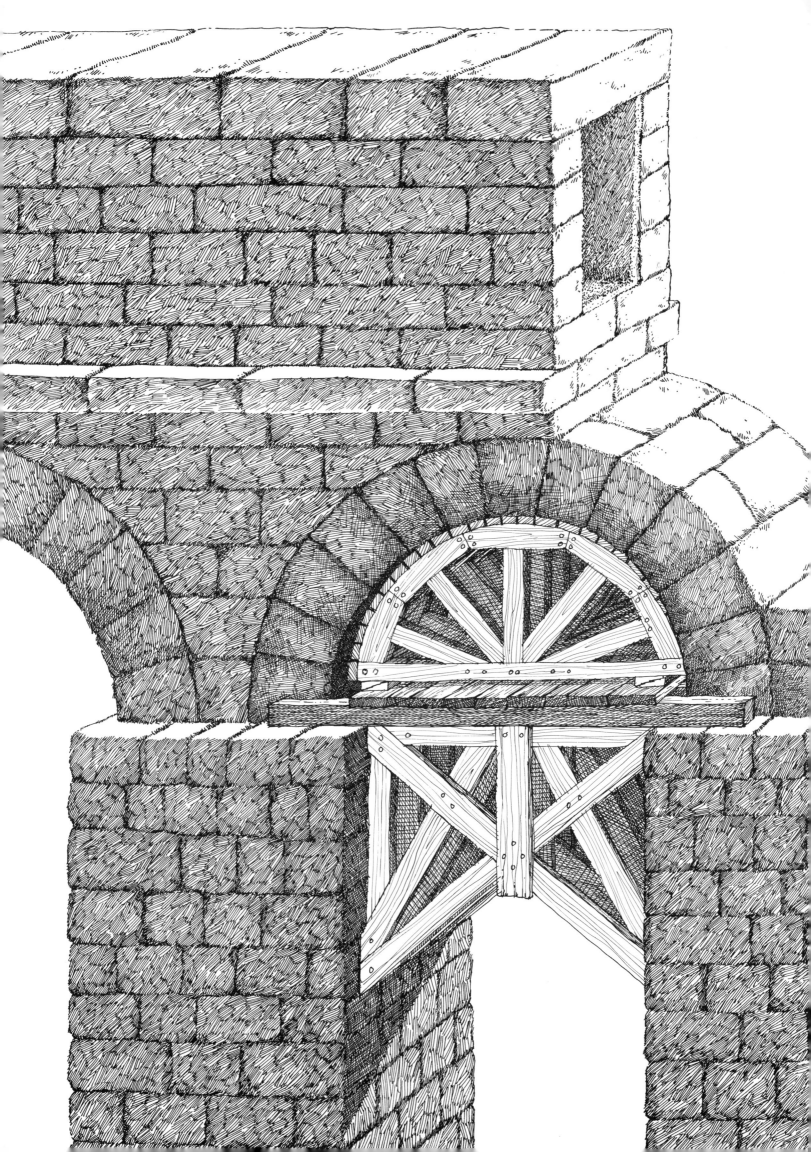

The foundations and piers were constructed of stone-faced concrete — stone set in mortar on the outside with layers of concrete on the inside. To make the concrete, the masons first laid a course of rough stones across the area to be filled. The mortar men then covered the stones with a layer of mortar to bind them together. When the mortar had set, the process was repeated.

When two piers were finished, an arch was constructed between them. The aqueduct, itself a rectangular stone pipe about four feet wide and six feet high, was then built on top. The inner surface of the pipe was lined with hard cement to prevent leaks.

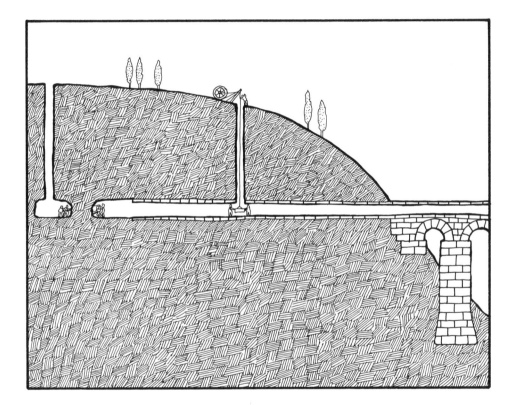

The route chosen for the aqueduct required that a short tunnel be dug through a hill. Every twenty yards vertical shafts were sunk from the surface of the hill to the level of the proposed aqueduct. The depths of the shafts were measured from the profile plan.

The laborers connected the ends of the shafts, and as a section was completed the masons lined it with stone and cement.

Appius Fluvius, the chief water engineer, rode out from the city once a week to inspect construction. The foremen and laborers lived in camp sites which moved with the aqueduct farther and farther from the city. For twenty miles the aqueduct ran alongside the main highway, and the laborers would often stop

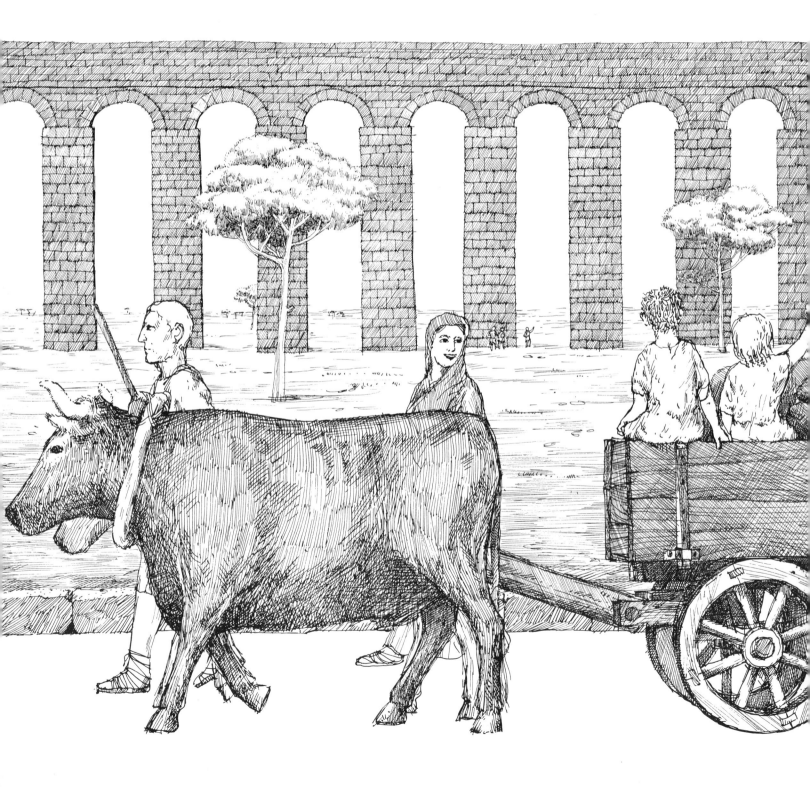

to watch the endless procession of merchants and farmers. About three years after construction began, large numbers of families could be seen traveling toward the city. Many belonged to the soldiers stationed in Verbonia. During the fifth year of construction the aqueduct turned away from the highway and two years later it was completed.

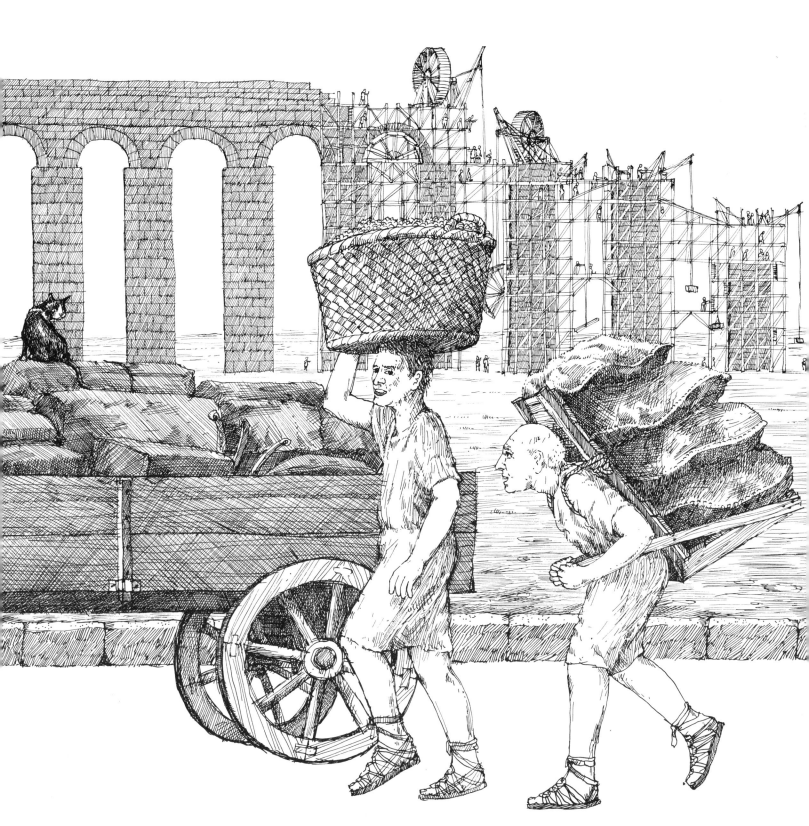

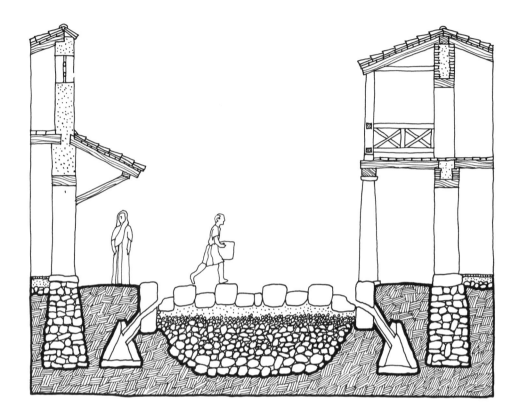

Before the wall of the city was finished, work began on the streets. Verbonia's streets were designed for people. Therefore adequate sidewalks were built and strict laws were written to control any movement of carts and chariots which could endanger the health and safety of people in the streets.

During the day all carts and chariots except those carrying building materials were banned from the streets. This meant that deliveries had to be made at night or in the early morning. Carts and horses were very noisy, so many of the streets on which people lived were made one way or dead end to reduce traffic.

The sidewalks on both sides of the streets were raised one and a half feet above the road surface. This precaution prevented vehicles from accidentally rolling into the path of pedestrians. Steppingstones were embedded in the middle of the road to connect the sidewalks. Animals and carts could straddle the stones — but only if they went slowly. In this way the stones helped to enforce the speed limit. When it rained, the streets were the gutters through which water ran into sewers under the sidewalks. The steppingstones enabled people to cross the street without getting their sandals drenched. The cardo and decumanus were finished first. Other streets were completed as the area around them developed.

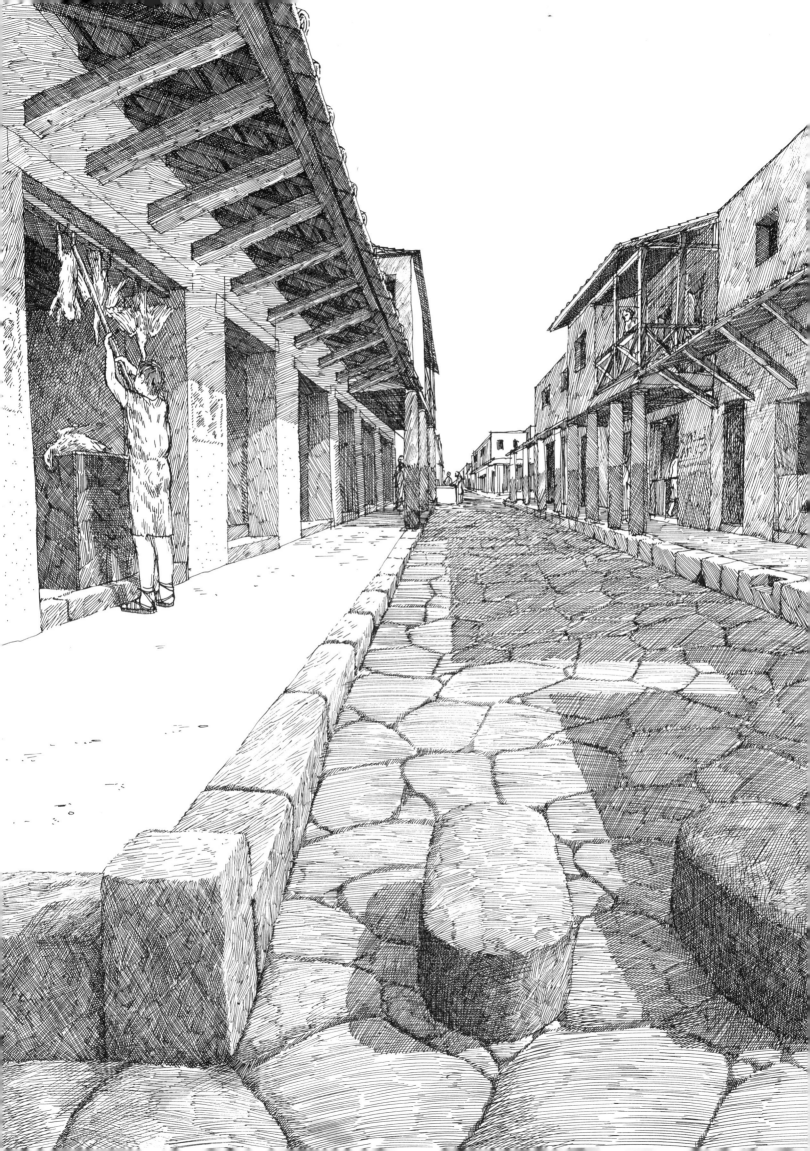

In 20 B.C. Appius and his staff started on the supply system that would distribute water throughout the city. The aqueduct was carried over the south wall and connected to two reservoirs. These were deep rectangular pools whose walls were brick-faced concrete — a wall of triangular bricks on the inside and outside enclosing layers of concrete. Every few feet the top of the wall was covered with three courses of large flat bricks. This allowed the contractor to adjust the level of the wall if it was not perfect.

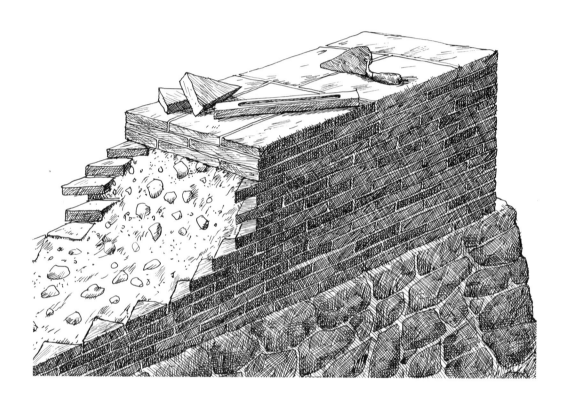

Each reservoir was covered by a concrete tunnel vault. The vaults were constructed over a semicircular wooden form supported on scaffolding between the sides of the pool. Brick reinforcing arches were first constructed over the form ten feet apart. The entire form was then lined with flat bricks and covered with a thick layer of concrete. When the concrete hardened and could stand by itself the form was moved into the next position. Using the same form over and over, the process was repeated until the reservoir was covered. The brick facing on the inside surface of the vault and walls was covered with hard cement. The outside of the vault was shaped like a pitched roof and covered with tiles.

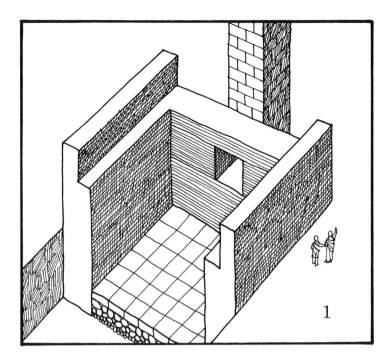

1

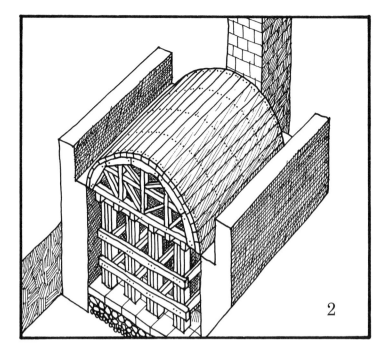

2

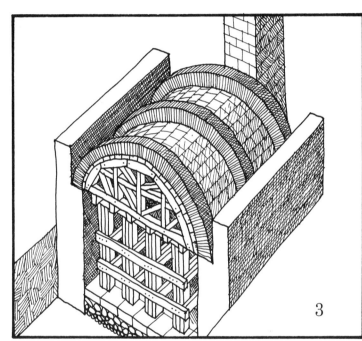

3

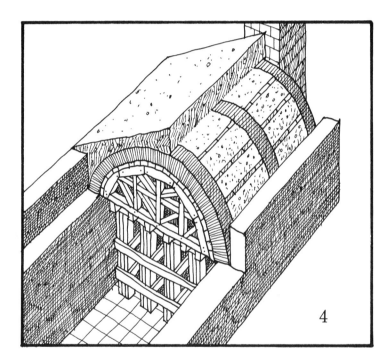

4

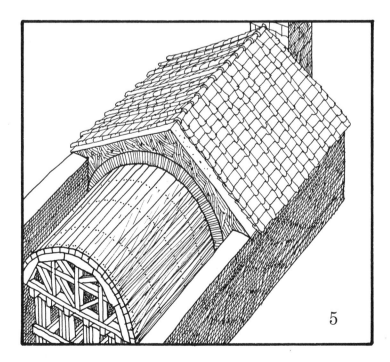

5

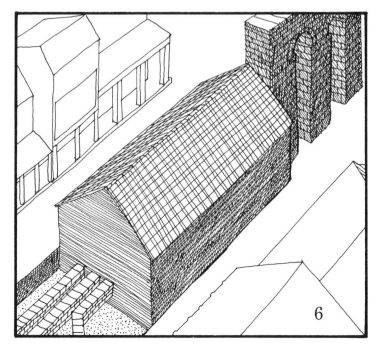

6

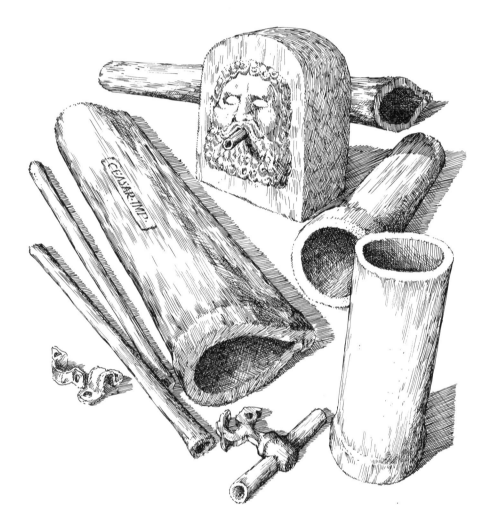

On the wall at one end of the reservoir were several gates channeling the water into lead pipes which ran either to public fountains, toilets, and baths, or to the homes of the wealthy. When there was a shortage of water, the gate leading to these homes was closed, and then, if necessary, the gate to the baths and toilets was closed as well. This insured that the public fountains supplying the majority of Verbonia's residents would be the last to run dry. The water for wealthy homes was first piped into a lead tank placed on one of many high brick towers. As it ran back down other pipes, the water gained enough pressure to feed all the houses to which the tower was connected.

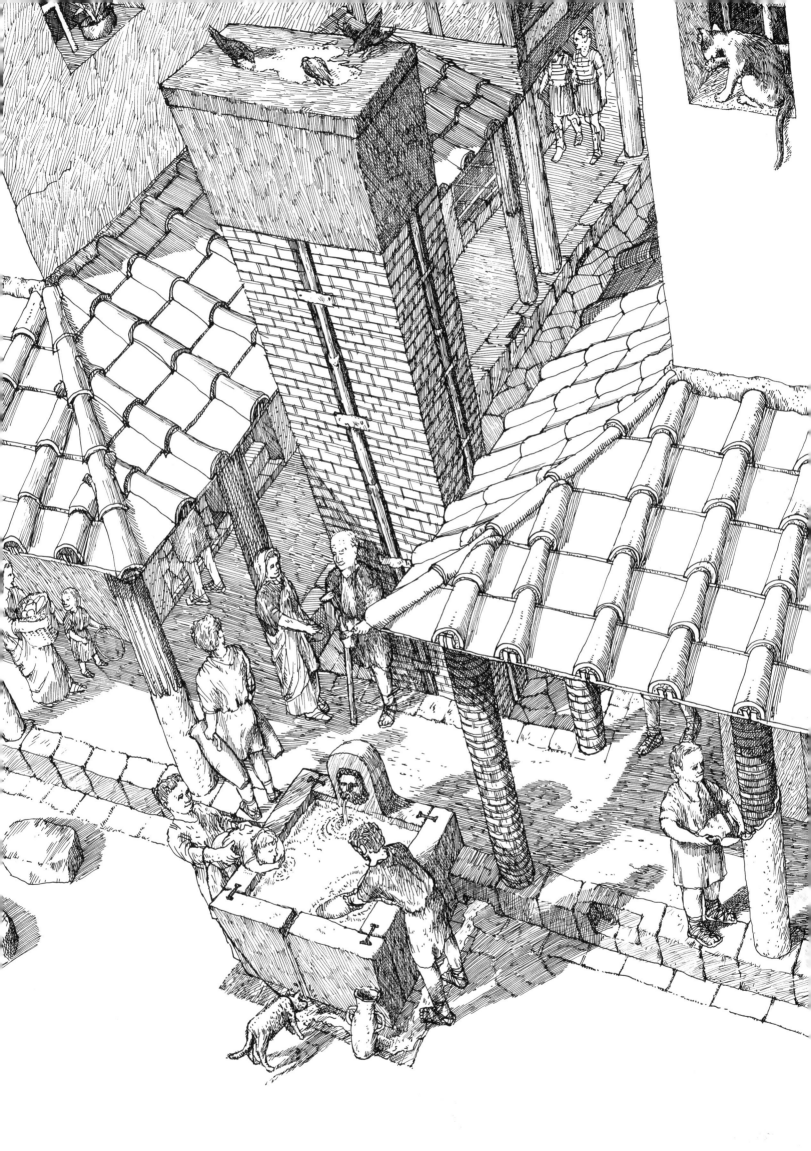

In order for the water supply system to be efficient, an equally efficient drainage system was required. Sewers originally constructed under the sidewalks for rainwater were enlarged. They were connected to both public and private buildings by clay pipes. Some of the sewers were six feet deep. They were all built of stone and mortar and their tops were removable stone slabs in case repairs were necessary. The slabs were covered by compressed dirt in which the lead supply pipes from the water towers were laid.

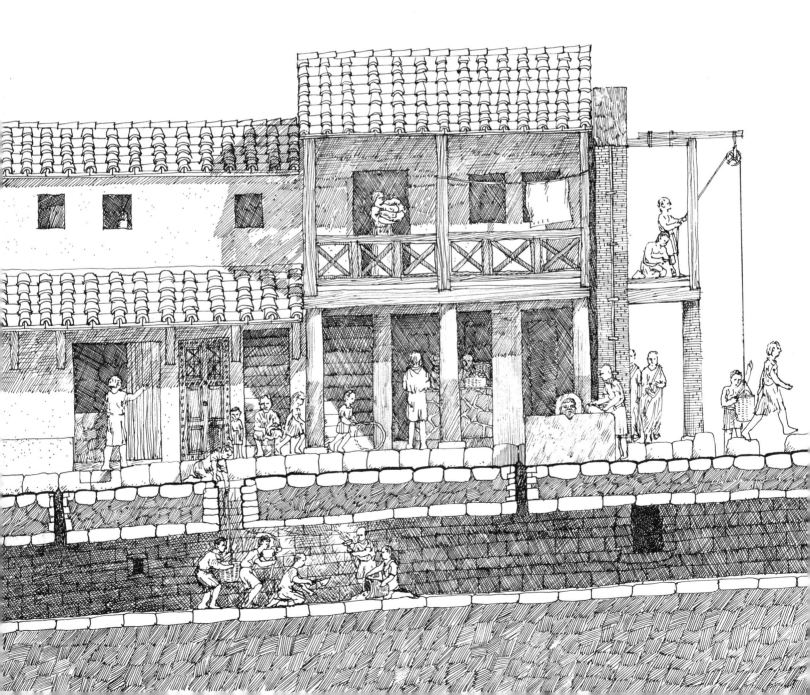

All the sewers were connected to two cloacae — tunnels large enough to walk in — which carried the water under the walls of the city and down to the river. Iron grills were installed inside them which let the water out but prevented anyone from getting in.

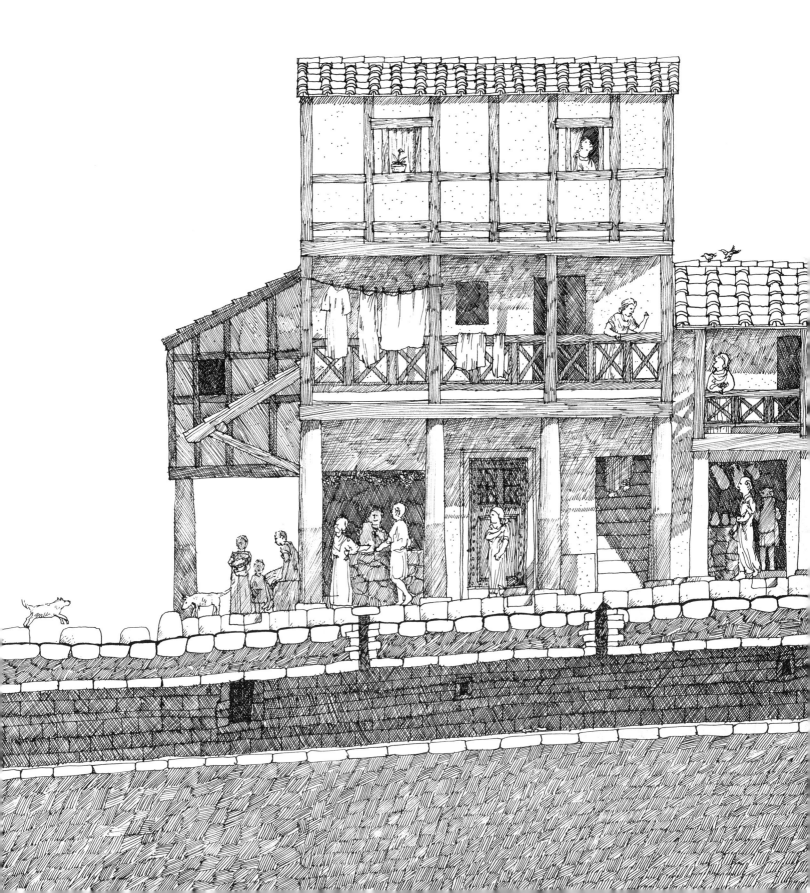

By 19 B.C. the city walls were finished and work began on the first and most important public areas of the city — the forum and the market.

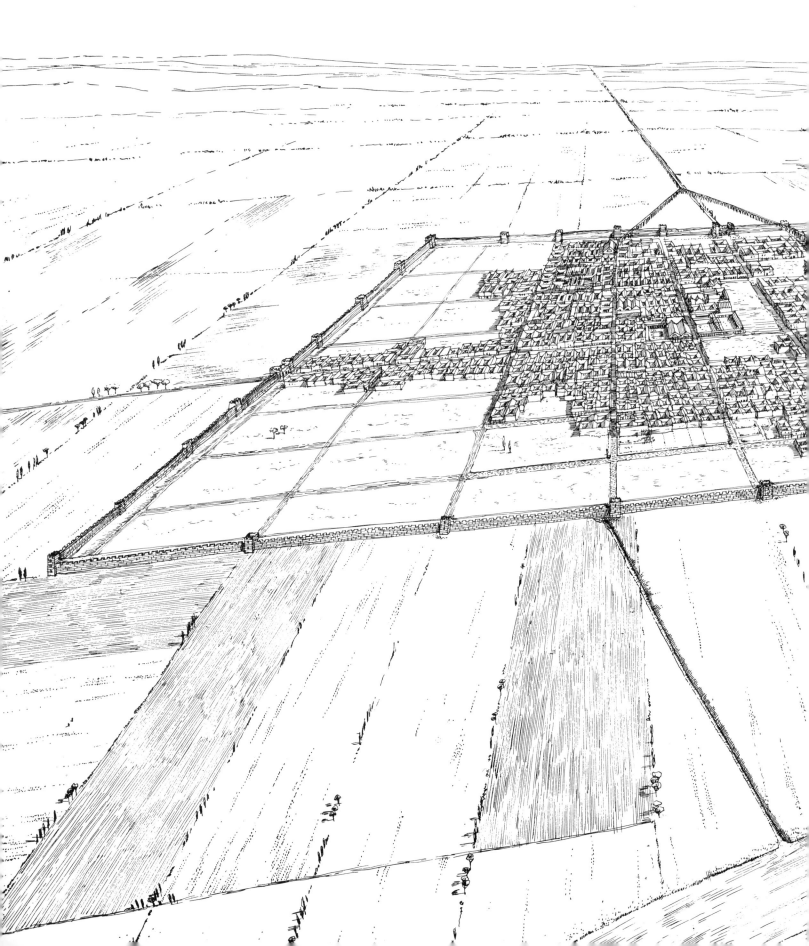

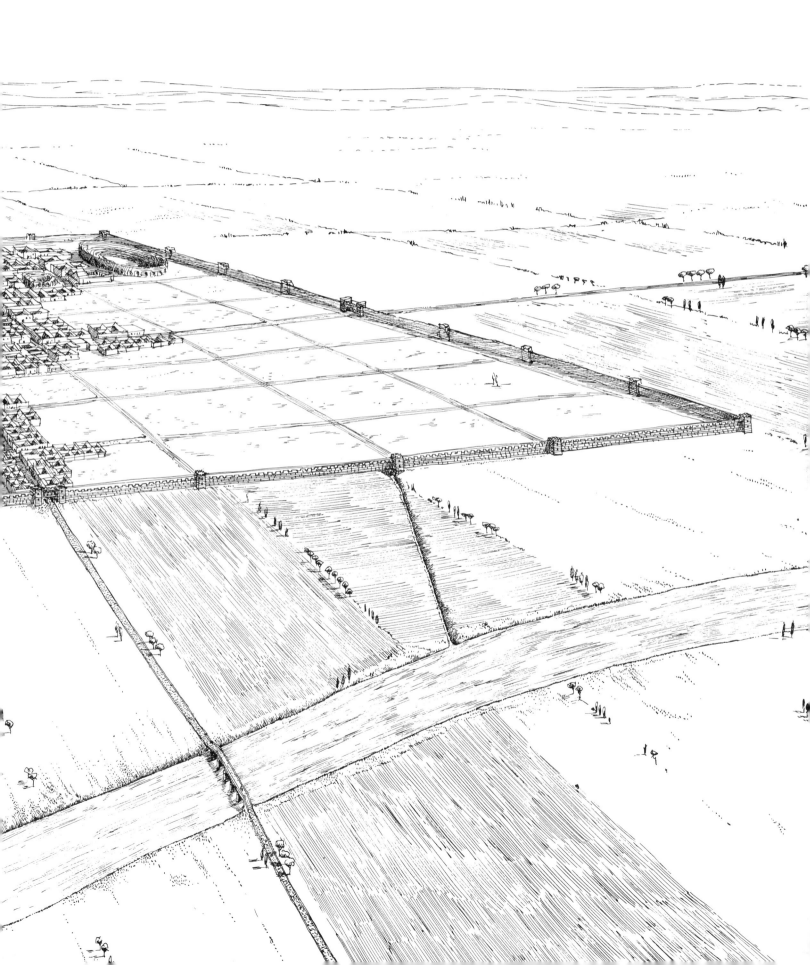

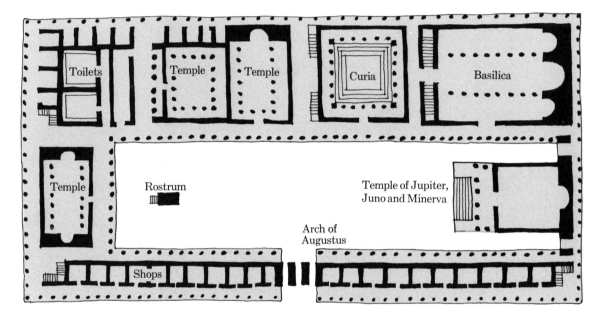

THE FORUM · PLAN

The forum was paved and covered two entire blocks. At one end the temple of Jupiter, Juno, and Minerva was built. Of all the temples to be built in the forum this was the most important. At the opposite end, facing the temple, was the rostrum. This was a raised platform from which speeches were made and decrees were read to the residents of the city. Along one side of the forum stood the Curia — the building in which the elected senators of the city met. Next to the Curia was the Basilica, the court of justice. The temple was constructed of polished limestone, while the other two buildings were brick-faced concrete covered with sheets of limestone. All the roofs were made of triangular wooden frames called trusses, covered by rows of clay tiles.

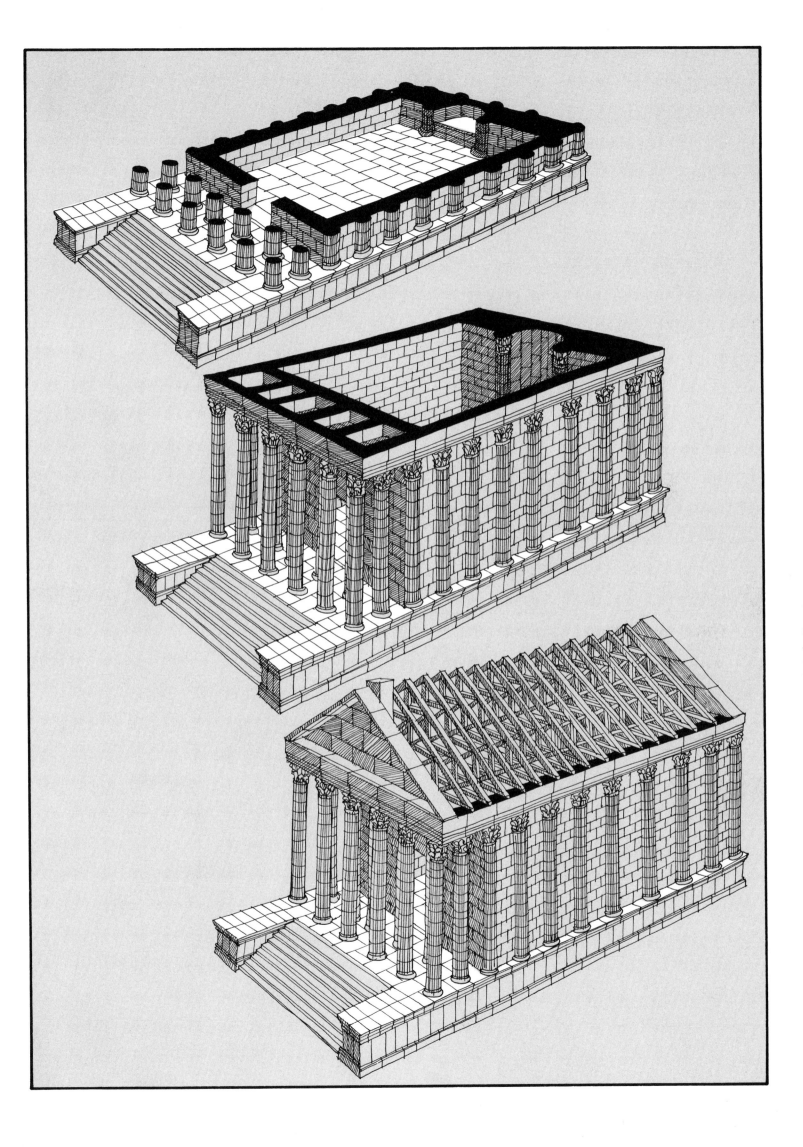

The buildings and the forum were surrounded by rows of columns called colonnades. The columns were either built of cylindrical stone blocks set on top of each other or they were constructed of brick and mortar covered by cement.

A long two-story structure enclosed on both sides by colonnades was built to separate the forum from the busy streets. On the lower level were little shops which faced the street. On the second level were offices and schoolrooms which faced the forum.

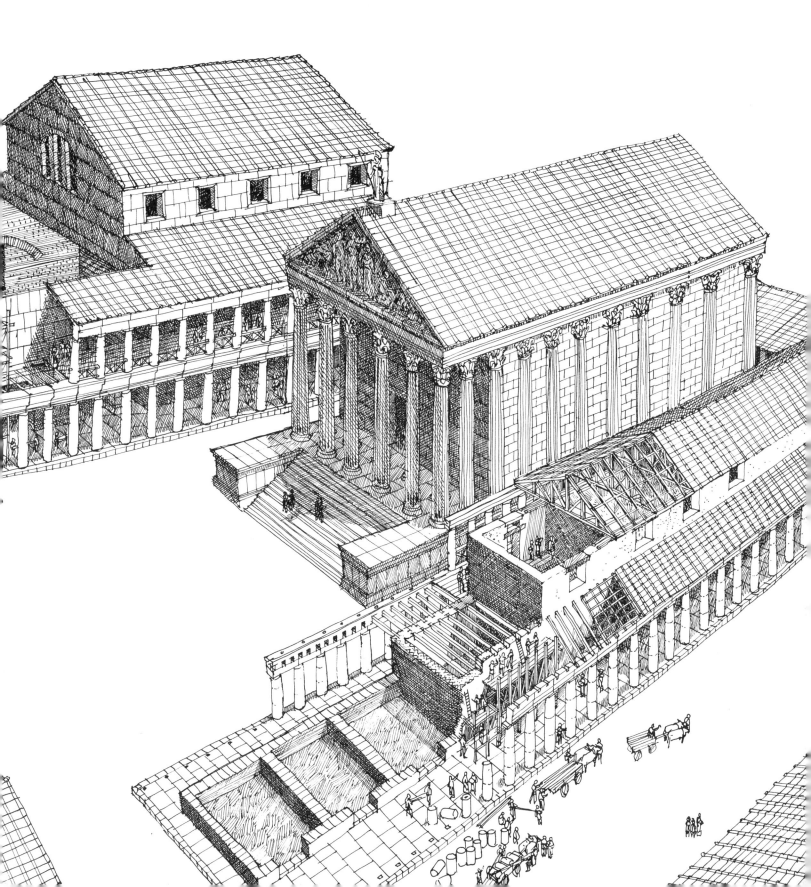

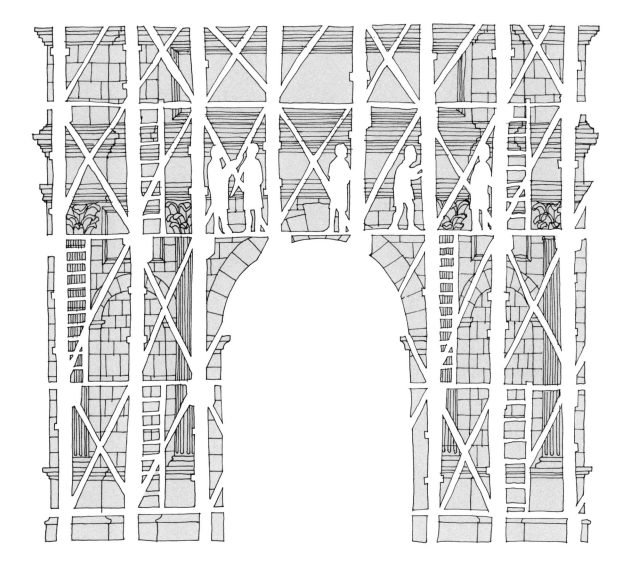

Over the main entrance to the forum, off the cardo, a large triumphal arch was constructed to the glory of the Emperor. It was made of brick-faced concrete and covered with sheets of colored marble. On special holidays processions would enter the forum through the arch.

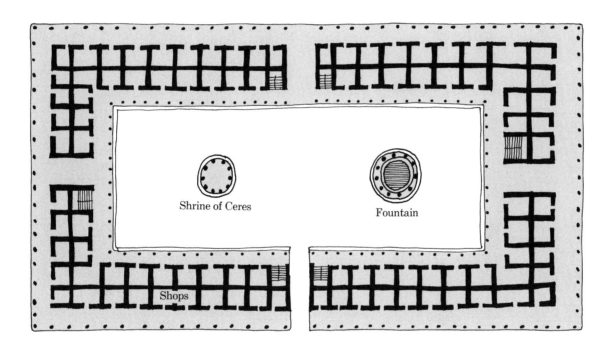

Shrine of Ceres

Fountain

Shops

THE CENTRAL MARKET · PLAN

Because new temples were always being enlarged or replaced the forum really wasn't finished for two hundred years. But the central market across the street was finished in less than five. This was not surprising since Verbonia's main function was that of a trading center.

The open area in which farmers and merchants set up their stands covered almost half a block and was surrounded on all four sides by colonnades similar to those of the forum. In the center was a public fountain and a shrine to Ceres, the goddess of agriculture.

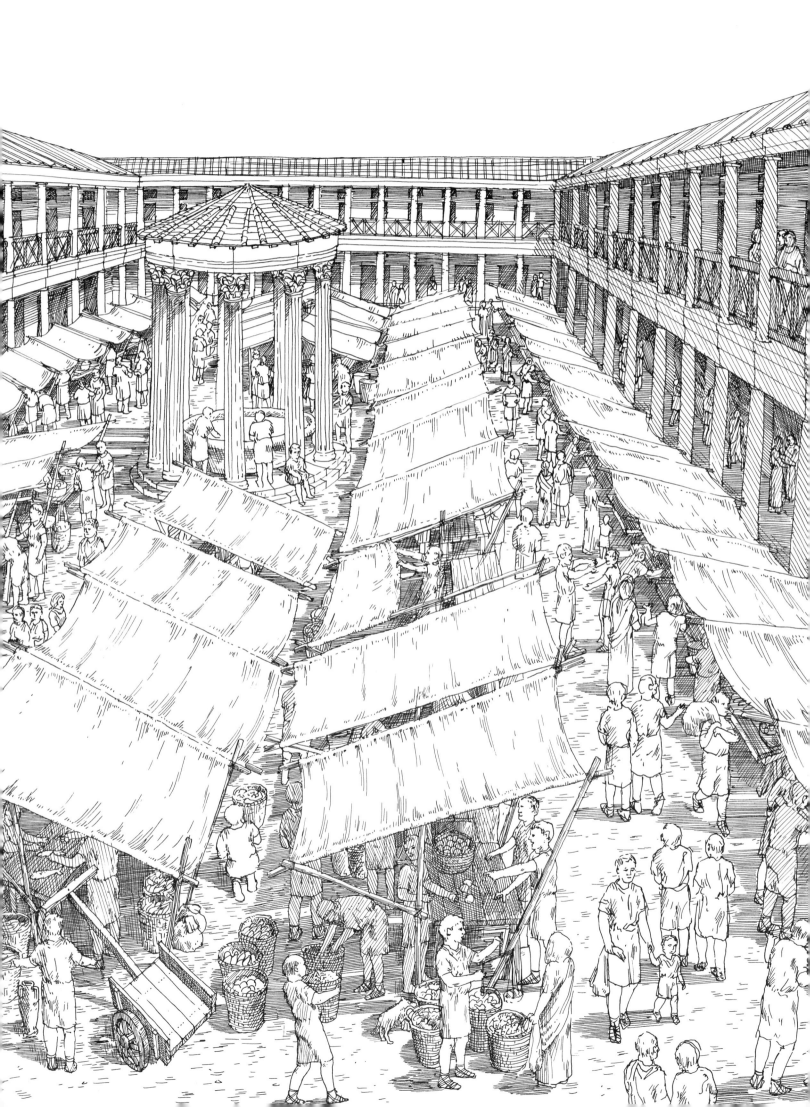

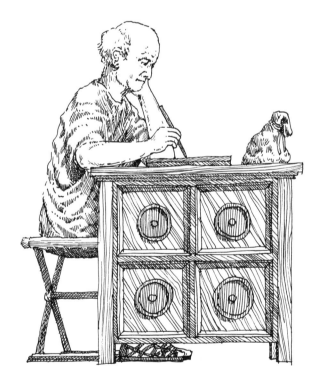

Many of the offices on the second level were rented by businessmen who kept similar offices in other cities, including Rome. These men bought much of the produce from the fields around the city and shipped it to markets all over the empire.

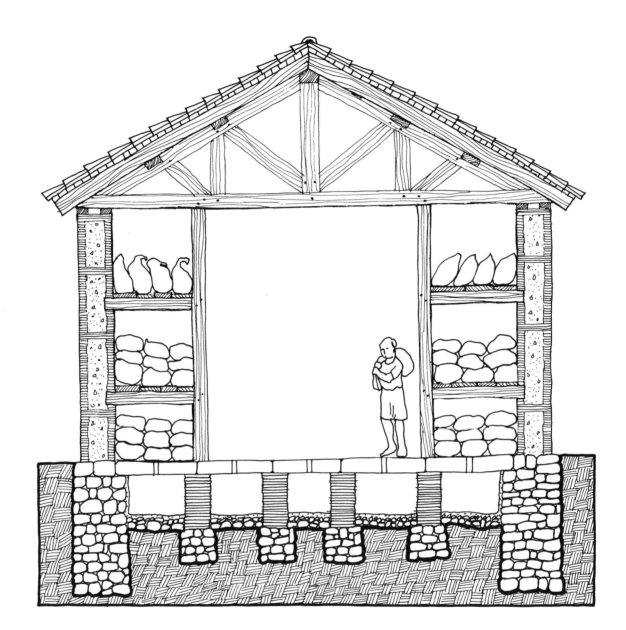

Warehouses, for storing grain, wine, and oil, were built along the streets close to the market. The wine and oil were stored in large clay pots called amphorae buried in the ground, which kept them cool. To prevent moisture from damaging the grain crop it was stored on a floor supported two feet above a lower floor by brick piers. Ventilation holes in the raised floor let air move freely around the sacks of grain. Some of the larger warehouses contained many storerooms located around an open courtyard. Since much of the crop was transported by boat, a dock and some warehouses were constructed along the riverbank.

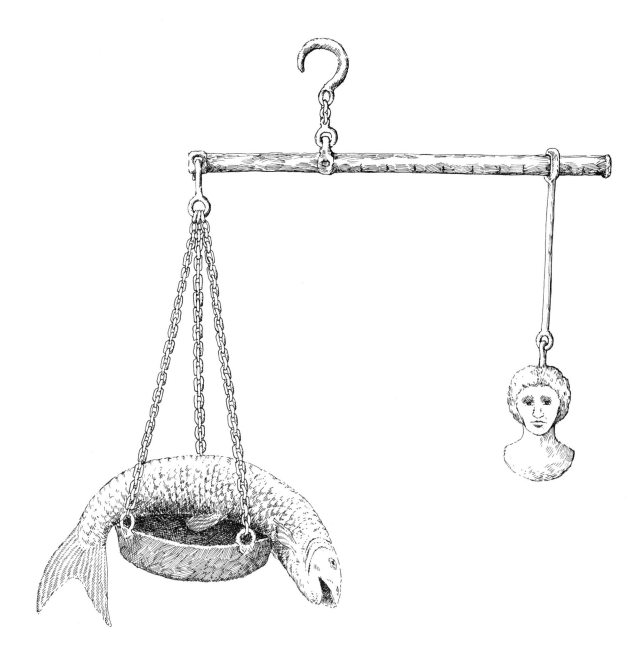

At first everyone shopped in the central market but as the population increased, the market, in spite of its size, became too small. In anticipation of this, the planners had set aside areas on the master plan for future markets. Although they looked very similar, one market specialized in fruit and vegetables, another in grain, and a third, near the north gate and closest to the river, sold only fish.

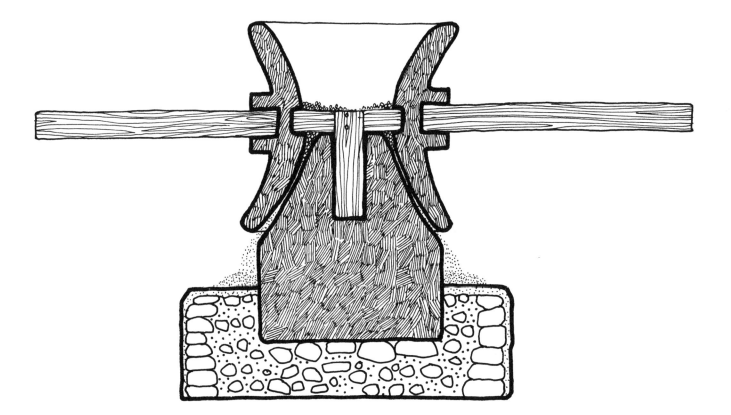

Along the streets that connected the markets, shops and workshops were built side by side. On one street Marcus Licinius, who came from Rome, built a bakery. Bread was one of the most important foods for the people of Verbonia and many bakeries were built throughout the city. The main ingredient in the bread was flour, which was obtained by grinding grain in stone mills. Each mill consisted of two main pieces. The outer piece was rotated around the inner piece by pushing on the projecting arms. The grain was crushed or milled as it passed through the narrow space between the two. The flour that came out at the bottom of the mill was mixed with water and made into dough. Salt and leaven were then added. The dough was kneaded and formed into flat circular loaves and baked in a large brick oven.

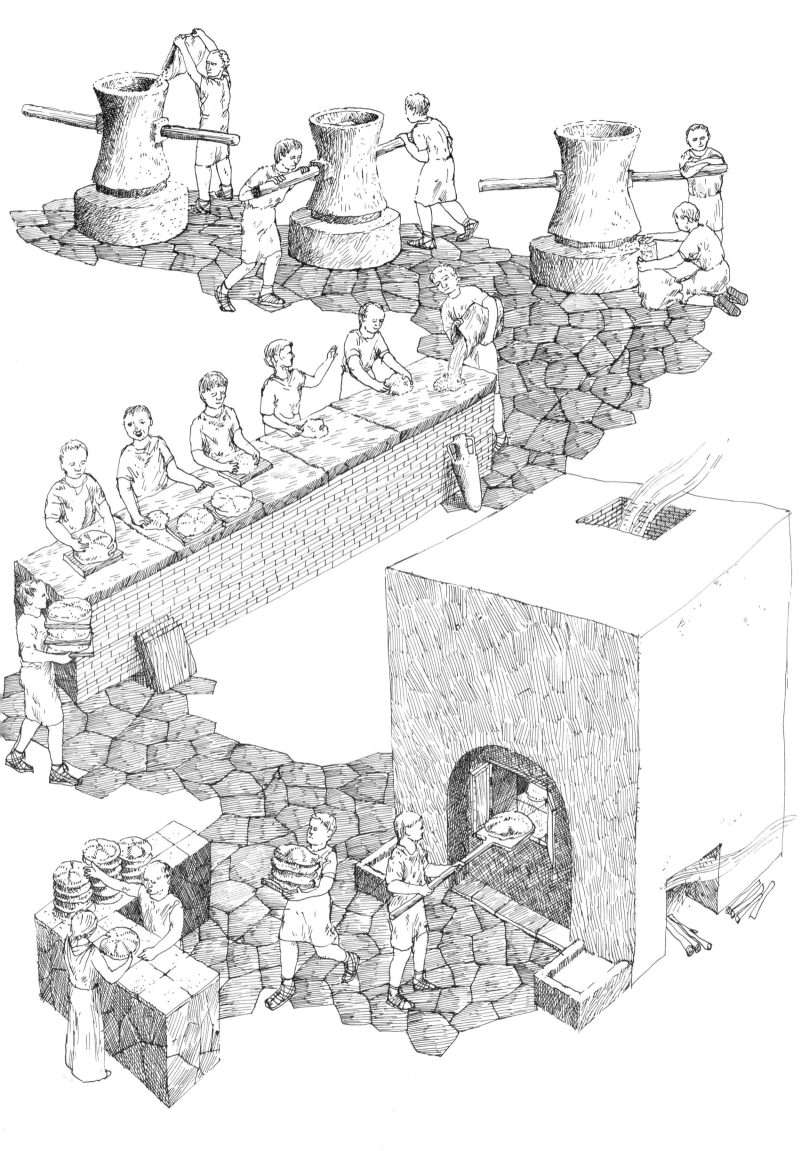

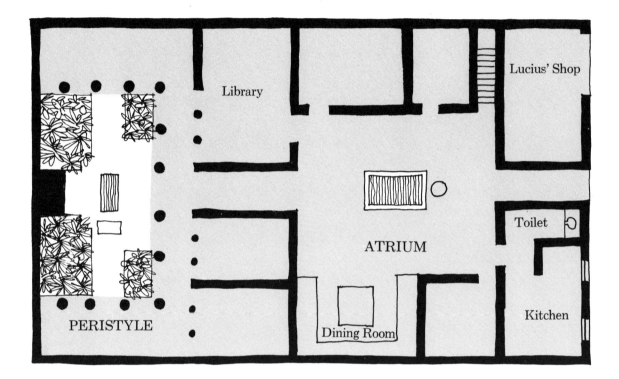

THE HOUSE OF MARCUS LICINIUS • PLAN

The contractor who built Marcus' bakery also built his house. Like those of his neighbors, Marcus' house was quite large. The exterior walls were brick-faced concrete. Some of the interior walls were the same, while others were vertical wooden frames filled with small stones and mortar. All the walls were covered with a thick coat of plaster called stucco and painted.

There were many areas shown on the plan but two were much larger than the others. The first, at the front of the house, was called the atrium and was connected to the sidewalk by a narrow passage. The second, in the rear of the house, was a garden surrounded by a colonnade. This area was called the peristyle. The dining room, library, kitchen, and storerooms were located around the atrium, while the bedrooms and servants' quarters were on a second level.

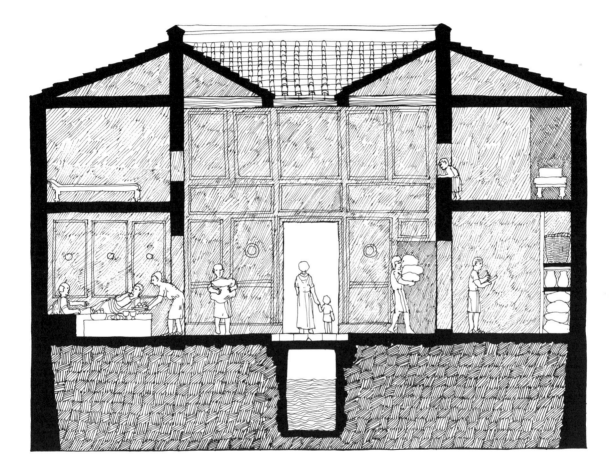

Most of the activities took place in the atrium because of its size and the light that came through a square opening in the roof. Under the opening, called a compluvium, a shallow pool, called an impluvium, was sunk into the floor. Rain which fell into the impluvium ran through a small hole and into an underground tank. When water was needed the cover was taken off the tank and a clay jug lowered into it.

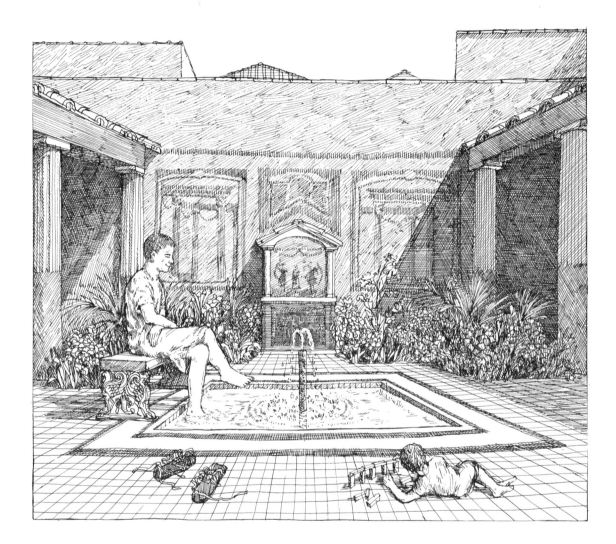

Marcus' favorite part of the house was the peristyle. It was quiet and private and very relaxing after a few hours in the bakery. It contained a fountain which could be turned off and on by a faucet. It also contained a shrine to the Lares — the gods who protected Marcus' house.

The floors of the atrium and peristyle were covered with mosaic — small black and white marble tiles that were pressed into wet cement in a variety of geometric patterns.

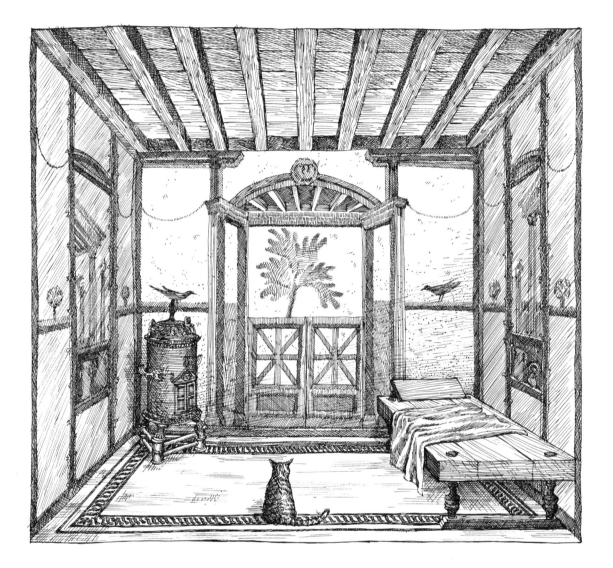

Because one house was built right up against another the only windows were located at the front facing the street. These were usually very small and covered with bars for security.

To brighten up the small dark rooms colorful pictures were painted on the walls. Many rooms contained jungle scenes full of wild animals and exotic plants. Imitation windows were painted in other rooms to make them seem less confining. In the winter the important rooms were heated by wood stoves.

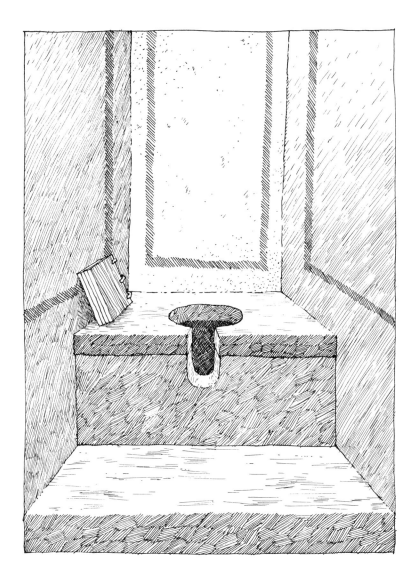

On one side of the passage between the sidewalk and the atrium a toilet was connected to the sewer pipe and flushed by a continuous stream of water. On the other side a room that opened onto the sidewalk was rented out to a jeweler named Lucius Julius, who knew that a jewelry shop in Marcus' neighborhood would be very profitable.

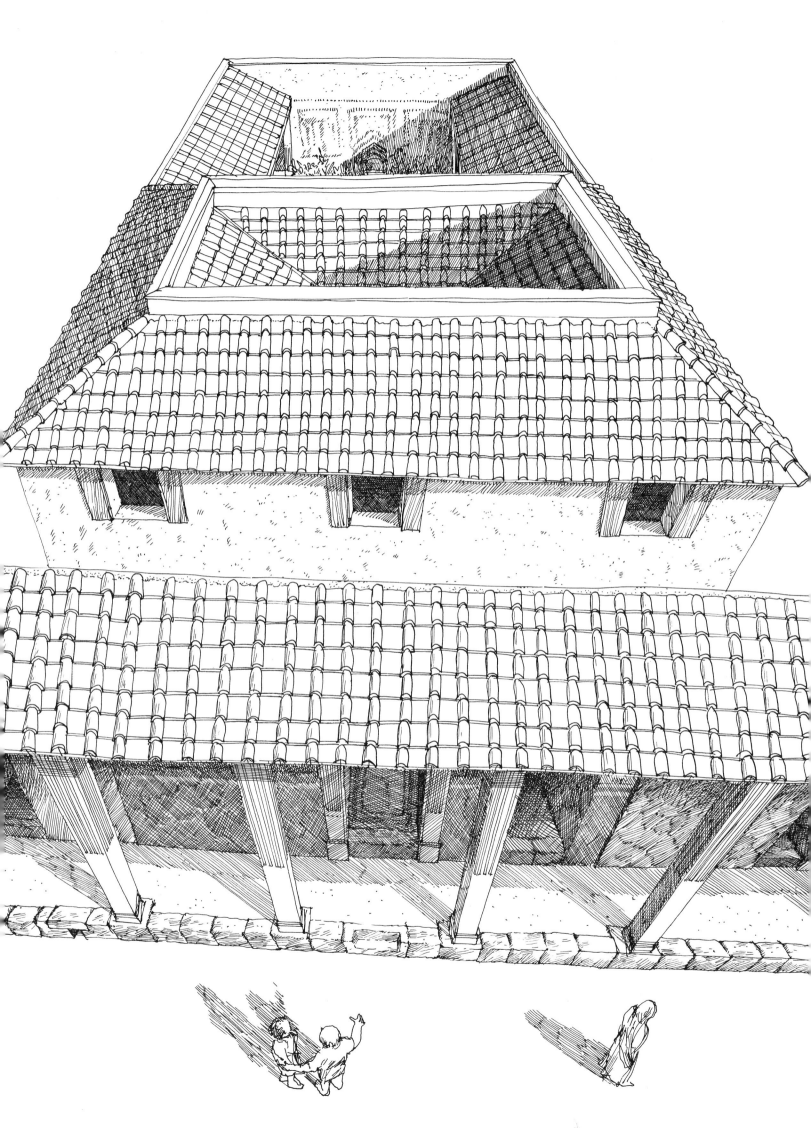

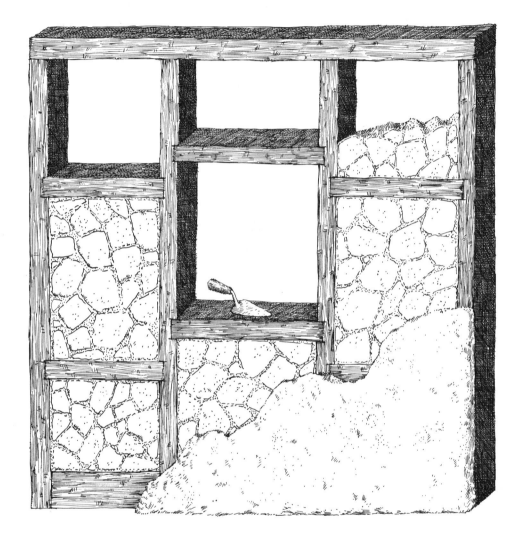

Lucius was a former slave who had learned his craft in Egypt and had taken the name of the man who bought and eventually freed him. He and his family lived in an apartment in another section of the city.

Both the interior and exterior walls of this building were constructed of heavy timber framework filled with stone and mortar and covered with stucco. Instead of an atrium the apartment building contained a small courtyard above which was a high open space. It was called a light shaft because it supplied the only natural light for the small inner rooms.

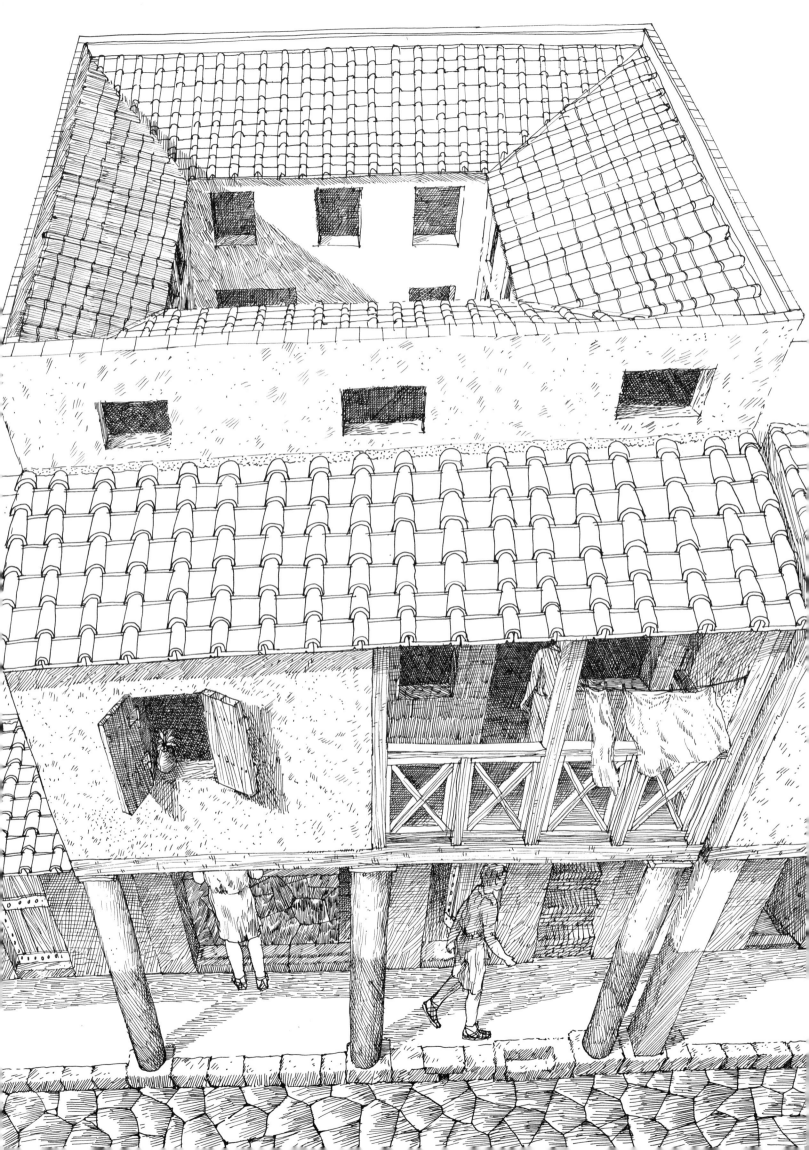

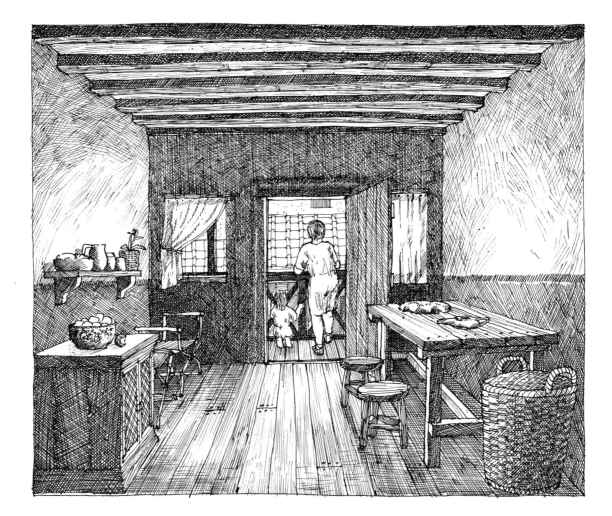

The few rooms of Lucius' apartment were quite small and the same one was often used for many purposes. The largest of the rooms opened onto a balcony overlooking the street.

On the ground floor of the building was a shop which sold olive oil. Besides amphorae buried in the ground for storing the oil the shop contained a press for squeezing the oil out of the olives.

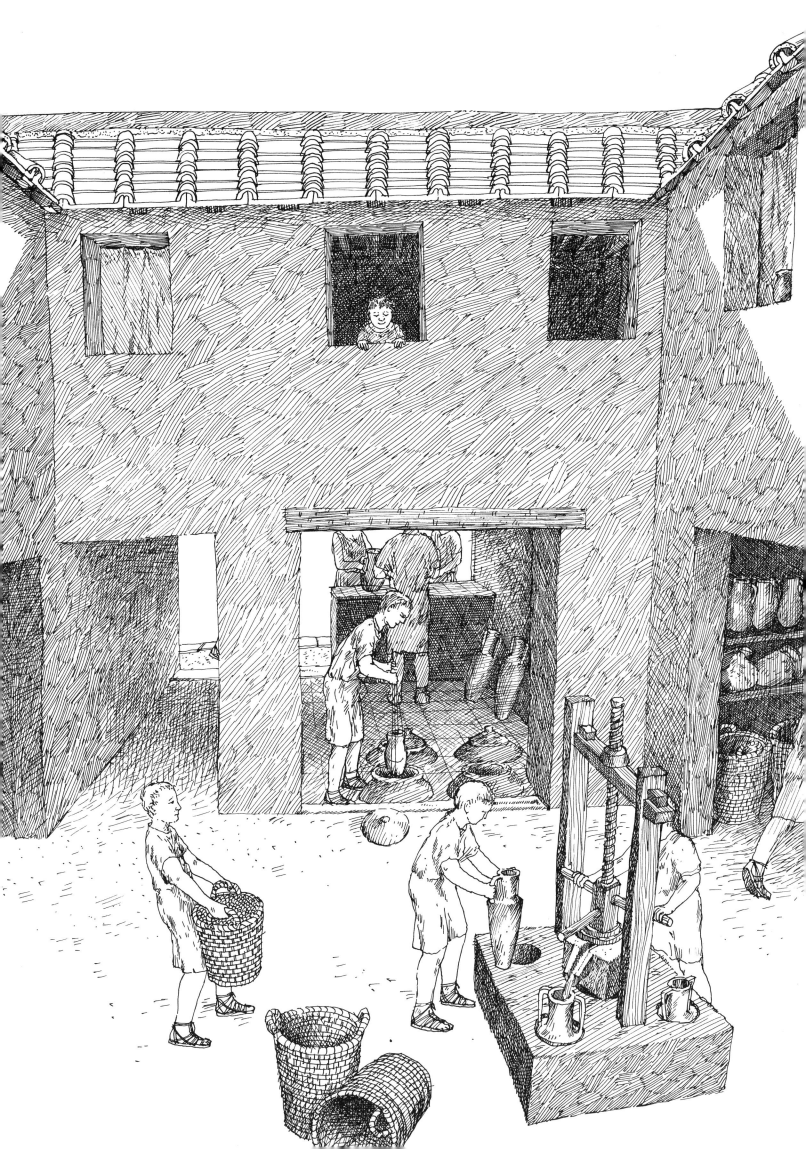

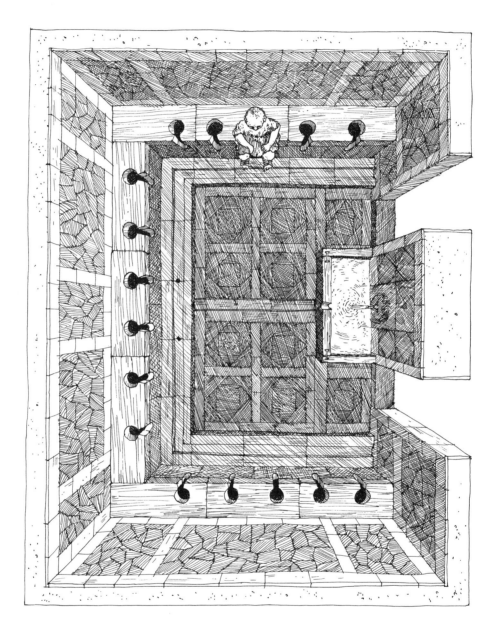

Some of the apartment buildings had small wells but few contained toilets; most of the residents used the public toilets located around the city.

All the buildings in Lucius' neighborhood contained two or more apartments. Many were owned by Marcus Licinius' neighbors and all contained shops open-

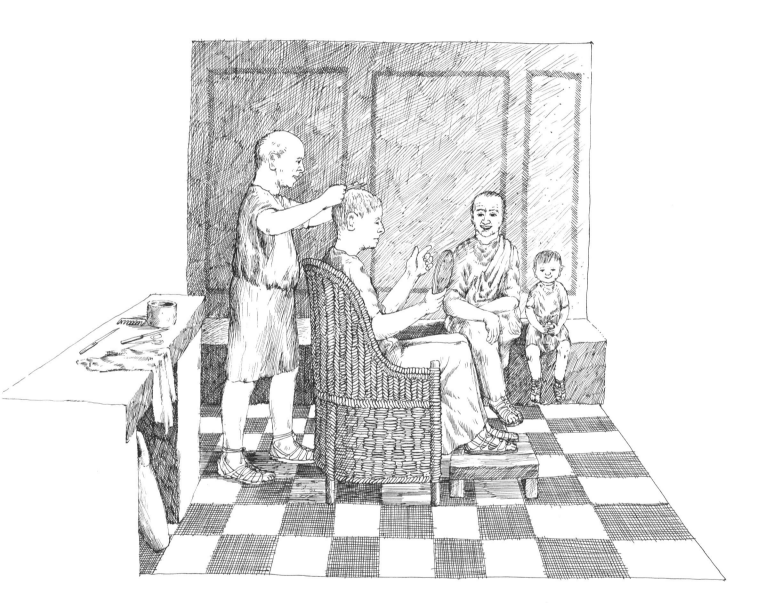

ing onto the sidewalk. One of those shops was rented by a barber named Quintus Aurelius. The success of Quintus' business was mostly due to his willingness to gossip. For spreading news Quintus and Verbonia's other barbers were almost as important as the government decrees read in the forum, and they were definitely faster.

By the time of Augustus' death in A.D. 14, the streets of Verbonia were lined with grocery shops, pastry shops, ceramic shops, furniture shops, clothing shops, drugstores, wine shops, and snack bars.

Many of the craftsmen on a particular street often specialized in the same or related crafts. Most of the shops along a small quiet street near the forum were

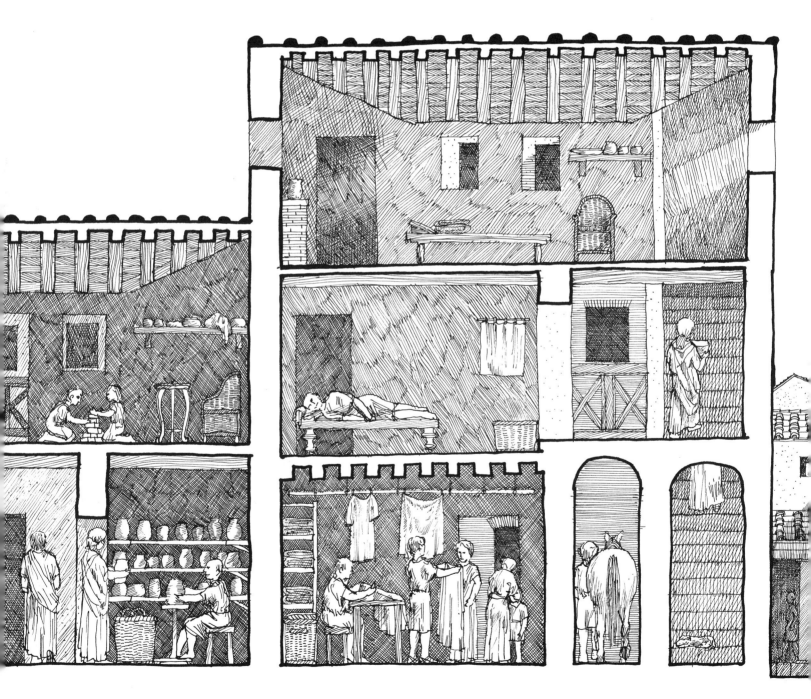

owned by highly skilled gold workers and the street eventually became known as "the street of gold." The craftsmen and their families lived in rooms behind or above their shops. As neighborhoods developed, families often got together to build shrines on their streets dedicated to the Lares.

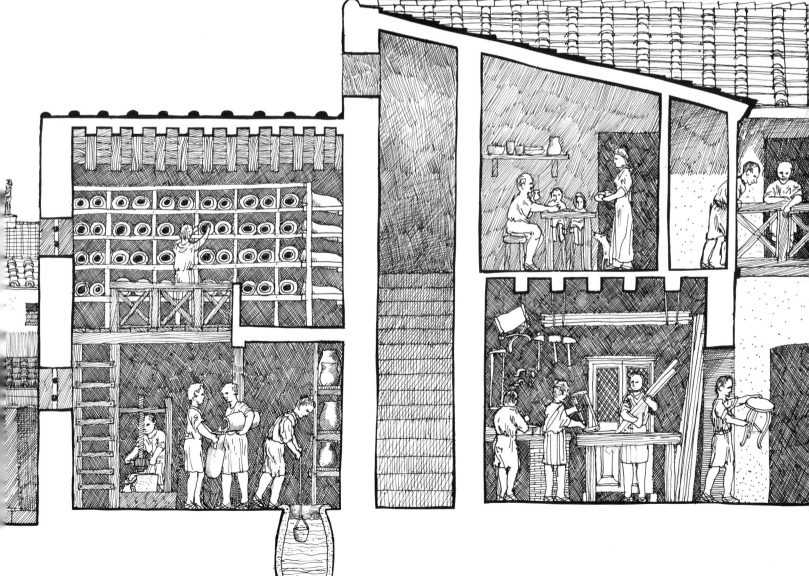

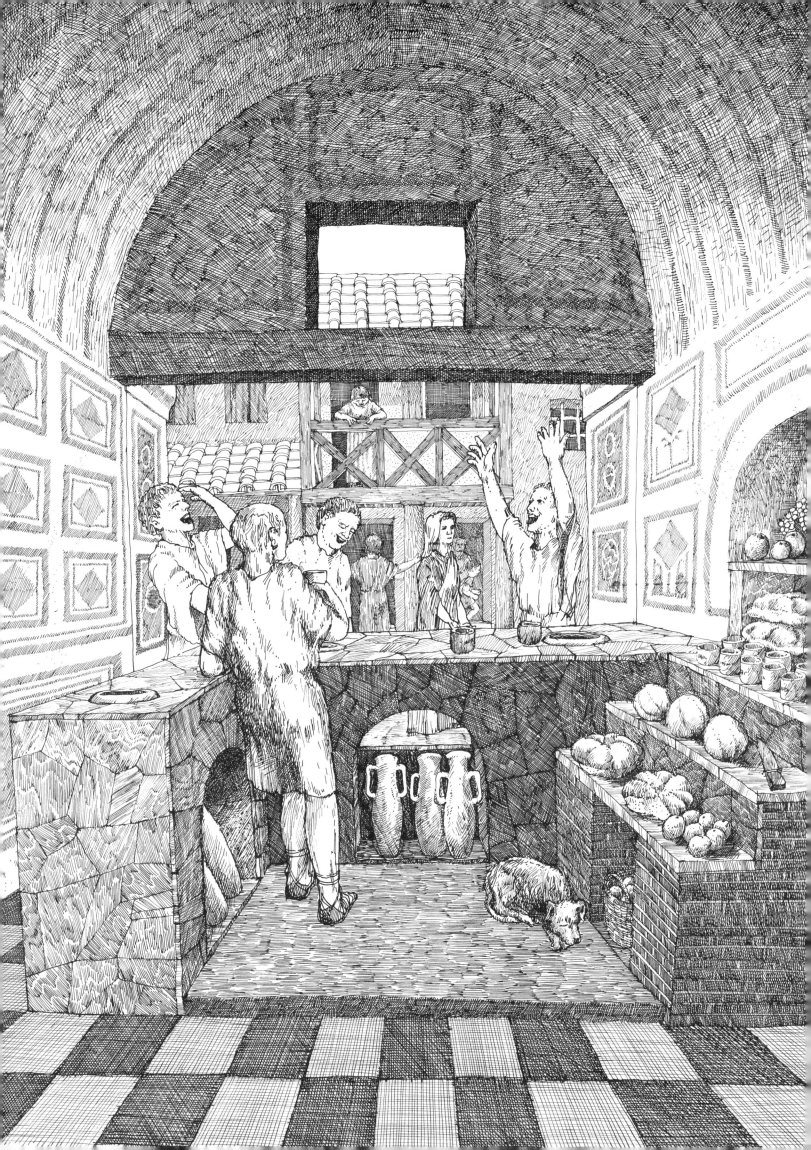

Most of the snack bars were owned by Servius Vitellius, who also owned a chain of snack bars in Ariminum. The snack bars opened onto the sidewalk and each contained a concrete serving counter decorated with pieces of colored marble. Clay jugs embedded in the counter contained hot and cold drinks to be sold. A row of clay drinking cups marked with Servius' name stood on a marble shelf next to the counter.

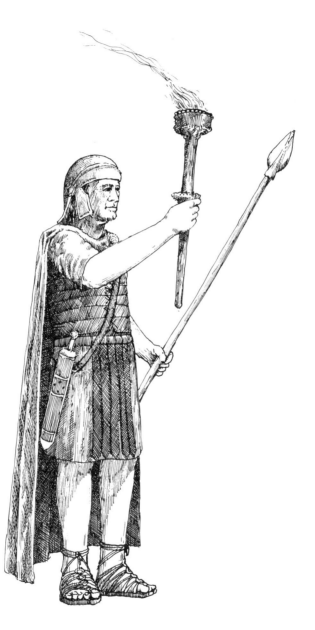

At night and during the hot afternoons all the shops could be closed by fitting wooden panels into grooves on the tops and bottoms of the doorways. A lock was used to secure them in place. At night the city provided torch-carrying watchmen who patrolled the streets checking the locks and doors of all the buildings.

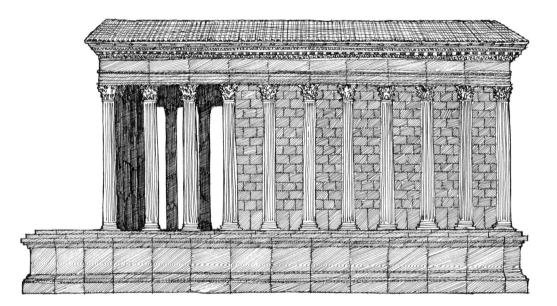

Upon his death Augustus became a god, and the Emperor Tiberius who succeeded him ordered the building of temples in Augustus' honor throughout the empire. As usual the citizens of each city, not the Emperor, paid for these temples.

The wealthy of Verbonia managed to take advantage of the situation by either renting some of their slaves to the contractor building the temple or by contributing enough money to insure that their names would be carved in some prominent place in the building.

Numerius Septimius, who owned a lot of farmland, was the wealthiest man in the city. Not only did he contribute willingly to the new temple, but he paid for the entire construction of a new market. So that everyone would know of his generosity he commissioned a marble statue of himself holding a bust of Ceres. It was carved in the workshop of Titus Statius, the best and largest stone cutting shop in the city. When it was finished it was transported by cart to the new market and erected near the fountain.

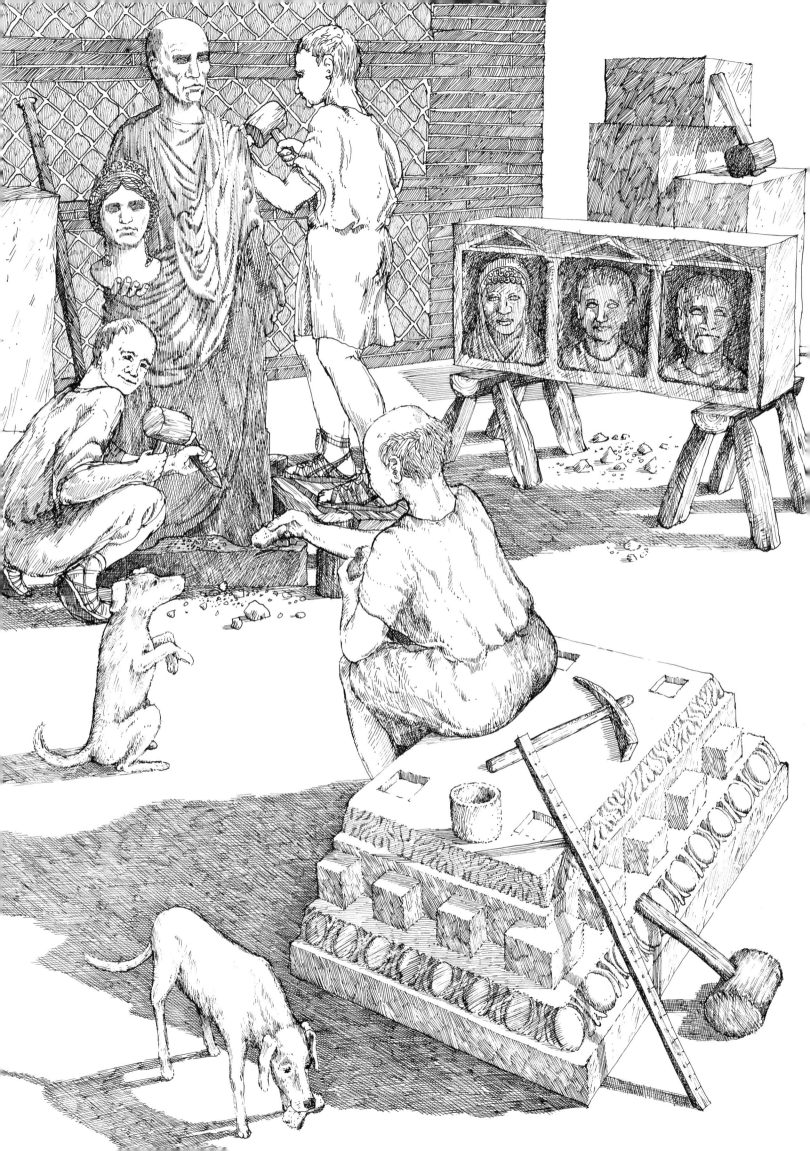

As open land within the walls gradually disappeared, the importance of careful planning became more and more evident — especially in two well-thought-

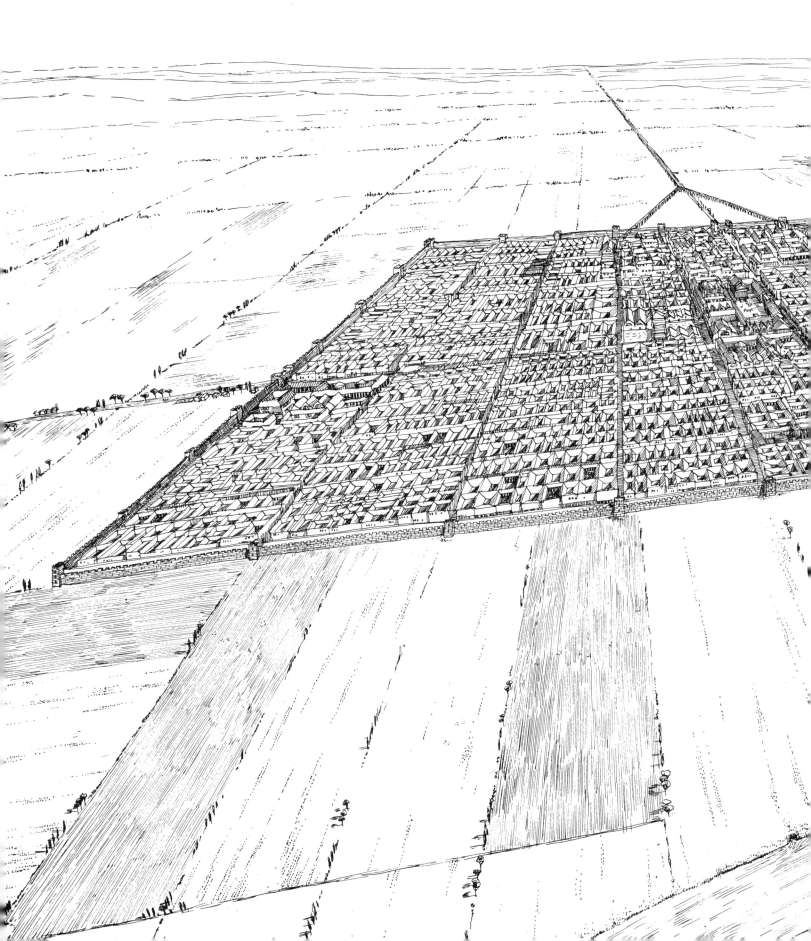

out ideas. The first was the street plan, which maintained order throughout, and the second was the setting aside of land for recreation and entertainment.

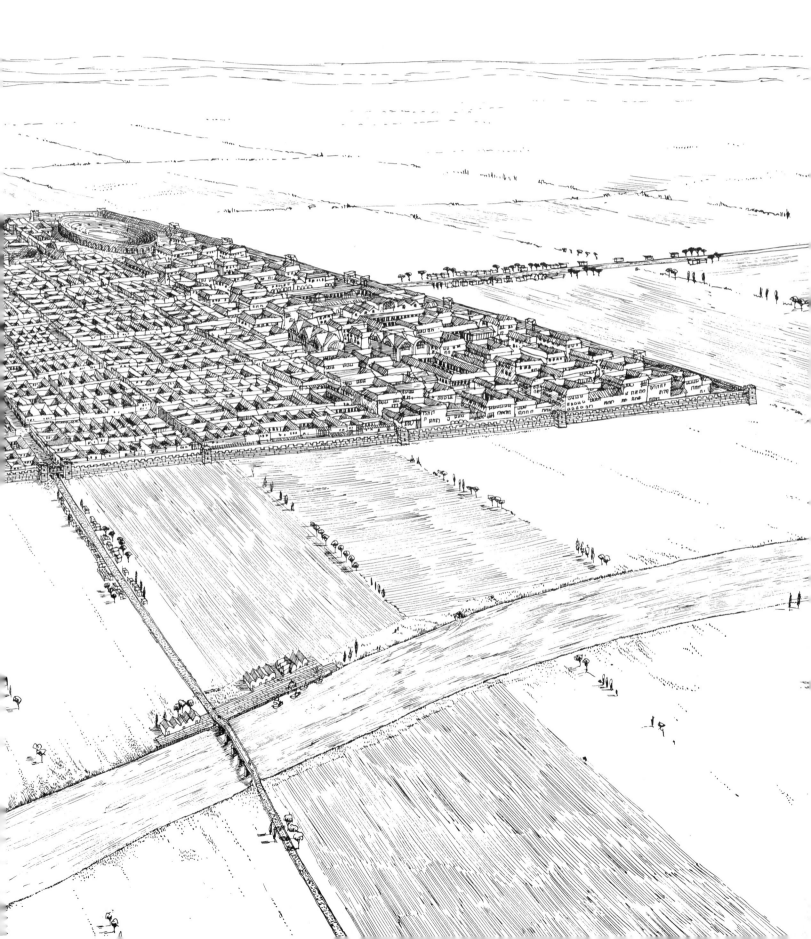

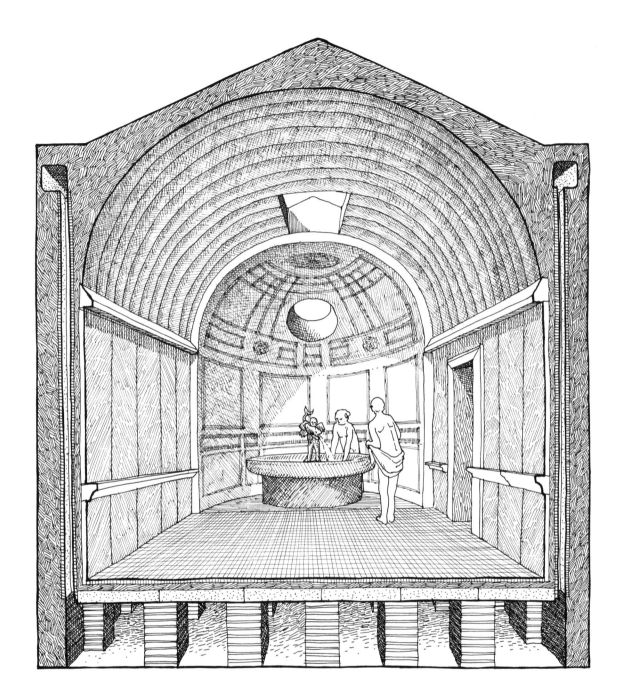

The public baths, called thermae, were not only for washing but also provided a place to meet, talk, exercise, gamble, and even read. Bathing was traditionally accomplished in three stages. First the Romans washed in hot water from a pool in the steamy caldarium. Then they relaxed in a warm-water pool in the tepidarium and finally ended the process with a dive into the cold-water pool of the frigidarium.

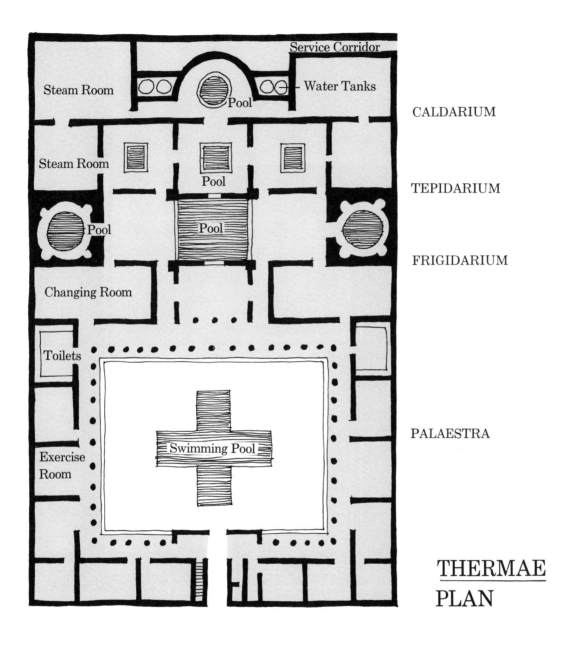

Steam Room

Water Tanks

Service Corridor

Pool

Steam Room

CALDARIUM

Pool

Steam Room

Pool

Pool

TEPIDARIUM

Pool

Pool

FRIGIDARIUM

Changing Room

Toilets

PALAESTRA

Swimming Pool

Exercise
Room

THERMAE
PLAN

Several small thermae were built during the reign of Augustus, but by A.D. 42 the population had reached 30,000 and the existing facilities were inadequate. The new Emperor Claudius ordered that a much larger thermae be built near the forum on the site of the original baths. A professional demolition company was hired and the old structure, along with a few apartment buildings, was torn **down.**

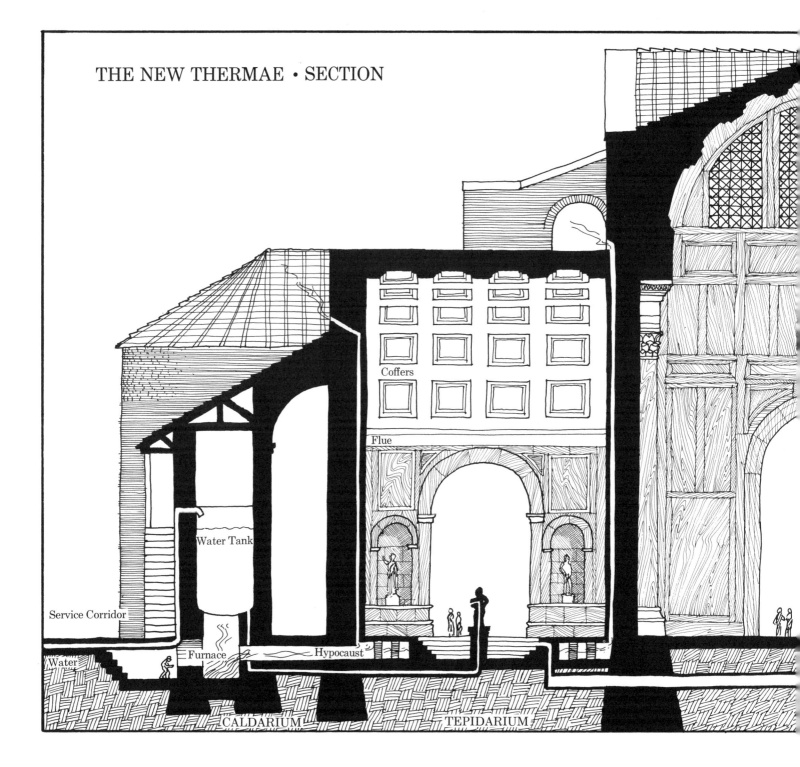

Coffers

Flue

Water Tank

Service Corridor

Water

Furnace

Hypocaust

CALDARIUM

TEPIDARIUM

The mosaic-covered stone floors of the caldarium, tepidarium, and steam rooms were supported two feet off the ground by brick piers, creating a space below the floor called a hypocaust. Hot gases from a furnace outside the building were piped into the hypocaust to heat the rooms. When the hypocaust was

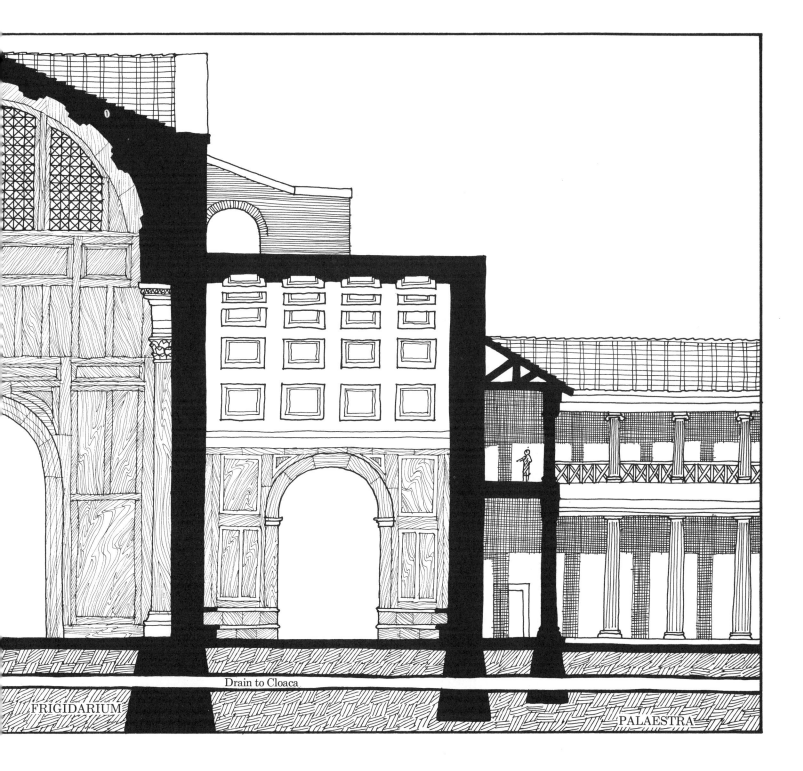

FRIGIDARIUM

Drain to Cloaca

PALAESTRA

full, the gas went up flues — clay pipes in the walls — heating the walls, and out through vents in the vaults.

Suspended over the furnace were large bronze tanks in which water was heated for the baths. The hot water ran into the pool of the caldarium and the overflow, cooling as it went, was piped into the pool of the tepidarium.

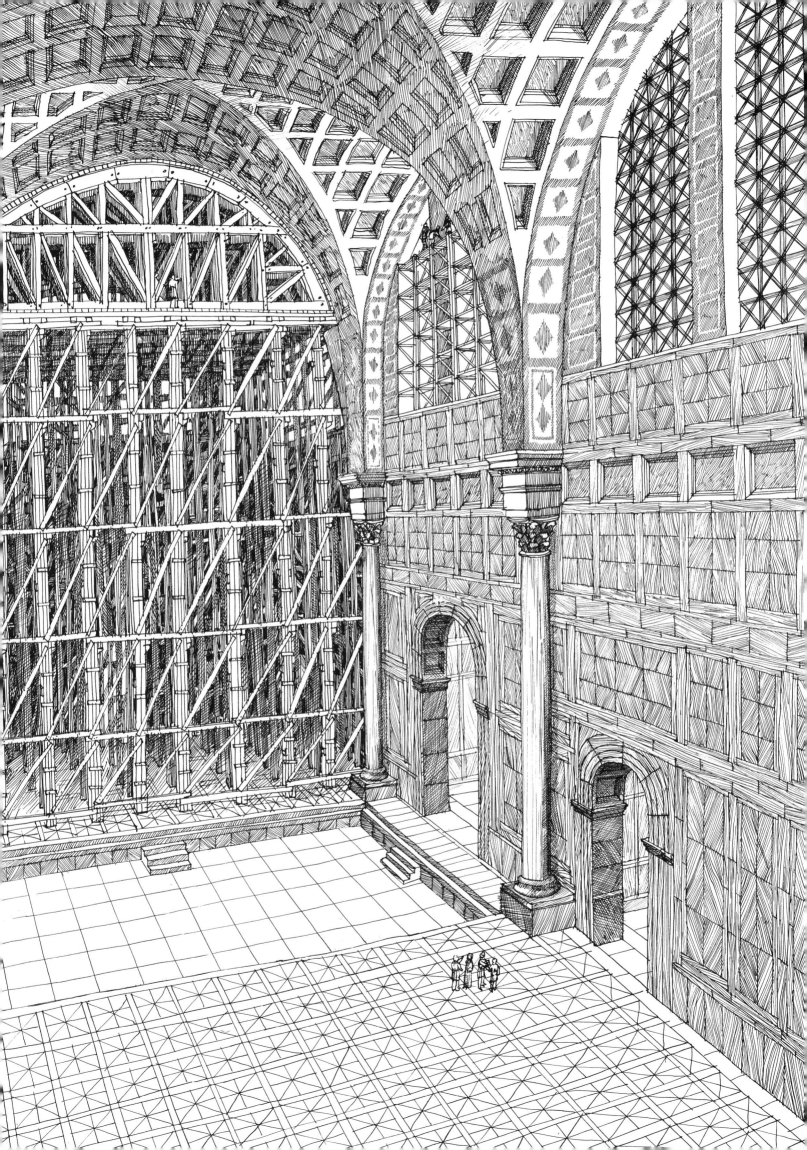

The caldarium, tepidarium, changing rooms, steam rooms, exercise rooms, snack bars, and toilets all had tunnel-vaulted ceilings. The larger area of the frigidarium was covered by a series of groin vaults which are created when two tunnel vaults cross each other at a right angle. Each of the cold-water pools in the frigidarium was covered by a dome ceiling with a round opening in the top, called an oculus, to let light in.

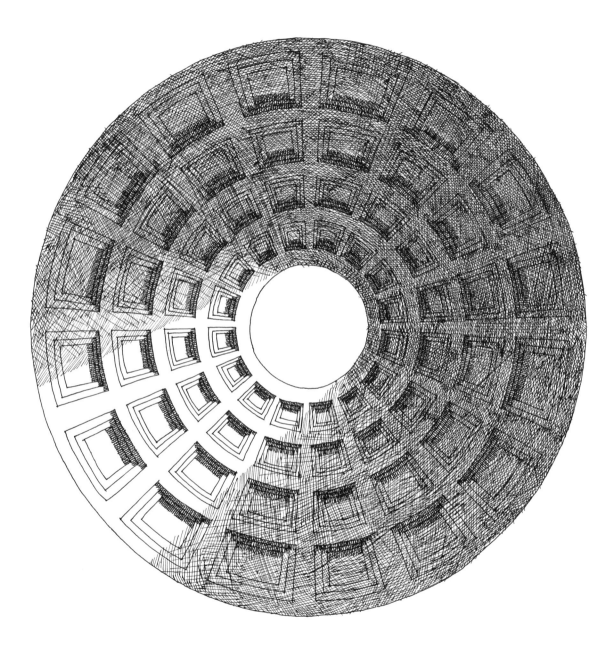

During the construction of both the domes and the vaults, wooden shapes called coffers were fastened on top of the forms. When the concrete had set, the form and coffers were lowered, leaving indentations in the surface of the ceiling which lightened but did not weaken it. This allowed the supporting walls or piers to be somewhat thinner.

Next to the thermae, a grassed area containing a swimming pool was enclosed by a two-story colonnade. This area was called the palestra and was used for exercising and wrestling, among other things. Behind the second floor colonnade and over the entrance a library was built with a collection of scrolls for those who wished to read.

To supply the increased amount of water needed for the larger baths and growing population a second aqueduct was constructed directly on top of the first.

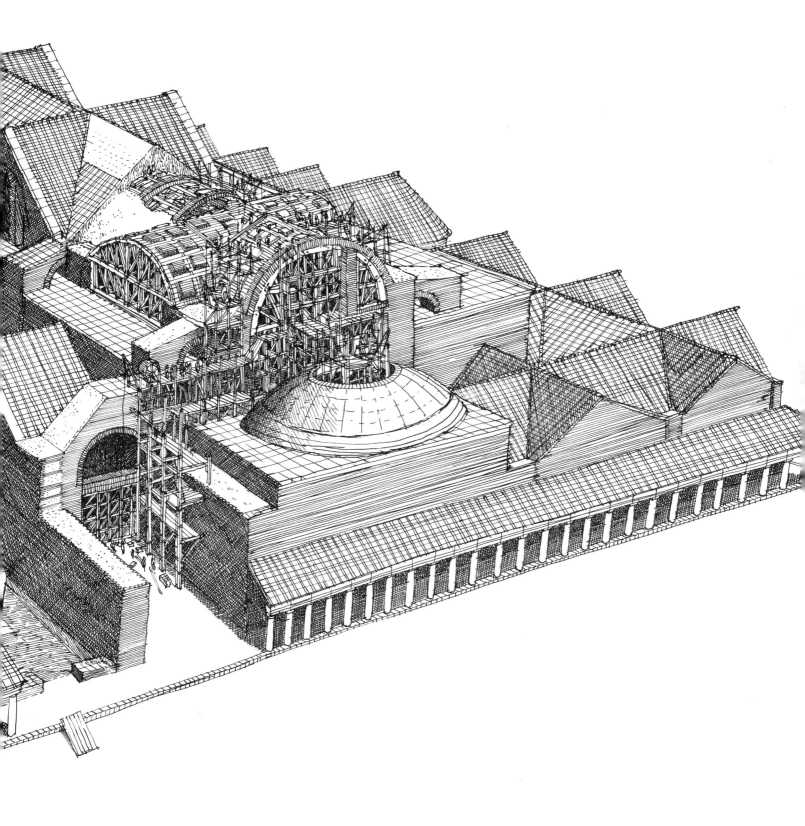

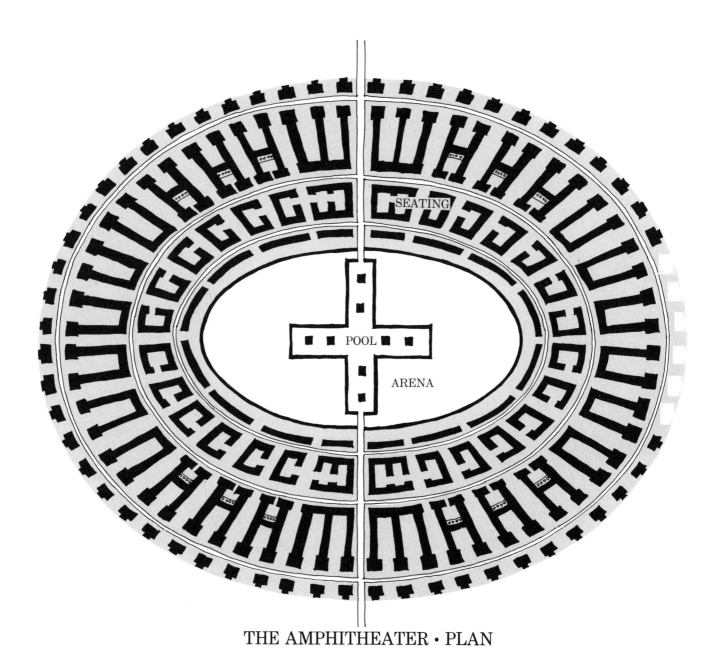

THE AMPHITHEATER · PLAN

The last public area to be fully developed was the city's entertainment center. In A.D. 44 the senate voted to build a more permanent amphitheater and theater. Until that time a sloped earth mound lined with stone seats and reinforced by a ring of arches had enclosed both the arena and the stage of the theater.

The original oval shape of the amphitheater was maintained and enlarged. The stone seats now rested on two layers of tunnel-vaulted passages radiating out from the center. These passages were connected by other passages which ran around the arena.

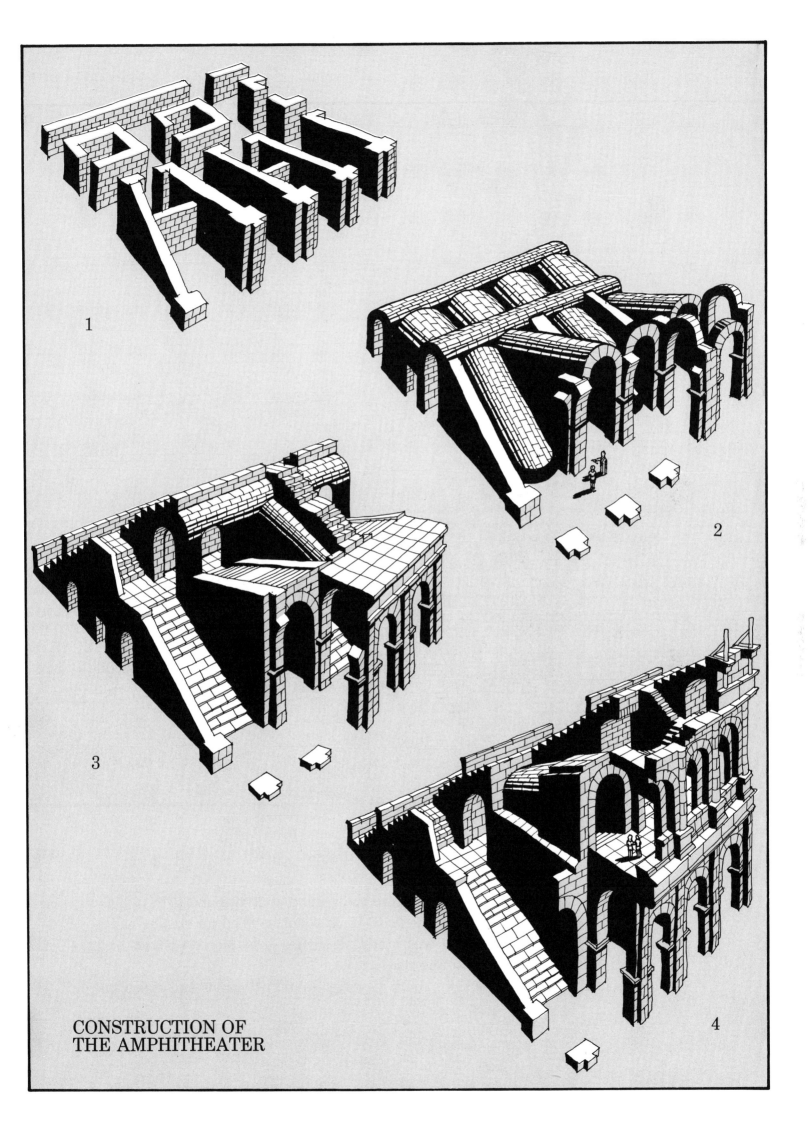

1

2

3

CONSTRUCTION OF
THE AMPHITHEATER

4

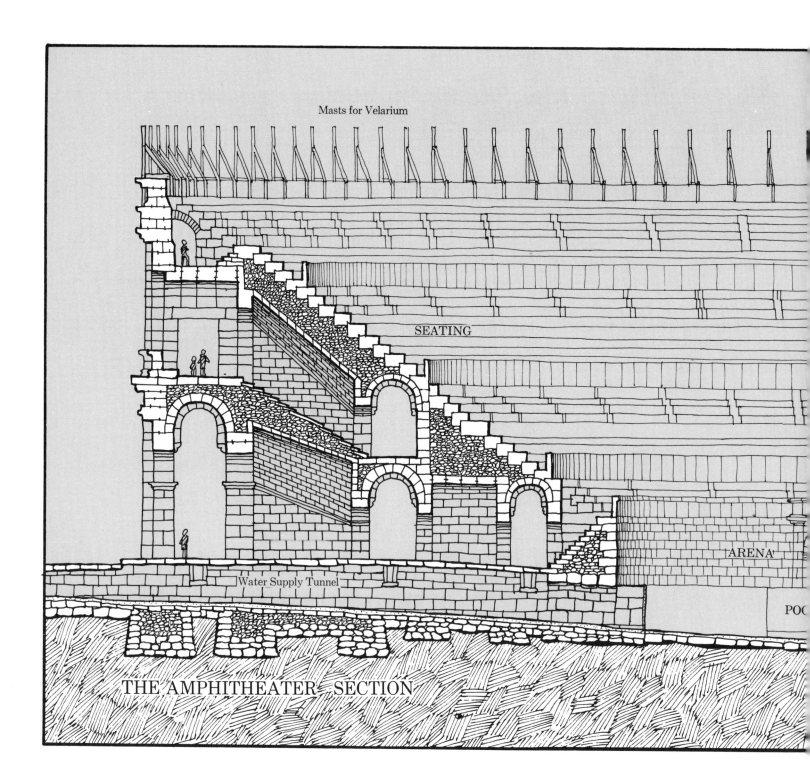

Masts for Velarium

SEATING

Water Supply Tunnel

ARENA

POO

THE AMPHITHEATER SECTION

The arena was sunk several feet into the ground and surrounded by a high wall. Deep pools were built in the floor which could be filled for staging naval battles. When they weren't needed, they were covered by wooden boards and emptied through a canal into the cloaca.

Besides toilets and a snack bar the passages contained ramps and stairways

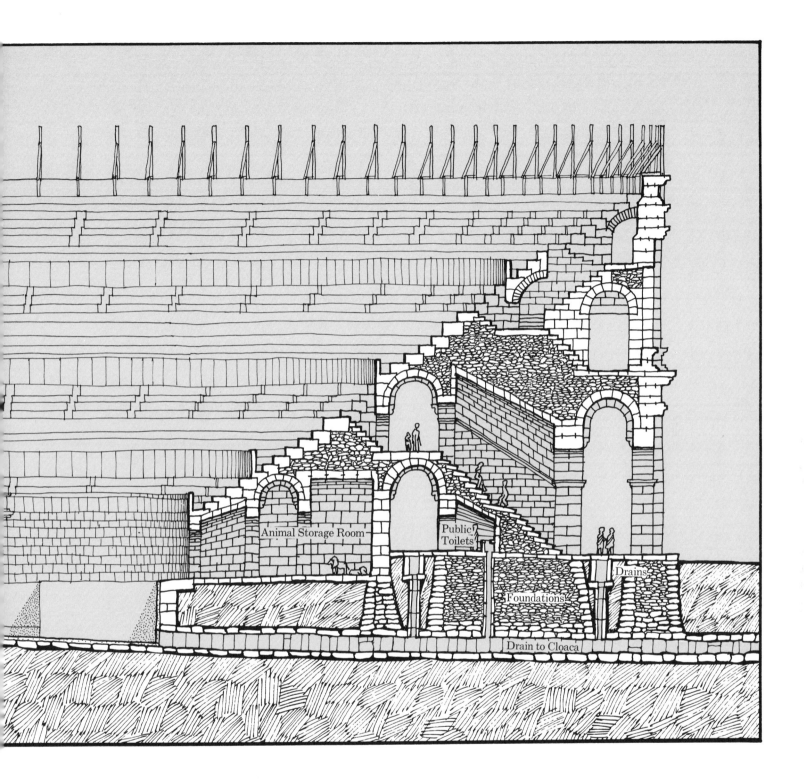

Animal Storage Room

Public Toilets

Drains

Foundations

Drain to Cloaca

which enabled the entire twenty thousand spectators to enter or leave the structure in less than ten minutes. Wild animals and equipment used in the performances were kept under the lowest seats in rooms which opened onto the arena. The most popular performances involved the deaths of either animals, slaves, or gladiators — men paid to fight each other.

Two rows of arches, one on top of the other, formed the exterior wall of the amphitheater. This wall was constructed of carefully cut stones clamped together with iron and bronze pins. The passages and vaulting were all constructed of stone and concrete. A rope net was suspended above the entire

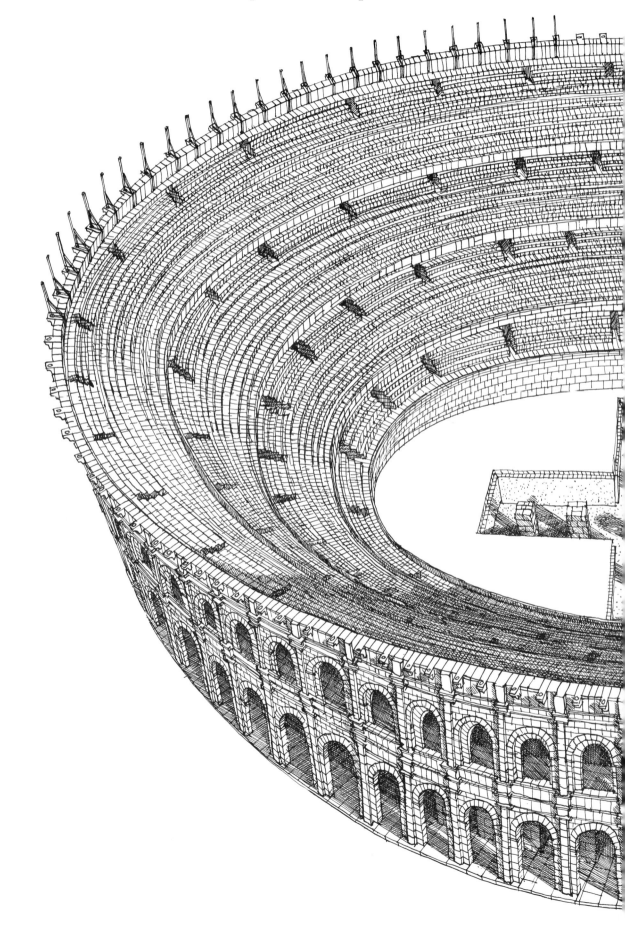

seating area from wooden masts. If the sun was too hot a canvas roof called a valarium was drawn over the seating area. When it rained during a performance everyone took shelter in the passages.

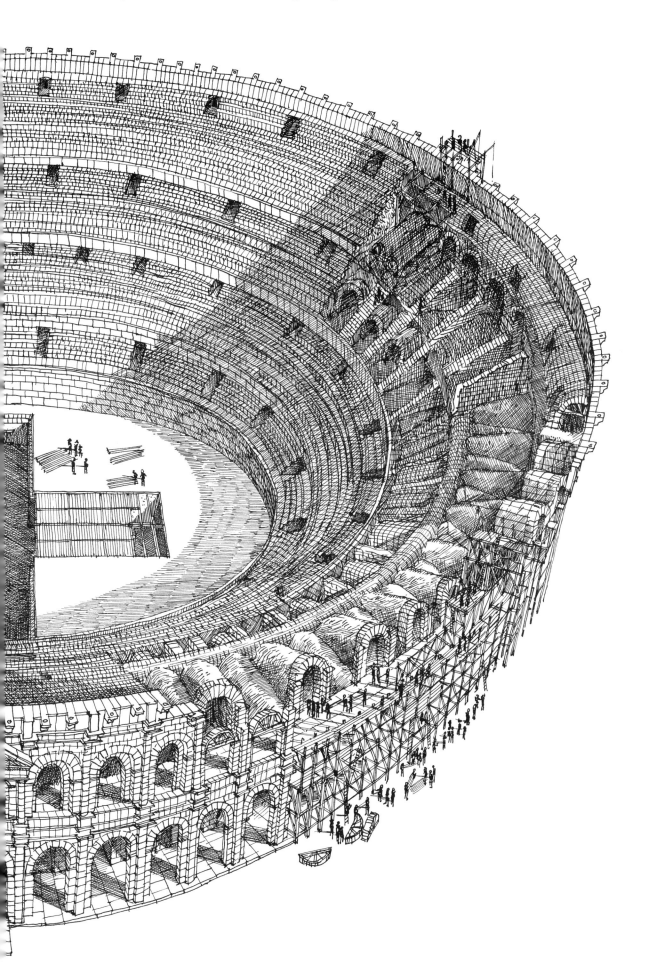

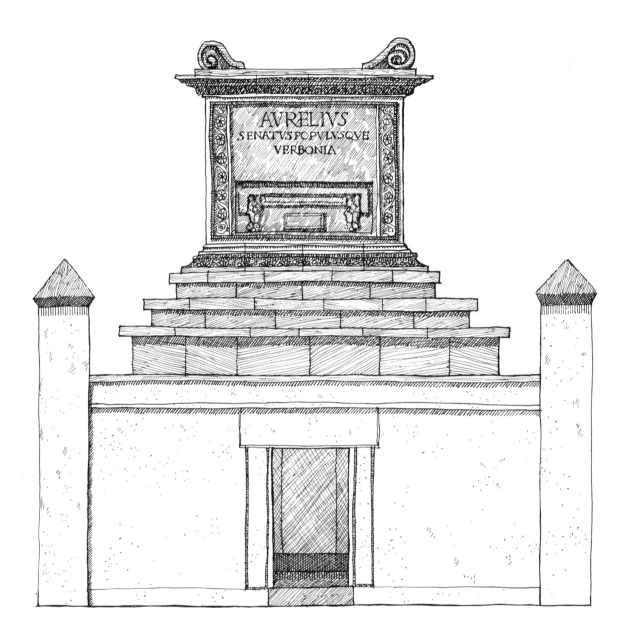

During the construction of the amphitheater some formwork was accidentally moved before the concrete in the vault had completely set, killing twenty-five slaves, their foreman, and a senator observing the work from the ground. The bodies of the slaves were taken on two carts to a field four miles outside the city and buried in a large pit. The bodies of the senator and foreman were cremated and the ashes sealed in urns. The senator's urn was placed in his elaborate family tomb, much closer to the city but still outside the walls as required by law. The foreman's urn was buried in a public but still respectable graveyard, where his family erected a tombstone in his memory.

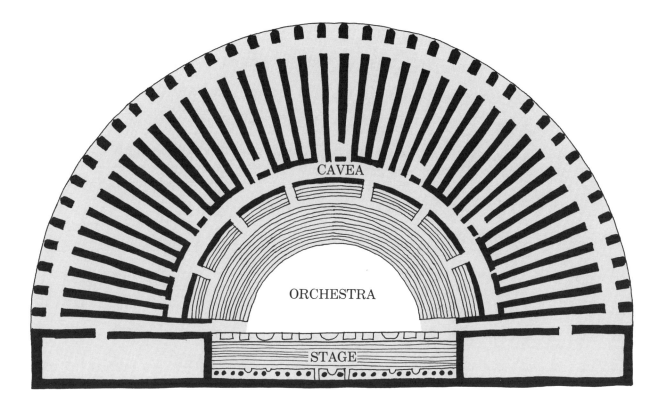

CAVEA

ORCHESTRA

STAGE

THE THEATER · PLAN

Because the senator had always enjoyed plays, his family donated a large sum of money toward the construction of the new theater. The seats were built around a steep semicircular pit called a cavea. Like the seats of the amphitheater they were supported by a network of concrete tunnels. A long wooden stage was constructed across the diameter of the cavea. At both sides of the stage rooms were built for changing and storing costumes.

A curtain could be raised from under the stage for scenery changes. Behind the stage the wall called the frons scaenae was covered with marble columns and architectural ornamentation. This wall reached the same height as the colonnade that was built around the last row of seats in the cavea. Sometimes the actors

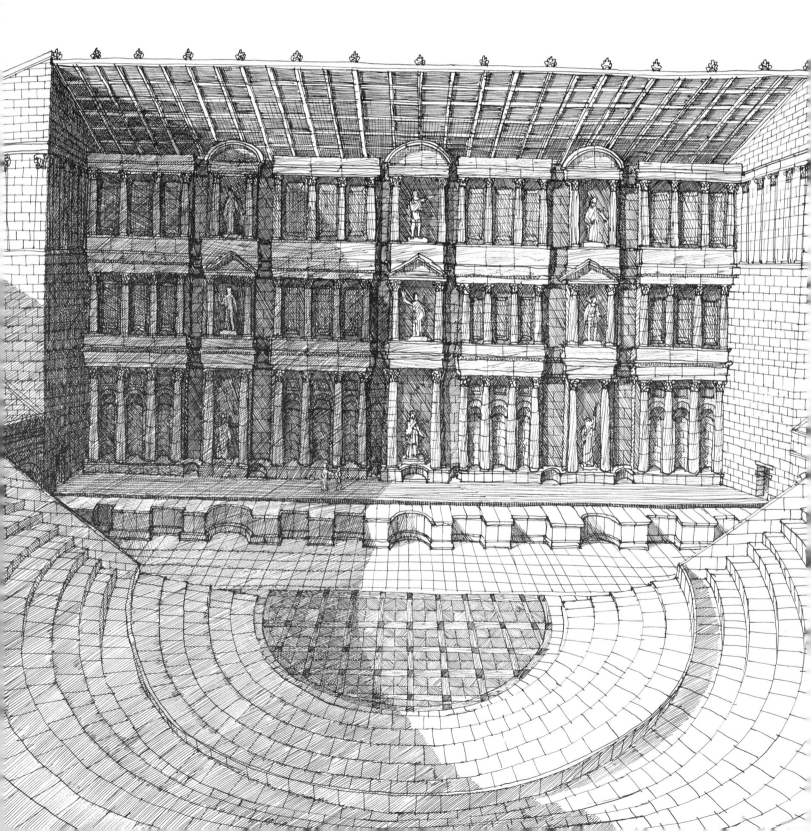

performed in the orchestra — the flat semicircular area directly in front of the stage. The most important people sat either on wide seats around the orchestra or in balconies over the side entrances. The theater, too, could be covered by a valarium.

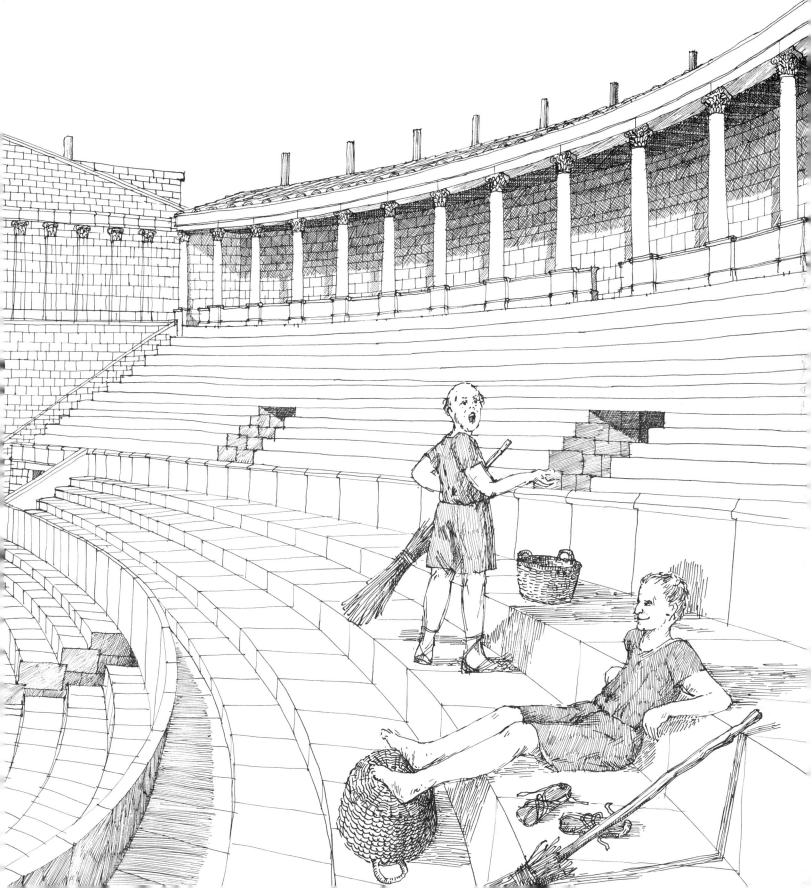

By A.D. 75 both the amphitheater and theater were finished and a festival which lasted twenty-five days was held to celebrate the occasion.

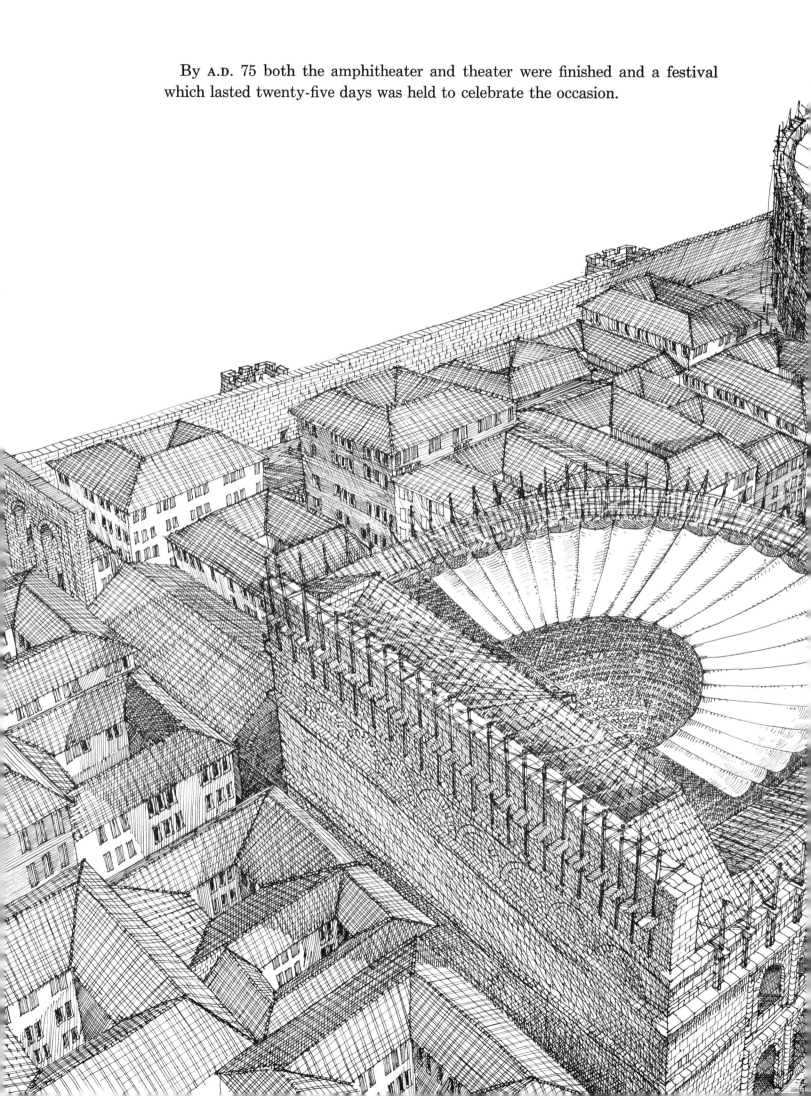

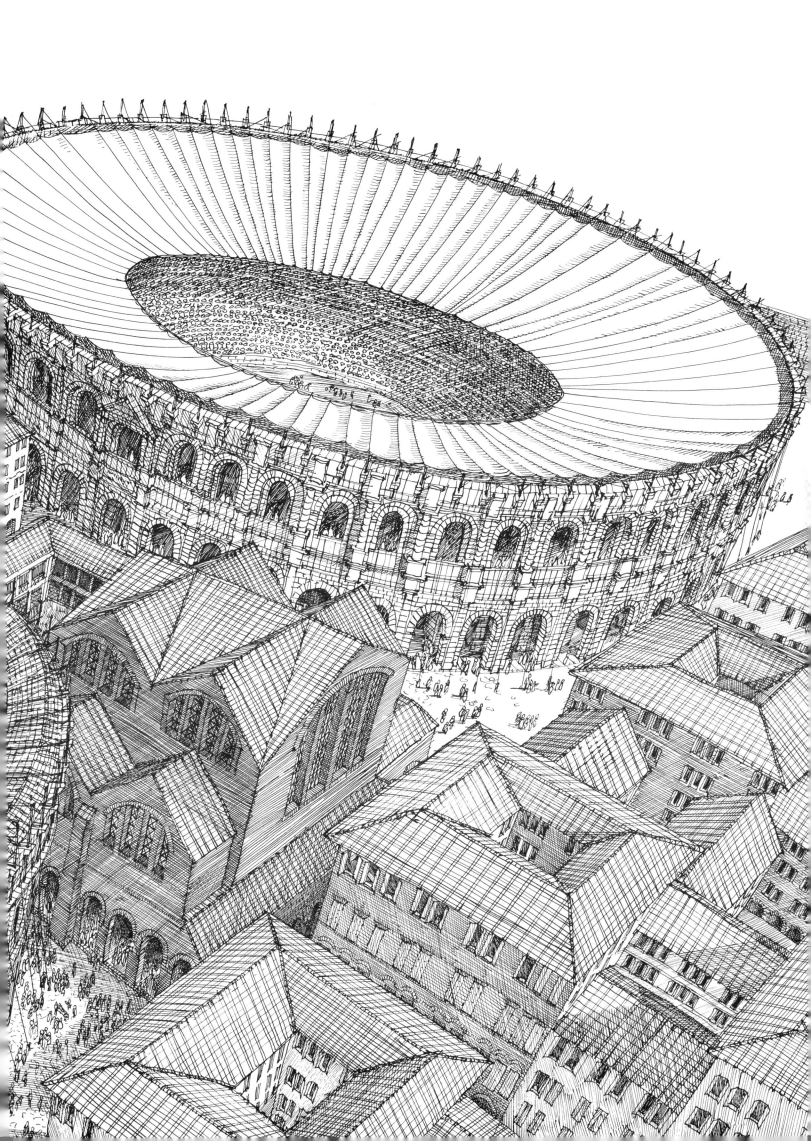

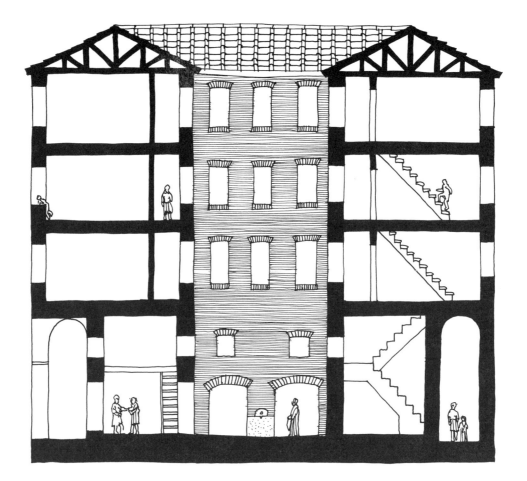

As Verbonia's population steadily climbed, most landlords replaced their small apartment buildings with large apartment blocks. Some, as high as five stories, contained twenty families. To take advantage of this height, which could still be no more than twice the width of the street, the senate passed a law limiting the first apartment blocks to insulae along the northern and western sides of the city. In the winter these buildings would shield the city from the cold wind that blew down the valley.

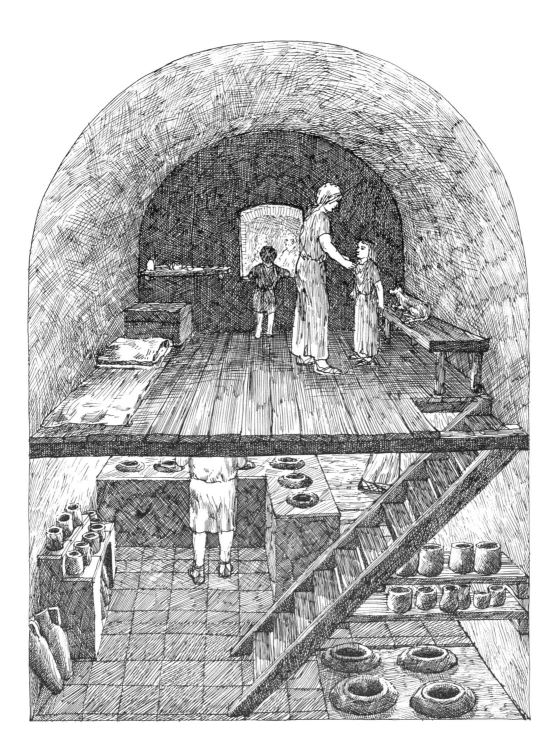

As in earlier buildings, the apartments in each block were built around a light shaft. The lowest level of the buildings was a series of tunnel-vaulted rooms built side by side and opening onto the sidewalk. These spaces were rented by shopkeepers who constructed a wooden platform on which to live eight feet above the floor. Stables and storerooms around the central courtyard were also rented out.

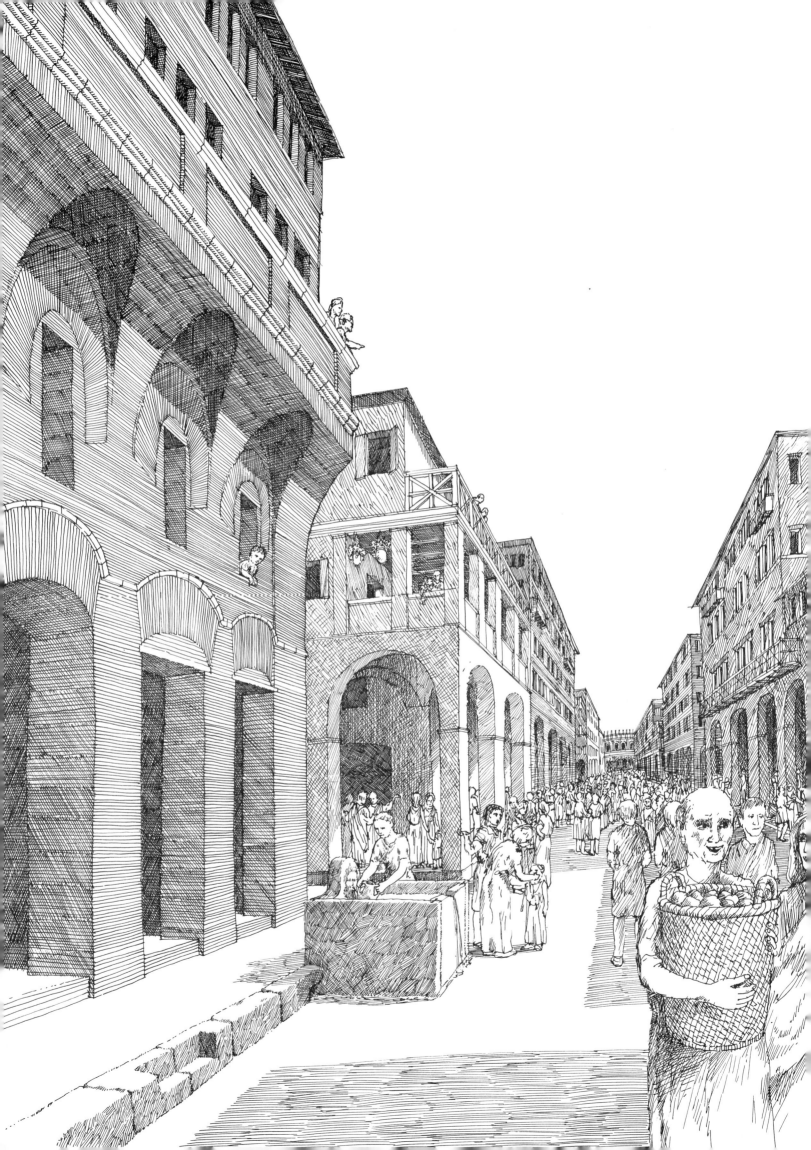

By A.D. 100 Verbonia's population was almost fifty thousand. Many of the insulae now contained up to eight large apartment blocks and only the wealthiest residents of the city could afford privately owned houses. As the demand increased, old thermae, markets, and temples were torn down and replaced by larger, more adequate structures. The two aqueducts still satisfied the city's

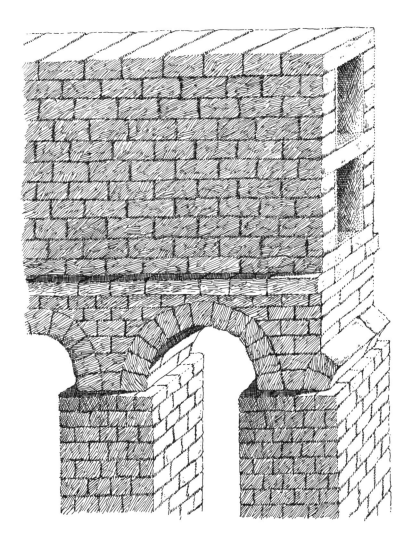

water needs and the one-hundred-and-twenty-year-old sewer system was still operating flawlessly. Because of the efficient organization of farmland and the large number of markets and bakeries, food continued to remain in good supply. The streets, although busy, were not overcrowded. They were still safe and comfortable outdoor areas as originally intended in the master plan.

One hundred and twenty-five years after its founding, Verbonia had reached its limit. With the empire stronger than ever the walls once constructed to keep the enemy out were now serving a more important function — that of keeping the city in.

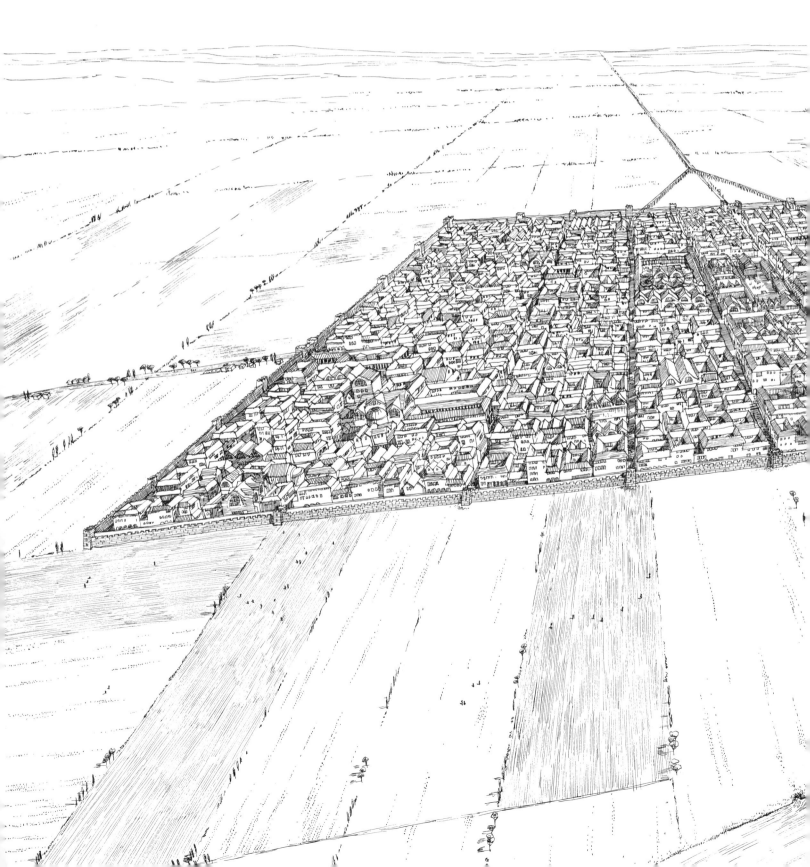

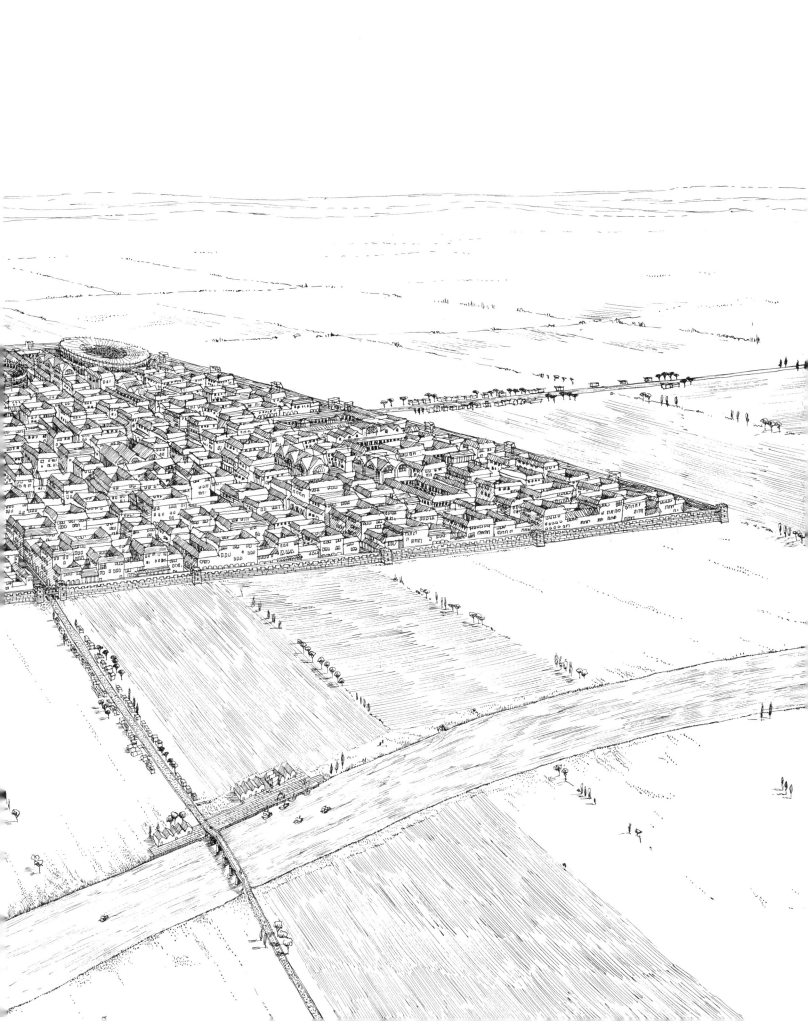

GLOSSARY

AMPHITHEATER
An oval arena completely surrounded by gradually rising rows of seats.

ATRIUM
The largest interior space in a Roman house. It is completely covered by a roof except for the central section which is left open to the sky.

AQUEDUCT
A pipeline specifically built to carry water.

AXLE
The shaft on which a wheel revolves.

CALDARIUM
The heated area of the thermae containing hot water pools.

CARDO
The main north-south road through a Roman city.

CASTRUM
A Roman military camp usually square or rectangular in shape.

CAVEA
The steep semicircular seating area of the theater.

CENTERING
A temporary wooden arch over which a brick or stone arch is constructed. When the mortar sets between the bricks or stones of the permanent arch, the centering is removed.

CHOROBATE
A long wooden surveying instrument used for general siting as well as determining the profile of the land.

CLOACA
A large underground sewer in the form of a tunnel.

COFFERDAM
A water tight enclosure constructed in a river or lake. The water is pumped out of the cofferdam enabling laborers to work directly on the river or lake bed.

COFFERS
Recessed areas in a concrete vault or dome which reduce the weight of the roof.

COLONNADE
A row of columns supporting a horizontal beam or a roof.

COMPLUVIUM
The opening in the roof of the atrium.

CONCRETE
An extremely strong building material made by combining stones of varying sizes and mortar.

CRENELATIONS
The alternating high and low sections of stonework along the top of a defensive wall. The defender is protected behind the high sections while firing his weapon over the lower sections.

DECUMANUS
The main east-west road through a Roman city.

FORGE
A workshop in which metal is heated in a furnace and hammered into shapes for tools and instruments.

FORUM
The government and religious center of a Roman city consisting of an open meeting area surrounded by buildings and colonnades.

FRIGIDARIUM
The area of the thermae containing cold water pools.

GROIN VAULT
The vault created by the intersection of two tunnel vaults at right angles to each other.

GROMA
A surveying instrument consisting of a pole and a horizontal cross from which hang four weighted strings. When the strings hang parallel to the pole the instrument is known to be perfectly vertical and the roads and walls could then be accurately laid out on the ground by siting along the arms of the cross.

HYPOCAUST
The chamber under a raised floor into which hot gases were piped in order to heat the floor.

IMPLUVIUM
The pool in the floor of the atrium which collected the water that fell through the compluvium.

INSULA
A Roman city block, usually square or rectangular in shape.

KEYSTONE
The central locking stone at the top of an arch.

MORTAR
A mixture of sand, lime and water used to cement stones and bricks together. When it dries it becomes very hard.

OCULUS
A round opening or window.

PERISTYLE
The open courtyard or garden in a Roman house surrounded by a colonnade.

PIERS
A free-standing brick, stone or concrete structure similar to a column but usually thicker, used to support an arch.

PILE
A tree trunk stripped of bark and pointed at one end that is then driven into a river bed or marshy area in the construction of a cofferdam or is used to create a sturdy base for a pier.

POMERIUM
The open strip of land along the inner face of the wall around a Roman city. It served as the sacred boundary within which the land was thought to be protected by the gods.

PORTCULLIS
A metal-clad timber grill which could be lowered to seal off the gates of the city.

POZZOLANA
A gravelly substance mixed with regular mortar, enabling it to harden under water.

PROFILE MAP
A drawing which outlines the surface of the land showing the height and depth of hills and valleys.

ROSTRUM
A raised platform from which speeches are delivered.

STUCCO
Heavy plaster.

TEPIDARIUM
The heated area of the thermae containing hot water pools.

THERMAE
Roman public baths.

TRUSS
A wooden frame used to bridge a space too wide to be bridged by a single beam.

TUNNEL VAULT
A continuous semicircular ceiling or roof.

VALARIUM
A canvas roof drawn over a theater or amphitheater to protect the spectators from the sun.

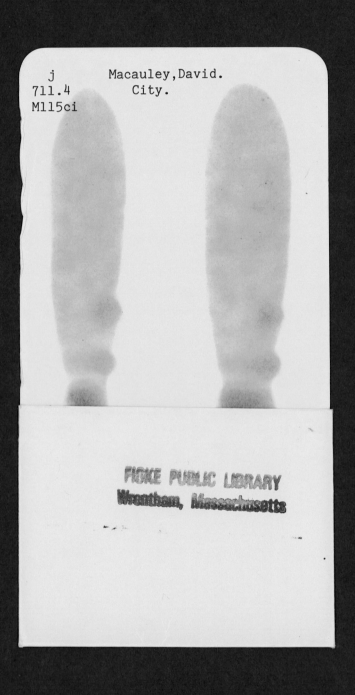